www.harcourt-international.com

Bringing you products from all Harcourt Health Sciences companies including Baillière Tindall, Churchill Livingstone, Mosby and W.B. Saunders

- ▶ **Browse** for latest information on new books, journals and electronic products

- ▶ **Search** for information on over 20 000 published titles with full product information including tables of contents and sample chapters

- ▶ **Keep up to date** with our extensive publishing programme in your field by registering with eAlert or requesting postal updates

- ▶ **Secure online ordering** with prompt delivery, as well as full contact details to order by phone, fax or post

- ▶ **News** of special features and promotions

If you are based in the following countries, please visit the country-specific site to receive full details of product availability and local ordering information

USA: www.harcourthealth.com

Canada: www.harcourtcanada.com

Australia: www.harcourt.com.au

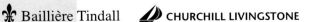 Baillière Tindall   CHURCHILL LIVINGSTONE   Mosby   W.B. SAUNDERS

Obstetric and Gynecologic Dermatology

SECOND EDITION

Commissioning Editor: Sue Hodgson
Project Development Manager: Tim Kimber
Project Manager: Kim Howell
Designer: Jayne Jones
Page Layout: Jim Hope

Obstetric and Gynecologic Dermatology

SECOND EDITION

Martin M. Black MD FRCP FRCPath

Professor of Dermatological Immunopathology,
St John's Institute of Dermatology,
Guy's, King's and St Thomas' School of Medicine,
St Thomas' Hospital,
London, UK

Marilynne McKay MD MS FAAD

Professor Emerita of Dermatology and Gynecology,
Emory University School of Medicine,
Atlanta, USA
Chairman,
Department of Dermatology,
Lovelace Health Systems,
Albuquerque, NM, USA

Peter R. Braude BSc MB BCh MA PhD FRCOG

Professor of Obstetrics and Gynaecology,
Head of Division of Women's and Children's Health,
Guy's, King's and St Thomas' School of Medicine,
Guy's and St Thomas' Hospitals,
London, UK

Samantha A. Vaughan Jones MD MRCP

Consultant Dermatologist,
St Peter's Hospital,
Chertsey, UK

Lynette J. Margesson MD FRCPC

Assistant Professor of Obstetrics and Gynecology, and Medicine,
Dartmouth Medical School,
Hanover, NH, USA

Mosby

London   Edinburgh   New York   Philadephia   St Louis   Sydney   Toronto   2002

Mosby International Limited

© Mosby International Limited 2002

M is a registered trademark of Mosby International Limited

The right of Martin M. Black, Marilynne McKay, Peter R. Braude, Samantha Vaughan Jones and Lynette J. Margesson to be identified as editors of this work has been asserted by them in accordance with the Copyright, Designs and Patents Act 1988

First edition 1995
Second edition 2002

ISBN 0 723 43182 5

British Library Cataloguing in Publication Data
A catalogue record for this book is available from the British Library

Library of Congress Cataloging in Publication Data
A catalog record for this book is available from the Library of Congress

Note
Medical knowledge is constantly changing. As new information becomes available, changes in treatment, procedures, equipment and the use of drugs become necessary. The editors/authors/contributors and the publishers have, as far as it is possible, taken care to ensure that the information given in this text is accurate and up to date. However, readers are strongly advised to confirm that the information, especially with regard to drug usage, complies with the latest legislation and standards of practice.

Existing UK nomenclature is changing to the system of Recommended International Non-proprietary Names (rINNs). Until the UK names are no longer in use, these more familiar names are used in this book in preference to rINNs, details of which may be obtained from the British National Formulary.

The
publisher s
policy is to use
**paper manufactured
from sustainable forests**

Printed in China by RDC Group Limited

Contents

Contents

Contributors

Martin M. Black MD FRCP FRCPath
Professor of Dermatological Immunopathology
St John's Institute of Dermatology
Guy's, King's and St Thomas' School of Medicine
St Thomas' Hospital
London, UK

Peter R. Braude BSc MB BCh MA PhD FRCOG
Professor of Obstetrics and Gynaecology
Head of Division of Women's and Children's Health
Guy's, King's and St Thomas' School of Medicine
Guy's and St Thomas' Hospitals
London, UK

Annemiek de Ruiter FRCP
Consultant in Genitourinary Medicine
St Thomas' Hospital
London, UK

Diana Hamilton-Fairley MD FRCOG
Consultant Obstetrician and Gynaecologist
Guy's and St Thomas' Hospitals
London, UK

Christine Harrington MD FRCP
Consultant Dermatologist (Retired)
Royal Hallamshire Hospital
Sheffield, UK

Ira R. Horowitz MD
Willaford Ransom Leach Professor and Vice Chairman
Department of Gynecology and Obstetrics
Director, Division of Gynecologic Oncology
Emory University School of Medicine
Atlanta, GA, USA

Rachel E. Jenkins BSc MD MRCP
Consultant Dermatologist
West Suffolk Hospital
Bury St Edmonds, UK

Diana N. J. Lockwood BSc MD FRCP
Consultant Leprologist
Hospital for Tropical Diseases
Senior Lecturer
London School of Hygiene and Tropical Medicine
London, UK

Eithne MacMahon MD MRCPI DCH MRCPath
Consultant Virologist and Honorary Senior Lecturer
Department of Infection
St Thomas' Hospital
London, UK

Lynette J. Margesson MD FRCPC
Assistant Professor of Obstetrics and Gynecology,
and Medicine
Dartmouth Medical School
Hanover, NH, USA

Pauline Marren MD MRCPI
Consultant Dermatologist
University College Hospital
Galway, Ireland

Barbara McAlpine MD
Dermatopathologist
Bethesda Dermatopathology Laboratory
Silver Spring, MD, USA

Marilynne McKay MD MS FAAD
Professor Emerita of Dermatology and Gynecology
Emory University School of Medicine
Atlanta, USA
Chairman
Lovelace Health Systems
Albuquerque, NM, USA

John M. Monaghan MB FRCS FRCOG
Senior Lecturer in Gynaecologic Oncology
Queen Elizabeth Hospital
Gateshead, UK

Sallie M. Neill MB ChB FRCP
Consultant Dermatologist
St Thomas' Hospital
Chelsea and Westminster Hospital
London, UK
Ashford and St Peter's Hospitals
Chertsey, UK

Catherine Nelson-Piercy MA FRCP
Consultant Obstetric Physician
St Thomas' Hospital
London, UK

Jenny Powell BA (Oxon) MRCP (UK)
Consultant Dermatologist
Oxford Radcliffe Hospital
Oxford, UK

C. Marjorie Ridley MA BM FRCP (Deceased)
Formerly Honorary Consultant
St Thomas' Hospital
Whittington Hospital
London, UK

Jeff K. Shornick MD MHA
Robert Wood Johnson Health Policy Fellow
Senator John D. Rockefeller IV
Hart Senate Office Building
Washington, DC, USA

Catherine J. M. Stephens MBBS MRCP
Consultant Dermatologist
Poole Hospital
Poole, UK

Samantha Vaughan Jones MD MRCP
Consultant Dermatologist
St Peter's Hospital
Chertsey, UK

Ursula Wesselman MD
Associate Professor of Neurology
and Biomedical Engineering
Johns Hopkins University School of Medicine
Baltimore, MD, USA

Fenella Wojnarowska BA MSc (Oxon) BM BCh (Oxon)
DM (Oxon) FRCP (UK)
Professor of Dermatology
Oxford Radcliffe Hospital
Oxford, UK

Preface to the second edition

The first edition of this text, which we believe was the first ever to focus specifically on the full range of dermatologic problems encountered in obstetric and gynecologic practice, was very well received. For the second edition, the sections on the vulva, inflammatory vulvar disease and vulvar tumors have, once again, been integrated into the sections dealing with obstetric manifestations of skin disease. This profusely illustrated color atlas presents numerous examples of common and unusual disorders. The format of the illustrations and text can aid the user in comparing images of similar-appearing skin problems. The text also outlines detailed and practical suggestions for therapy. For this reason, we believe that the atlas will be appreciated by consulting dermatologists and non-dermatologists alike.

All chapters have been thoroughly updated and each presents a basic, sensible approach to a complex subject. There are new sections on eczema in pregnancy, pediatric vulvar disorders and vulvar dysesthesia (former vulvodynia). The picture appendix on vulvar ulcers has been expanded to include pruritus vulvae and patient information sheets now include instructions for eczema as well as common vulvar disorders.

For this edition, we are again pleased to be joined by Dr Peter Braude and also by Dr Lynette Margesson and Dr Samantha Vaughan Jones. We are all proud of this combined effort, because we feel that this book will continue to be a useful reference for all clinicians who care about women's health.

Martin M Black
Marilynne McKay

Dedications

To my wife, Aniko.
M M Black

To two special mentors, the late Eduard G. Friedrich, Jr and the late C. Marjorie Ridley; my husband, Ronald S. Hosek; and my patients, who have taught me so much.
M McKay

To Beatrice, Philip and Richard – this should have been your quality time.
P R Braude

To Sean, Natalie and Claudia for the times I wasn't there. To Martin Black, my mentor. To my parents for all their continued support.
S. A. Vaughan Jones

This book is dedicated to my vulvar patients, who continue to amaze, inspire and teach me; and to my husband, Dr Bill Danby, who patiently edits all I write.
L. J. Margesson

1 Hormonal Changes during Puberty, Pregnancy, and the Menopause

Peter Braude
Diana Hamilton-Fairley

INTRODUCTION

This chapter summarizes the hormonal changes that occur during puberty, the menstrual cycle, pregnancy, and the menopause, and how these changes affect the skin physiologically.

All children go through the bewildering hormonal changes that the transition from child to adult necessitates. However, it is only the female who will continue to experience a changing hormonal milieu – either cyclically, with the monthly production of an egg followed by menses, or the effects of pregnancy if conception takes place. Then, for the last third of their lives, women face the consequences of a reduction in estrogen levels following the menopause. Although the hormonal events immediately preceding the menopause are turbulent, once the climacteric is reached, it too may cause its problems.

Most women are aware of the changes taking place in their skin at these different stages in their lives.

HYPOTHALAMIC–PITUITARY AXIS

An understanding of the interrelationship between the hypothalamus, the pituitary gland, and the ovary is imperative if the cyclical and long-term hormonal changes occurring in women are to be appreciated.

Situated above the pituitary gland, the hypothalamus initiates the release of the polypeptides that regulate ovarian function. The ovary cannot produce mature fertile oocytes (eggs) if the signals from the pituitary gland never start, cease prematurely, or are disordered. The female reproductive cycle is regulated precisely via biologic feedback mechanisms from the ovary, which alter the activity of the hypothalamus and pituitary. Normal physiologic changes in the functioning of the hypothalamic–pituitary axis result in the hormonal changes that occur during the four main reproductive endocrine phases of woman's life: puberty, menstruation, pregnancy, and the climacteric.

As menarche (the first period) is one event during the years of puberty, so menopause (the final period) marks one event during the years of declining reproductive function (the climacteric or menopause).

PUBERTY

Puberty describes the physiologic, morphologic, and behavioral changes that occur in a child as the gonads mature from the infantile to the adult state that affects most of the organs of the body in both sexes.

These physiologic changes can be divided into two main groups: growth and hormonal. Although the changes start at different chronologic ages in different individuals, the sequence of events is similar. In girls the start of puberty is strongly weight-related, with the mean bodyweight being 47 kg at menarche. Although the age of menarche has declined from 17 years in 1840 to 13.5 years in the 1940s, and is now 12.5 years in the USA, the mean bodyweight at menarche seems to have remained constant.

GROWTH SPURT

The adolescent growth spurt is an acceleration of growth in most skeletal dimensions. The peak height velocity (PHV) is 9–10 cm per year and lasts for about 2 years. There is no difference in the PHV of girls and boys, and both sexes grow between 25 and 28 cm during puberty. However, girls start their growth spurt 2 years earlier than boys, at which time they are 10 cm shorter than when boys start theirs. This accounts for the difference in adult height between the sexes.

This large increase in height is mediated by an increase in growth hormone (GH) production by the pituitary gland. The greatest increase in the frequency and amplitude of GH takes place at night in a similar fashion to luteinizing hormone (LH) pulses (**1.1**).

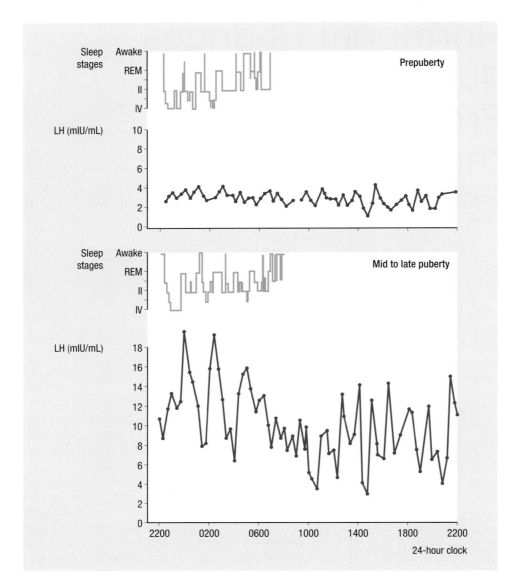

**Fig 1.1
Luteinizing
hormone levels
during puberty.**
Changes in the
pulse frequency
and amplitude of
luteinizing
hormone during
puberty.

HORMONAL CHANGES

The hormonal changes of puberty produce two main effects: maturation of the ovary so that reproduction can occur, and development of secondary sexual characteristics (breasts, axillary and pubic hair).

During childhood, serum levels of the gonadotrophins – LH and follicle-stimulating hormone (FSH) – are low. During early to mid puberty, however, there is a striking increase in the magnitude and frequency of LH pulses at night during sleep (1.1). In late puberty, there is an increase in magnitude during the day, but not as marked as at night. Only when puberty is complete do the LH pulses lose their diurnal variation and settle into an adult pattern, with pulses approximately every 90 minutes during the follicular phase, and between 120 and 180 minutes in the luteal phase.

These events are probably initiated by the maturation of the hypothalamus and the onset of secretion of gonadotrophin-releasing hormone (GnRH). However, it is impossible to prove the exact sequence of events initiating puberty because the experiments required would be unethical in humans.

The increase in both LH and FSH activity has a trophic effect on the ovary, stimulating the production of estradiol. The primordial follicles (the oocyte and surrounding support cells) present from birth, begin to mature into antral follicles lined by granulosa cells. This process of maturation takes about 10 weeks. LH acts mainly on the theca cells which surround the follicles, causing them to produce testosterone, which then is converted by an aromatase into estradiol in the granulosa cells under the influence of FSH.

The increase in estradiol secretion stimulates breast development. The five stages of breast development take about 4 years to complete (1.2). Menarche (the first menstruation) usually occurs once breast development is quite well advanced – between stages III and IV[1]. Rapid breast development or increase in breast

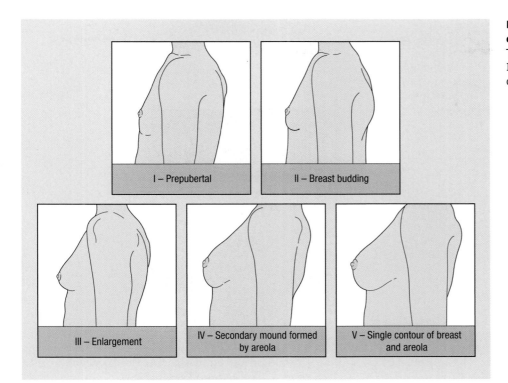

Fig 1.2 Breast development.
The Tanner stages I–V of breast development.

I – Prepubertal

II – Breast budding

III – Enlargement

IV – Secondary mound formed by areola

V – Single contour of breast and areola

size, commonly during pregnancy and less commonly on the oral contraceptive pill, may cause stretch marks to develop, especially in the lateral margins of the breast, which may be of concern, particularly to younger women.

Several other changes also occur, which are important in understanding the physiologic changes in the skin. The first is adrenarche. This is an increase in the production of adrenal androgens, dehydroepiandrosterone (DHEA) and its sulfate (DHEAS), which starts at about 8 years of age and continues until 13–15 years of age in both sexes. This increase is thought to stimulate the development of axillary and pubic hair, as hair growth and changes in sebum secretion are modulated predominantly by androgens in both sexes. Pubic and axillary hair growth usually starts before the breasts change following the increase in adrenal androgen levels, but reaches the mature stage at around the same time. The testosterone level increases in girls, as in boys, under the influence of LH, but most of it is converted into estradiol.

During puberty, the concentration of the main binding protein of the sex hormones (sex hormone-binding globulin, SHBG) declines in both sexes, despite the increase in estradiol concentrations in girls[2]. SHBG has a greater affinity for testosterone than for estradiol, with the result that, in most girls, more than 90% of circulating testosterone is bound to SHBG, thus limiting the effect that testosterone may have peripherally. The decrease in SHBG seems to be mediated by an increase in insulin concentration, which has been demonstrated in both sexes[3].

POLYCYSTIC OVARY SYNDROME

There is a group of girls who produce an excess of testosterone accompanied by morphologic changes in their ovaries, a phenomenon known as polycystic ovaries (PCO)[4]. Typically these girls never establish regular menstruation and have increased hair growth, usually of a male pattern, with an abdominal escutcheon, moustache, or other facial hair growth (1.3). They may also develop acne. Many girls with acne and/or hirsutism have polycystic ovary syndrome. These girls also have higher insulin concentrations and lower SHBG concentrations than their weight-matched contemporaries[5].

A lower SHBG concentration, together with an increased circulating testosterone level, will lead to an increased free testosterone level. It is the fraction of free testosterone that is thought to be active peripherally on the skin, sebaceous glands, and hair follicles.

ACNE

Testosterone has major effects on the hair follicle and sebum secretion. Acne vulgaris[6] (1.4) and hirsutism are never seen in prepubertal children with normal adrenal function, providing further evidence that puberty-related changes trigger these events. Although there is no evidence of increased androgen production in men with acne, most women with acne do have increased ovarian androgen production and a reduced SHBG concentration. Undoubtedly, genetic factors

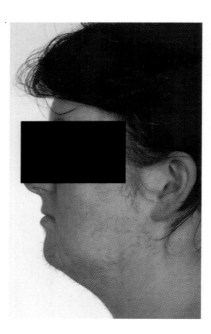

**Fig 1.3
Polycystic ovary
syndrome.**
Facial hirsutism
associated with
polycystic ovary
syndrome.

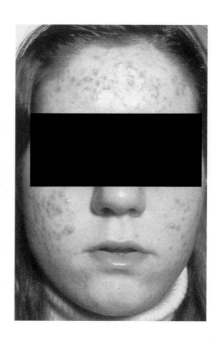

**Fig 1.4
Acne vulgaris.**

also play an important part in determining which girls will suffer and which will not. The pilosebaceous gland becomes more differentiated, increases in size, and changes its sebum composition. These changes are most marked on the scalp and around the nose, chin, and cheeks, as well as on the upper chest and back (*See Chapter 2*). Acne tends to reach a peak during puberty and before sexual maturity. It is therefore thought that the adrenal glands provide the initial stimulus.

THE MENSTRUAL CYCLE

The menstrual cycle is divided into two phases which are named as viewed from two different standpoints:

- The follicular and luteal phases – according to events in the ovary
- The proliferative and secretory phases – according to changes that take place in the endometrium

As endometrial changes are dependent on the hormonal changes occurring in the ovary, the terms follicular phase and luteal phase will be used in this chapter.

FOLLICULAR PHASE

A few days before the onset of menstruation, the level of FSH starts to rise under the stimulation of GnRH secreted from the hypothalamus (1.5). This causes several antral follicles to start producing estradiol. As these follicles fill with fluid produced by the granulosa cells, which lie as a single layer around each follicle, they become visible on an ultrasonographic scan. In

order to produce estradiol, the granulosa cells utilize testosterone produced by the theca cells, which lie as a second monolayer around the follicle.

In the early follicular phase, the granulosa cells carry receptors for FSH, whereas the theca cells are stimulated by LH. The estradiol produced by the ovary is released into the circulation. The pituitary has an abundance of estradiol receptors; their activation results in the inhibition of both LH and FSH production in the mid-follicular phase. The granulosa cells also produce inhibin, a protein that augments the negative feedback of estradiol on FSH. This protein is also produced by the corpus luteum following ovulation. As a result of this effect, the smaller follicles stop growing and undergo atresia.

By this stage, only one follicle (but, occasionally, two or more) has reached a diameter of about 10–12 mm, and is called the dominant follicle[7]. The granulosa cells of the dominant follicle develop LH receptors and so become receptive to both LH and FSH. The follicle increases in diameter by 2 mm per day. The estradiol concentration rises faster and the granulosa cells begin to accumulate in several layers over the oocyte.

OOCYTE RELEASE

When the follicle reaches a diameter of around 18–20 mm, and the estradiol concentration reaches 800–1000 pmol/L, the biofeedback on the pituitary is reversed. This results in a rapid rise in hormone concentrations, predominantly of LH and to a lesser extent of FSH. In turn, this leads to a luteinization of the granulosa cells and consequently they begin to produce progesterone in preference to estradiol. This change leads to the rupture of the follicle wall, and the oocyte is released into the peritoneum about 24–36 hours after the

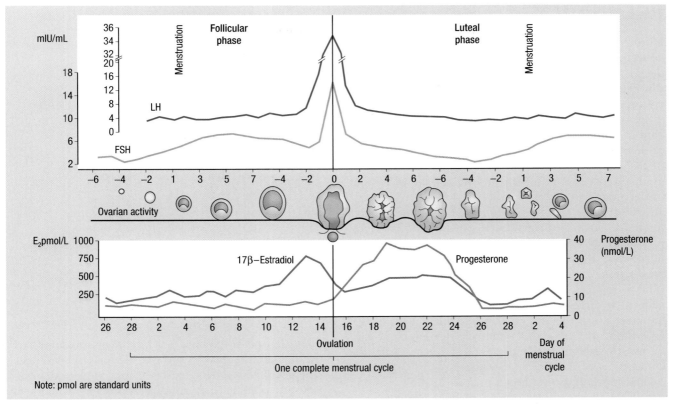

Fig 1.5 Hormonal changes of the menstrual cycle.

LH surge. The follicular phase ends with release of the oocyte, and varies in length from 12 to 16 days.

LUTEAL PHASE

Oocyte release marks the start of the luteal phase. Following release of the oocyte, the granulosa cells reseal the defect in the wall within a few hours, forming the corpus luteum. The granulosa (now luteal) cells produce progesterone, and this reaches a peak concentration 5–8 days after ovulation. The effect of progesterone on the endometrium is to increase the surface area of the endometrial glands and their blood supply by causing them to become spiral. They also start to produce large amounts of glycogen, an essential nutrient for the early days of embryo development if fertilization takes place.

If the oocyte is fertilized and implantation occurs, then progesterone levels remain high. These levels are maintained by human chorionic gonadotrophin (hCG) produced by the trophoblastic elements of the embryo as the primitive placenta invades the endometrium. If fertilization does not occur, the concentration of LH is insufficient to maintain production of progesterone by the corpus luteum. The levels decline and the endometrium becomes ischemic; its superficial layers slough off. This, together with bleeding from the spiral arterioles that supplied the endometrium, produces menstruation.

Thus, the cycle has come full circle to the hormonal and endometrial states found at its beginning. The whole process then begins again.

SKIN CHANGES

Skin changes during the menstrual cycle are usually temporary and of minor importance. They include an increase in sebum production before menses, which may lead to acneiform eruptions on the face and occasionally on the back.

Knowledge of the hypothalamic, pituitary, and ovarian hormonal changes is useful in understanding therapies to modify or ablate the hormonal mileu. There is a range of superactive GnRH analogs (buserelin, goserelin, nafarelin, etc.), which can be given by daily nasal spray or by monthly depot injections, whose effect (after a brief stimulation of FSH output) is competitively to block the GnRH receptor and thus abolish FSH and LH production. This effectively renders the woman reversibly menopausal, such that events attributable to the cyclicity of the menstrual cycle can be investigated, such as cyclic pain, eruptions, or progesterone sensitivity (*see Chapter 2*). This regimen should not be employed for more than 6 months at a stretch because of the estrogen-depleting effect and thus its potentially adverse effect on bone loss.

PREGNANCY

During the first few weeks of pregnancy, progesterone concentrations increase. Progesterone is initially produced by the corpus luteum, which is maintained by the production of hCG from the trophoblast of the conceptus.

hCG has been found in the maternal circulation almost immediately after fertilization and rises to a peak by 60–90 days of gestation. The concentration of hCG doubles every 2–3 days until this time, then gradually declines to a plateau level for the remainder of the pregnancy.

The corpus luteum continues to produce progesterone, 17-hydroxyprogesterone, estrone, and estradiol, producing a rise in the concentration of all these hormones. In addition, hCG is responsible for the production of inhibin and relaxin by the corpus luteum. Inhibin reduces FSH concentrations so that folliculogenesis is arrested once the embryo has become implanted into the endometrium. It may also act as a growth factor for the early embryo. Relaxin is thought to act in synergy with progesterone to reduce the contractility of the uterine myometrium.

The concentrations of both of these hormones rise in parallel with the concentration of hCG, but they are produced only for a limited period by the ovary. From around 7 weeks' gestation, they are produced by the decidual fetal membranes and placental tissues. Similarly, ovarian steroid hormone production declines from 7 weeks' gestation, with the placental unit taking over this function. This explains why pregnancies fail if the corpus luteum is removed before 8 weeks, but continue unharmed if the pregnancy has reached 9 weeks' gestation.

THE PLACENTA

The placenta is a complex organ. Not only does it provide nutrients and excrete waste products from the fetus, but it also modifies the maternal metabolism at various stages of pregnancy via hormones. The placenta reaches structural maturity by the end of week 12 of pregnancy. The functional unit is the chorionic villus, which consists of a central core of loose connective tissue and abundant capillaries. These connect to the fetal circulation and provide a large surface area in contact with the maternal uterine circulation. Around this central core are two layers of trophoblast, an outer syncytium (syncytiotrophoblast), and an inner layer of discrete cells (cytotrophoblast).

The fetus and placenta form an interdependent partnership which regulates the endocrine–metabolic processes during pregnancy. This fetal–placental unit therefore becomes an endocrine system, producing a large number of different hormones (**Table 1.1**).

Table 1.1 Hormones Produced by the Fetal–Placental Unit.

Peptides	Inhibin
	Relaxin
	Human placental lactogen
Neuropeptides	Gonadotrophin-releasing hormone
	Corticotrophin-releasing hormone
	Thyroid-releasing hormone
Steroid hormones	Progesterone
	Androgens
	Estradiol
	Estrone
	Estriol
Peptide growth factors	Insulin-like growth factors I and II

Several placental products have been measured over the years in the search for a marker for placental insufficiency. These include estriol and human placental lactogen (hPL), the concentrations of which rise steadily throughout pregnancy. But, as their normal ranges are very large, they have not proved clinically useful in predicting the outcome of pregnancy.

Following the baby's birth, all the hormone levels return to normal within a few days. The production of hCG, progesterone, estriol, estradiol, and hPL during pregnancy is shown in **1.6**. Despite our ability to measure these hormones during pregnancy, the role that they play in maintaining pregnancy and/or initiating parturition is still poorly understood.

THE CLIMACTERIC AND THE MENOPAUSE

The menopause (cessation of menses) marks the end of a woman's reproductive life. The average age for the end of menses in the UK is 50.3 years. During the perimenopausal years (the climacteric), there is an increase in circulating FSH levels and a decrease in estradiol concentrations.[8] The negative feedback of estradiol on FSH still occurs, but the resting concentration of FSH is higher than in younger women. The concentrations of FSH at the mid-cycle surge and in the late luteal phase are also greater. LH levels tend to remain within the normal range until the cessation of menses. Ovulatory cycles may still occur with increased levels of FSH, providing evidence that the ovary gradually becomes less responsive to gonadotrophins. The timing of menses may become more irregular, and most cycles become anovulatory, as the ovaries become depleted of antral follicles[9,10] and no longer respond to FSH.

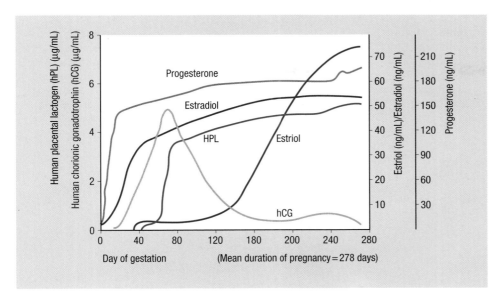

Fig 1.6
Hormonal changes during pregnancy.
Changes in the production of progesterone, estradiol, estriol, human chorionic gonadotrophin, and human placental lactogen.

Estradiol levels decline until they are so low that the endometrium no longer undergoes proliferation, and becomes atrophic. The endometrium is no longer shed and menses cease. As well as a decline in estradiol levels, androgen levels also decrease from an average of 1.6 to 0.5 nmol/L. This reduction in androgen levels has been used to explain the decrease in libido sometimes experienced by postmenopausal women.

As a secondary effect of reduced estradiol concentrations, FSH and LH levels rise owing to a lack of negative feedback on the pituitary gland. While the postmenopausal ovary produces minimal estradiol, it continues to produce quite significant amounts of testosterone and, to a lesser extent, androstenedione, produced by the stromal cells of the ovary.

These androgens, predominantly adrenal androstenedione, are converted peripherally by aromatase into estrone. The extent to which this happens depends on age and weight (fat mass). Heavier women have higher conversion rates and circulating estrogen concentrations than slim women. The average percentage of conversion in menopausal women is 2.8%, double that found in premenopausal women. The relative change in balance between estrogen and androgen production in older women[11] may account for the increased incidence of hirsutism in this group.

SKIN CHANGES

The predominant process is progressive atrophy of the dermis and architectural changes leading to folds and wrinkles. The extent to which this occurs varies from individual to individual and depends on genetic and environmental factors. The generalized aging process of the skin involves the vagina and vulva too. Estradiol is essential to the maintenance of the elasticity and lubrication of the vagina. Most of the changes in the vulva and vagina associated with the menopause are secondary to low estradiol concentrations, as they can be reversed by the topical application of estradiol. In areas such as the vulva and vagina, which are protected from ultraviolet light, the epidermis becomes very thin. There is a reduced number of capillaries within the skin and elastotic changes occur in the arterioles. With time, the withdrawal of estrogens causes the vaginal skin to lose its folds, and the vaginal epithelium becomes thin and friable, making it more susceptible to trauma, with the result that it bleeds. This is a very common cause of postmenopausal bleeding, especially in the older woman.

The atrophic changes that affect the vulva predispose it to trauma, often secondary to excessive itching. This may lead to ulceration or scar formation as the wounds heal. In a few women, this leads to fusion of the labia majora (1.7, 1.8).

CONCLUSION

A woman's skin is affected by the many hormonal changes that occur during her lifetime. The degree to which each individual is affected depends on genetic and environmental factors. There is sound research to support the hormonal basis for some skin changes. An appreciation of the prevailing hormonal milieu is important in understanding the etiology of certain skin-related complaints. However, it is equally important not to apportion a physiologic explanation for many other conditions that come and go – often regardless of changes in the woman's serum endocrinology. This is particularly true in pregnancy.

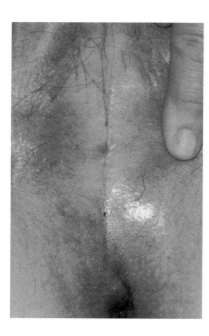

Fig 1.7 Fused labia. This condition occurred secondary to postmenopausal skin changes.

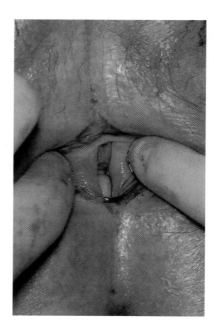

Fig 1.8 Surgical correction of fused labia. The same patient as in **1.7**, after surgical opening performed.

REFERENCES

1 Tanner, J.M. and Whitehouse, R.H. Clinical longitudinal standards for height, weight, height velocity, weight velocity, and stages of puberty. *Arch. Dis. Child.* 1976; **51**: 170–179.

2 Cunningham, S.K., Loughlin, T., Culliton, M. *et al.* Plasma sex hormone binding globulin levels decline during the second decade of life irrespective of pubertal status. *J. Clin. Endocrinol. Metab.* 1984; **58**: 915–918.

3 Smith, C.P., Archibald, H.R., Thomas, J.M. *et al.* Basal and stimulated insulin levels rise with advancing puberty. *Clin. Endocrinol.* 1988; **28**: 7–14.

4 Balen, A.H., Conway, G.S., Kaltsas, G. *et al.* Polycystic ovary syndrome: the spectrum of the disorder in 1741 patients. *Hum. Reprod.* 1995; **10**: 2107–2111.

5 Burghen, G.A., Givens, J.R., and Kitabchi, A.E. Correlation of hyperandrogenism with hyperinsulinism in polycystic ovarian disease. *J. Clin. Endocrinol. Metab.* 1980; **50**: 113–116.

6 Brown, S.K. and Shalita, A.R. Acne vulgaris. *Lancet* 1998; **351**: 1871–1876.

7 Gougeon, A. Ovarian follicular growth in humans: ovarian ageing and population of growing follicles. *Maturitas* 1998; **30**: 137–142.

8 Lee, S.J., Lenton, E.A., Sexton, L. and Cooke, I.D. The effect of age on the cyclical patterns of plasma LH, FSH, oestradiol and progesterone in women with regular menstrual cycles. *Hum. Reprod.* 1988; **3**: 851–855.

9 Faddy, M.J. and Gosden, R.G. A mathematical model of follicle dynamics in the human ovary. *Hum. Reprod.* 1995; **10**: 770–775.

10 Richardson, S.J. and Nelson, J.F. Follicular depletion during the menopausal transition. *Ann. N.Y. Acad. Sci.* 1990; **592**: 13–20.

11 Rannevik, G., Jeppsson, S., Johnell, O. *et al.* A longitudinal study of the perimenopausal transition: altered profiles of steroid and pituitary hormones, SHBG and bone mineral density. *Maturitas* 1995; **21**: 103–113.

2 Perimenstrual Skin Eruptions; Autoimmune Progesterone Dermatitis; Autoimmune Estrogen Dermatitis

Martin M. Black
Catherine J.M. Stephens

INTRODUCTION

The activity of many skin diseases fluctuates in relation to the menstrual cycle. Some eruptions are confined to the premenstrual period and are considered as part of the premenstrual syndrome. Furthermore, many chronic dermatoses also flare premenstrually. Since the menstrual cycle is controlled by the sex hormones, premenstrual deterioration is thought to be an effect of progesterone, the predominant circulating hormone of the premenstrual period. Hypersensitivity to progesterone can be demonstrated in some of these cases, when the condition is known as autoimmune progesterone dermatitis[1]. However, hypersensitivity to estrogens may also occur (autoimmune estrogen dermatitis), although it is rarer than with progesterone[2].

SEX HORMONES AND THE SKIN

The skin is highly sensitive to the effects of the sex steroid hormones, to both estrogen and progesterone, as well as to androgens.

Estrogens have been shown to suppress sebaceous activity but have little or no effect on the apocrine glands. They increase dermal hyaluronic acid levels with a consequent increase in the water content of the dermis and slow the breakdown of dermal collagen, possibly by increasing the conversion of soluble collagen to the insoluble form. Estrogens also stimulate epidermal melanogenesis, accounting for the transient hyperpigmentation that commonly occurs premenstrually, particularly around the eyes and nipples, and they have also been shown to slow the rate of hair growth. Estrogens alone appear to possess anti-inflammatory properties and will reduce the cutaneous response in delayed hypersensitivity reactions.

The way in which natural progesterone affects the skin is less clear. The vascularity of the skin is greatly increased during the second half of the menstrual cycle and there is increased sebaceous gland activity, producing seborrhea and, frequently, mild premenstrual acne. Although the mechanism of action is not known, these are both likely to be effects of progesterone.

THE PERIMENSTRUAL DERMATOSES

THE PREMENSTRUAL SYNDROME

Perimenstrual eruptions fall into three categories. An eruption recurring cyclically, and confined to the premenstrual period, may be considered part of the premenstrual syndrome (PMS) (Table 2.1).

A specific endocrine etiology for PMS has not yet been defined. Changes in endorphins, prostaglandins and prolactin[3] have all been implicated, but because of the temporal association of symptoms with the luteal phase of the menstrual cycle an abnormality of progesterone is strongly suspected[3]. Several hypotheses for a progesterone-related effect have been proposed, but not proven, including progesterone deficiency[4], a relative imbalance of estrogen and progesterone levels, and a progesterone allergy[5].

Table 2.1 The Premenstrual Syndrome.

Seborrhea, acne vulgaris
Edema, weight gain
Nausea, vomiting
Constipation, frequency of micturition
Breast fullness/tenderness
Headache, migraine
Excitability, irritability
Lethargy, malaise, depression

Acne vulgaris is one of the most common disorders treated by dermatologists. It is a disease of the pilosebaceous unit leading to the formation of open and closed comedones, papules, pustules, nodules, and cysts. The noninflammatory lesions are open comedones (blackheads) and closed comedones (whiteheads). Papules and pustules constitute the superficial inflammatory lesions, and cysts and nodules, and occasionally deep pustules, make up the deep lesions. In most patients several types of acne lesions are present simultaneously. In *mild acne*, scattered comedones and/or papules with a few pustules predominate. In *moderate acne* more papules and pustules are present (**2.1**), whereas nodulocystic lesions usually predominate in *severe acne*.

Mild facial acne is reported by up to 70% of women during the premenstrual period, often accompanied by excessive greasiness of the scalp. Perioral dermatitis, which is common in teenage girls, is quite frequently cyclical. In addition, edema of the hands and feet, and more rarely patchy pigmentation of the skin, may occur transiently as part of PMS.

If premenstrual acne requires treatment, a topical antiseptic–keratolytic preparation (e.g. benzoyl peroxide) or antibiotic (e.g. clindamycin 1% solution) is usually helpful, but suppression of ovulation, and thus the postovulatory surge of progesterone, can also be effective. The choice of oral contraceptive pill is also important, as some synthetic progestogens (e.g. norethisterone, levonorgestrel) tend to make acne worse (**2.2**). For any acne-prone patient, a combined pill containing gestodene, desogestrel, or norgestimate is recommended. These progestogens appear not to have a stimulatory effect on sebaceous glands. Conversely, they raise levels of sex hormone-binding globulin, so reducing the level of free testosterone, producing a clinical antiandrogenic effect[6].

Although a progestogen is frequently prescribed for symptoms of premenstrual syndrome in which a functional deficit of natural progesterone is suspected[4], it currently has no place in the management of premenstrual acne.

PREMENSTRUAL EXACERBATION OF EXISTING DERMATOSES

Many women complain of cyclical premenstrual worsening of existing dermatoses (**Table 2.2**). This is a common phenomenon. Inflammatory disorders, particularly of the face, become more active and irritable

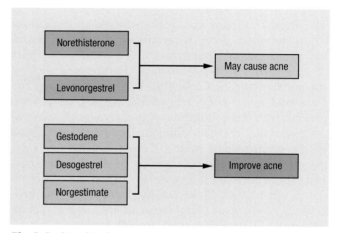

Fig 2.2 Synthetic progestogens used in the combined oral contraceptive pill which may affect acne.

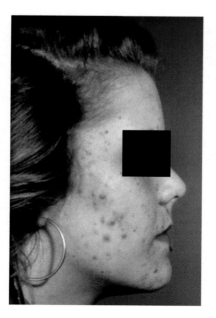

Fig 2.1 Acne vulgaris.
Premenstrual flares are extremely common.

Table 2.2 Chronic dermatoses that may flare premenstrually.
Acne vulgaris
Acne rosacea
Lupus erythematosus
Psoriasis
Atopic eczema
Lichen planus
Dermatitis herpetiformis
Pompholyx
Urticaria
Erythema multiforme
Pruritus vulvae
Pemphigoid gestationis

premenstrually, in part due to the hormonal effects of increased cutaneous vascularity, seborrhea, and dermal edema. Acne vulgaris **2.1**, rosacea (**2.3**), and the various forms of lupus erythematosus (**2.4**) are notable examples. Premenstrual flares are also well recognized in young women with psoriasis, atopic eczema (**2.5**), lichen planus, dermatitis herpetiformis[7], pompholyx, and urticaria. Pemphigoid (herpes) gestationis may persist postpartum, classically falling into a pattern of premenstrual exacerbations[8]. Herpes simplex and aphthosis, although frequently recurrent, are often not strictly cyclical.

Increased cutaneous vascularity and the increased metabolic rate that occurs premenstrually will aggravate pruritic conditions (e.g. eczema and pruritus vulvae) and, in general, tolerance of a dermatosis is often lowered in women with premenstrual tension at this time of the cycle.

AUTOIMMUNE PROGESTERONE DERMATITIS

Autoimmune progesterone dermatitis (AIPD) is a rare condition characterized by recurrent premenstrual exacerbations of a dermatosis in which sensitivity to progesterone can be demonstrated[1].

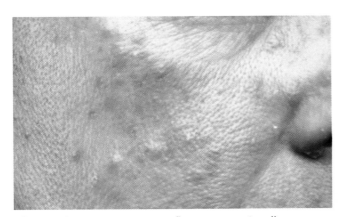

Fig 2.3 Acne rosacea may flare premenstrually.

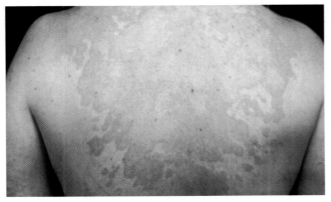

Fig 2.4 Subacute cutaneous lupus erythematosus.

HISTORY

The first case report of a cyclical eruption in which an allergy to endogenous sex hormones was suggested was by Géber[9], who in 1921 reported a case of menstrual urticaria in which the eruption could be reproduced by autoinjection of premenstrual serum. The concept of sex hormone sensitization was extended in 1945 when Zondek and Bromberg[10] described several patients with conditions related to menstruation and the menopause, including cases of cyclical urticaria. They demonstrated positive delayed hypersensitivity reactions to intradermal progesterone in affected patients but not in healthy controls, evidence of passive cutaneous transfer of skin reagins, and clinical suppression by desensitization.

In 1951, Guy et al.[11] reported a patient with premenstrual urticaria who reacted strongly to intradermal injections of extracts of corpus luteum and was later successfully treated by desensitization. The term autoimmune progesterone dermatitis was eventually introduced in 1964 by Shelley et al.[12], who were also the first to document a partial response to estrogens, and cure by oophorectomy.

CLINICAL MANIFESTATIONS

Various clinical morphological features are described including eczema (**2.6**)[13–15], erythema multiforme (**2.7, 2.8**)[10,15–18], urticaria (**2.9**)[11,15,19–21], pompholyx[15–22], stomatitis[23], and a dermatitis herpetiformis-like eruption (**2.10**)[7] (**Table 2.3**). The eruptions do not appear to differ morphologically or histologically from the non-cyclical variants. The condition is confined to ovulating women. Onset is usually in early adult life, occasionally

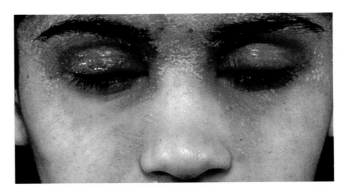

Fig 2.5 Atopic eczema is frequently less manageable premenstrually. Here, the dermatitis involves the eyelids as well as more typical areas such as the antecubital and popliteal fossae.

11

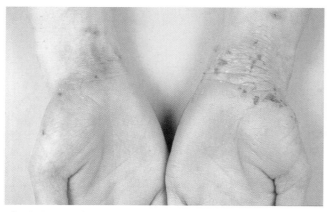

Fig 2.6 Autoimmune progesterone dermatitis.
Flexural lichenified eczema.

Table 2.3 Autoimmune Progesterone Dermatitis.

Eczema
Erythema multiforme
Urticaria
Pompholyx
Stomatitis
Dermatitis herpetiformis
Nonspecific papular erythema

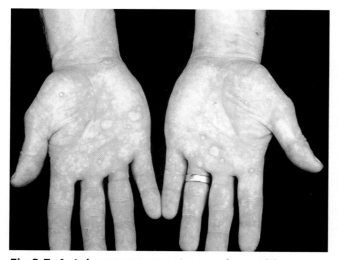

Fig 2.7 Autoimmune progesterone dermatitis.

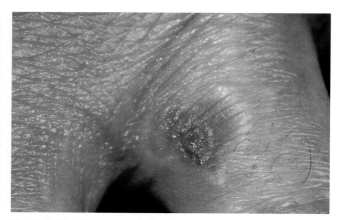

Fig 2.8 Erythema multiforme.

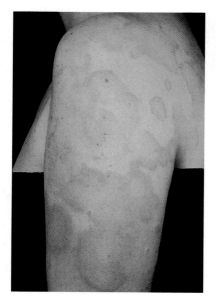

Fig 2.9 Autoimmune progesterone dermatitis. Polycyclic-urticarial lesions.

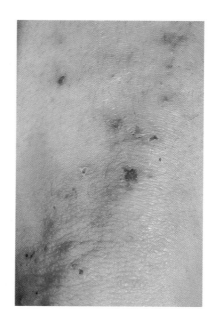

Fig 2.10 Autoimmune progesterone dermatitis. Excoriated papules over the elbows resembling dermatitis herpetiformis.

after a normal pregnancy, and the duration is very variable, with spontaneous remissions occurring. Two-thirds of patients have been exposed to exogenous progesterone in the form of the oral contraceptive pill prior to the eruption[15,24]. Typically the dermatosis appears to flare during the second half of the menstrual cycle, peaks premenstrually, and regresses spontaneously with the menstrual flow. Skin lesions are less florid, or the skin may be clear during the first half of the cycle. By definition, the eruption recurs clinically during every ovulatory cycle.

MECHANISM OF SENSITIZATION

The mechanism by which women become sensitive to their own progesterone is not known. One frequently quoted hypothesis is that previous use of exogenous progestogens induces allergy to endogenous progesterone. It is suggested that synthetic progesterone is sufficiently antigenic to act as a stimulus for antibodies which then cross-react with natural progesterone and perpetuate the immune response premenstrually[15]. However, not all women with AIPD have been exposed to synthetic progestogens. Schoenmakers *et al.*[25] suggested that steroid cross-sensitivity could be an alternative sensitizing mechanism after demonstrating cross-sensitivity on cutaneous testing between hydrocortisone and 17-hydroxyprogesterone in five of 19 corticosteroid-sensitive women, two of whom had features of AIPD. Stephens *et al.*[26] were, however, unable to demonstrate steroid cross-sensitivity in five patients with AIPD and obtained no positive reactions to 17-hydroxyprogesterone.

PREGNANCY

In three cases, onset or a worsening of the eruption has been reported during pregnancy[18,27,28], as well as premenstrual exacerbations. This is not unexpected, as progesterone and estrogen levels rise steadily throughout pregnancy. Two cases were associated with spontaneous abortion. However, spontaneous improvement or clearing during pregnancy has been reported in other cases[13,19,20].

Pregnancy is known to ameliorate many allergic states; therefore it is suggested that there is a low maternal immunological reaction during pregnancy, probably due to the raised cortisol levels that occur. It is also possible that the gradual rise in the hormone levels during pregnancy brings about hormonal desensitization in some individuals.

EVIDENCE FOR PROGESTERONE SENSITIVITY

All patients with AIPD show cyclical premenstrual exacerbations of the eruption (**2.11**), which, with the use of accurate diary cards, may be shown to correspond to the postovulation rise in serum progesterone concentration. In addition, the eruption is frequently resistant to conventional therapy, irrespective of clinical type, but responds to anovulatory drugs. This implies sex hormone sensitivity, but not necessarily an antibody-mediated reaction to progesterone.

Hypersensitivity to progesterone may be demonstrated by controlled intradermal tests, intramuscular or oral progesterone challenge, or the demonstration of circulating antibodies to progesterone[14,29] or the corpus luteum[19,29]. Two cases have been associated with a serum binding factor to 17-hydroxyprogesterone[30,31].

PROGESTERONE INTRADERMAL TESTS

Intradermal tests using synthetic progesterone are reported to show an immediate positive urticarial reaction in some cases, but more frequently a delayed hypersensitivity reaction. Intradermal tests, although frequently used, in the authors' experience are unpredictable because of the insolubility of progesterone in water, and the fact that all diluents are highly irritant. Reactions are often difficult to interpret, and false-positive reactions can occur (**2.12**). Furthermore, skin necrosis at test sites, producing scarring, often occurs (**2.13**). However, a persistent late reaction confined to test sites implies progesterone sensitivity.

Recommended Procedures for Progesterone Intradermal Tests

Various dilutions of progesterone solution 0.2 mL, plus controls of diluent alone, are injected intradermally

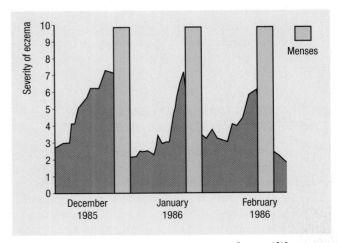

Fig 2.11 Autoimmune progesterone dermatitis.
Patient's diary cards confirm recurrent premenstrual exacerbations of eczema.

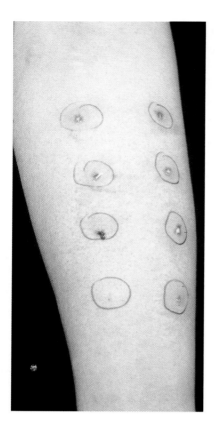

Fig 2.12 Progesterone intradermal testing demonstrating irritant reactions with necrosis at test sites. Such results cannot be interpreted.

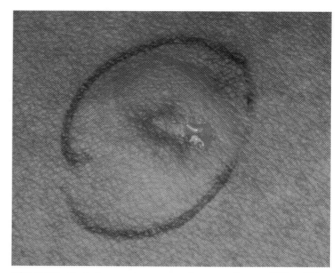

Fig 2.13 Autoimmune progesterone dermatitis. Skin necrosis commonly occurs at sites of progesterone intradermal testing.

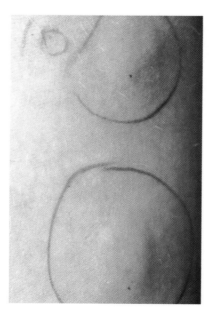

Fig 2.14 Positive progesterone intradermal test results. Persistent wheal and flare at two progesterone test sites.

into the anterior aspect of the forearm to produce a well-defined raised bleb. Pure progesterone powder is solubilized using a 60% ethanol–saline mixture to produce 1%, 0.1% and 0.01% test solutions. Ethanol–saline (60%) alone and normal saline should be used as controls.

Estrogen sensitivity may be investigated concurrently using ethinylestradiol and the same diluent. Readings should be made every 10 minutes for half an hour then every 30 minutes for the first 4 hours, and at 24 and 48 hours. Immediate irritant reactions to diluent alone may occur, in which case all early reactions at test sites should be discounted.

A positive reaction to progesterone is said to occur if a persistent wheal-and-flare reaction is present exclusively at the progesterone test sites, between 24 and 48 hours (**2.14**).

INTRAMUSCULAR AND ORAL PROGESTERONE CHALLENGE

Challenge with intramuscular progesterone has been reported in six cases and produced a flare of the eruption in all six patients. Testing should be undertaken during the first half of the menstrual cycle when the eruption would normally be quiescent, and the patient observed carefully as severe exacerbations of urticaria with angioedema, although extremely uncommon, have been reported. The authors have used Gestone (Ferring) 25 mg/mL successfully for intramuscular challenge.

Placebo-controlled oral challenge may also be of value, again if performed during the first half of the menstrual cycle. Dydrogesterone 10 mg daily for 7 days or levonorgestrel 30 µg made up to 500 mg capsules with lactose, one per day for 7 days followed by 7 days of lactose-only capsules may be used. Oral challenge is less reliable, as the eruption may not flare dramatically and may therefore be difficult to interpret.

CHALLENGE FOLLOWING CHEMICAL OOPHORECTOMY

The optimum test for AIPD, to be recommended only if the patient is so severely affected as to be considering surgical oophorectomy, is to perform a chemical oophorectomy using subcutaneous injections of a luteinizing hormone-releasing hormone (LHRH) antagonist over a 6-month period, and document clearance of the eruption alongside hormonal confirmation of absence of ovulation. Goserelin 3.6 mg by subcutaneous injection may be used for this purpose. If progesterone challenge then produces a flare of the eruption, this is substantial evidence for progesterone sensitivity.

TREATMENT

The majority of patients with AIPD encountered have failed to respond to conventional treatment modalities, although oral prednisone (prednisolone) in moderately high doses may bring about control[13,17,22]. Many patients, however, respond well to conjugated estrogens, presumably as a result of suppression of ovulation and hence the postovulatory rise in progesterone level. In practice, however, estrogen therapy is often not appropriate in view of the patient's age. When estrogen therapy is unsuccessful, the antiestrogen anovulatory drug tamoxifen may be tried. Tamoxifen 30 mg has caused complete remission,[13,18,26,32] but with consequent amenorrhea. A lower dose was achieved in one patient, with return of menstruation but not the rash. No side effects were encountered. The anabolic androgen danazol (200 mg twice daily started 1–2 days before the expected date of menses, and continuing for 3 days thereafter) has proved highly effective in two patients.

In severe cases, when the patient is unable to tolerate medical treatment, oophorectomy will clear the eruption and cure the disease[12,34]. Suppression of AIPD urticaria by chemical oophorectomy using the LHRH analog buserelin has been reported[35].

In the authors' experience, many cases of AIPD slowly settle spontaneously after a period of successful treatment.

AUTOIMMUNE ESTROGEN DERMATITIS

It is known that estrogen sensitivity can cause a clinical syndrome very similar to AIPD. The range of clinical expression includes papulovesicular eruptions, eczema, urticaria, localized pruritus (vulval or anal), and generalized pruritus. The condition is rarer than AIPD, but the hallmark of autoimmune estrogen dermatitis is the cyclical premenstrual flare[2]. In some cases, the inflammatory papulovesicles are localized to the neck, upper trunk, and arms. This localization may reflect estrogen receptor density, which is highest in the skin of the face and surrounding areas[36].

Intradermal tests are necessary to establish the diagnosis. It is essential that intradermal test materials are injected subepidermally to raise a superficial bleb and minimize rapid lymphatic removal. Shelley et al.[2] recommend using sterile aqueous suspensions of pure estrone (0.1 mL in a 1:1000 dilution) to be injected with a tuberculin syringe with a 27-gauge needle. Persistence of a papule for more than 24 hours is considered a positive test result. Oral challenges may also be done with ethinylestradiol, but a positive result may only support the concept of an estrogen-aggravated dermatitis. To show true sensitization, intradermal skin tests are needed.

Autoimmune estrogen dermatitis has been demonstrated in a patient presenting with urticaria in early pregnancy[37].

As with APID, treatment of autoimmune estrogen dermatitis has been successful with tamoxifen (10 mg twice daily), which may need to be administered only intermittently to control the eruption. Ultimately, the condition is likely to go into remission.

REFERENCES

1 Herzberg, A.J., Strohmeyer, C.R. and Cimillo-Hyland, V.A. Autoimmune progesterone dermatitis. *J. Am. Acad. Dermatol.* 1995; **32**: 335–338.

2 Shelley, W.B., Shelley, E.D., Talanin, N.Y. et al. Estrogen dermatitis. *J. Am. Acad. Dermatol.* 1995; **32**: 25–31.

3 Strickler, R.C. Endocrine hypothesis for the aetiology of premenstrual syndrome. *Clin. Obstet. Gynaecol.* 1987; **30**: 377–383.

4 Dalton, K. *The Premenstrual Syndrome and Progesterone Therapy.* 2nd ed. Year Book Medical Publishers, Chicago, 1984.

5 Maxson, W.S. The use of progesterone in the treatment of PMS. *Clin. Obstet. Gynaecol.* 1987; **30**: 465–477.

6 Anonymous. Starting oral contraceptives – which, when and how? *Drug Ther. Bull.* 1992; **30**: 41–44 (erratum in *Drug Ther. Bull.* 1992; **30**: 56).

7 Leitao, E.A. and Bernhard, J.D. Perimenstrual nonvascular dermatitis herpetiformis. *J. Am. Acad. Dermatol.* 1990; **22**: 331–334.

8 Holmes, R.C. and Black, M.M. The specific dermatoses of pregnancy – a reappraisal with specific emphasis on a proposed simplified clinical classification. *Clin. Exp. Dermatol.* 1982; 7: 65–73.

9 Géber, H. Einege daten zur pathologie dur urticaria menstruationalis. *Dermatol. Z.* 1921; **32**: 143–150.

10 Zondek, B. and Bromberg, Y.M. Endocrine allergy: allergic sensitivity to endogenous hormones. *J. Allergy* 1945; **16**: 1–16.

11 Guy, W.H., Jacobs, F.M. and Guy, W.B. Sex hormone sensitisation (corpus luteum). *Arch. Dermatol.* 1951; **63**: 377–378.

12 Shelley, W.B., Prencel, R.W. and Spoont, S.S. Autoimmune progesterone dermatitis: cure by oophorectomy. *JAMA* 1964; **190**: 35–38.

13 Stephens, C.J.M., Wojnarowska, F.T. and Wilkinson, J.D. Autoimmune progesterone dermatitis responding to tamoxifen. *Br. J. Dermatol.* 1989; **121**: 135–137.

14 Jones, W.N. and Gordon, V.H. Autoimmune progesterone eczema: an endogenous progesterone hypersensitivity. *Arch. Dermatol.* 1969; **99**: 57–59.

15 Hart, R. Autoimmune progesterone dermatitis. *Arch. Dermatol.* 1977; **113**: 426–430.

16 Stone, J. and Downham, T. Autoimmune progesterone dermatitis. *Int. J. Dermatol.* 1981; **20**: 50–51.

17 Torras, H., Fenaudo, H. and Mallolas, J. Postovulation dermatitis (dermatitis caused by progesterone). *Med. Cutan. Ibero Lat. Am.* 1980; **8**: 15–21.

18 Wojnarowska, F., Greaves, M.W. and Peachey, R.D. Progesterone induced erythema multiforme. *J. R. Soc. Med.* 1985; **78**: 407–408.

19 Farah, F.S. and Shbaklu, Z. Autoimmune progesterone urticaria. *J. Allergy Clin. Immunol.* 1971; **48**: 357–361.

20 Georgouras, K. Autoimmune progesterone dermatitis. *Aust. J. Dermatol.* 1981; **22**: 109–111.

21 Tromovitch, T. and Heggli, W. Autoimmune progesterone urticaria. *Calif. Med.* 1967; **106**: 211–212.

22 Anderson, R.H. Autoimmune progesterone dermatitis. *Cutis* 1984; **33**: 490–491.

23 Berger, H. Ulcerative stomatitis caused by endogenous progesterone. *Ann. Intern. Med.* 1955; **42**: 205–208.

24 Stephens, C.J.M. and Black, M.M. Perimenstrual eruptions: autoimmune progesterone dermatitis. *Semin. Dermatol.* 1989; **8**: 26–29.

25 Schoenmakers, A., Vermorken, A., Degreef, H. and Dooms-Goossens, A. Corticosteroid or steroid allergy. *Contact Dermatitis.* 1992; **26**: 159–162.

26 Stephens, C.J.M., McFadden, J.P., Black, M.M. and Rycroft, R.J.G. Autoimmune progesterone dermatitis. Absence of contact sensitivity to glucocorticoids, oestrogen and 17-OH-progesterone. *Contact Dermatitis.* 1994; **31**: 108–110.

27 Mayou, S.C., Charles-Holmes, R., Kenney, A. and Black, M.M. A premenstrual eruption treated with bilateral oophorectomy and hysterectomy. *Clin. Exp. Dermatol.* 1988; **13**: 114–116.

28 Bierman, S.M. Autoimmune progesterone dermatitis of pregnancy. *Arch. Dermatol.* 1973; **107**: 896–961.

29 Veda, T., Matuda, M., Yambe, H. *et al.* Two cases of autoimmune progresterone dermatitis. In Wilkinson, D.S., Mascaro, J.M. and Orfanos, C.E. (eds) *Clinical Dermatology. The CMD Case Collection*, pp. 214–215. Schattauer Stuggart, New York, 1987.

30 Pinto, J.S., Sobrinho, L., da Silva, M.B., Porto, M.T., Santos, M.A., Balo-Banga, M. and Arala-Chaves, M. Erythema multiforme associated with autoreactivity to 17 hydroxyprogesterone. *Dermatologica* 1990; **26**: 159–162.

31 Cheesman, K.L., Gaynor, L.V., Chatterton, R.T., Jr. and Radvany, R.M. Identification of a 17-hydroxyprogesterone-binding immunoglobulin in the serum of a woman with periodic rashes. *J. Clin. Endocrinol. Metab.* 1982; **55**: 597–599.

32 Nabai, H. and Rahbari, H. Autoimmune progesterone dermatitis treated with tamoxifen. *Cutis* 1994; **54**: 161–162.

33 Shahar, E., Bergman, R. and Pollack, S. Autoimmune progesterone dermatitis: effective prophylactic treatment with danazol. *Int. J. Dermatol.* 1997; **36**: 708–711.

34 Ródenas, J.M., Herranz, M.T. and Tercedor, J. Autoimmune progesterone dermatitis: treatment with oophorectony. *Br. J. Dermatol.* 1998; **139**: 508–511.

35 Yee, K.C. and Cunliffe, W.J. Progesterone-induced urticaria: response to buserelin. *Br. J. Dermatol.* 1994; **130**: 121–123.

36 Hasselquist, M.B., Goldberg, N., Schroeter, A. *et al.* Isolation and characterisation of the estrogen receptor in human skin. *J. Clin. Endocrinol. Metab.* 1980; **50**: 76–82.

37 Lee, A.Y., Lee, K.H. and Lim, Y.G. Oestrogen urticaria associated with pregnancy. *Br. J. Dermatol.* 1999; **141**: 774.

3 Physiologic Skin Changes of Pregnancy

Marilynne McKay

HYPERPIGMENTATION

Localized or generalized hyperpigmentation occurs to some extent in 90% of pregnant women. These changes are most prominent in patients with darkly pigmented skin, although they occur to some degree in fair-skinned individuals. Perhaps the most familiar example is the darkening of the lower abdominal midline, the linea alba. This is described in obstetric textbooks as an early change of pregnancy, but it may not be apparent until several months' gestation, especially in a first pregnancy. The midline streak usually proceeds from the symphysis pubis to the umbilicus, and can extend to the xiphoid process (3.1–3.4). It tends to appear earlier in subsequent pregnancies.

The nipples and areolae become pigmented (3.2–3.4), as do the external genitalia and the axillae (3.5). Darkening of the neck is particularly bothersome to some patients (3.6), but this gradually fades postpartum, along with other pigmentary changes. Striae ('stretch marks') are common, and may darken in susceptible individuals (3.7), along with other scars, nevi, and freckles. Vulvar melanosis may also develop during pregnancy (3.8).

PIGMENTARY DEMARCATION LINES

Some dark-skinned people (male and female) have pigmentary demarcation lines (also called Voight or Futcher lines) along the outer portion of the upper arms and/or posterior legs. These may not have been noticed by the patient until the general darkening of pigment during pregnancy makes them more prominent (3.9, 3.10).

MELASMA

Melasma (formerly called chloasma, or the 'mask of pregnancy') is macular hyperpigmentation of the face (3.11). Although the malar pattern is considered typical, the entire central face is affected in most patients, including the forehead, cheeks, upper lip, nose, and chin. It occurs in the second trimester in three-quarters of pregnant women and in one-third of those taking oral contraceptive pills (OCPs). Melasma is thought to be due to hormonal influences, and is worsened by sun exposure. It usually fades within a year after pregnancy or discontinuation of OCPs.

Melasma is persistent in approximately 30% of patients, whether induced by pregnancy or estrogen containing OCPs. Epidermal pigment (accentuated by Wood's light examination) is most responsive to bleaching with topical hydroquinone creams and tretinoin.

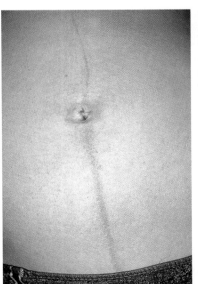

Fig 3.1 Hyperpigmentation. Darkening of the linea alba from the symphysis pubis to the xiphoid process during pregnancy.

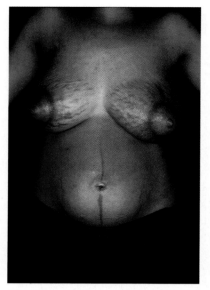

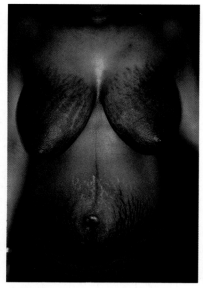

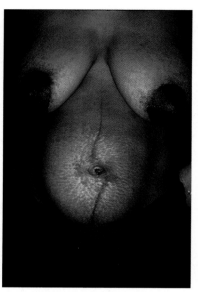

Figs 3.2–3.4 Hyperpigmentation. Three different patterns of skin darkening in African Americans, as seen immediately postpartum. Note the differences in striae formation on the abdomen and breasts, as well as patterns of pigmentation of the linea nigra, nipples, and areolae.

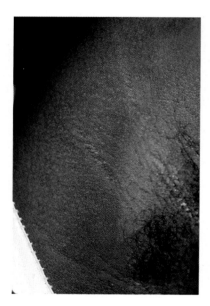

Fig 3.5 Hyperpigmentation. Pseudoacanthotic pigmentation of the axilla in another African American woman, who also had darkening of the vulva.

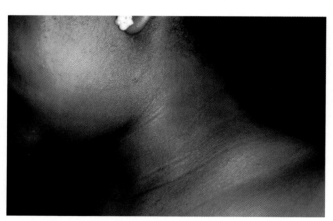

Fig 3.6 Hyperpigmentation. Darkening of the neck in an African American woman. This is cosmetically distressing to some patients, but will fade slowly.

STRIAE DISTENSAE

The so-called 'stretch marks', which occur in almost all pregnant women during the second and third trimester, are linear, pink-to-purplish, atrophic lines that develop at right angles to the skin tension lines on the abdomen, breasts, buttocks, thighs, and groin (3.12,3.13). They are the same as those seen in patients with Cushing's syndrome, steroid therapy, and rapid changes in body-weight. The red coloration typically becomes flesh-colored or pale with time (with or without topical creams of various kinds) but, although the atrophic lines may be thinner after delivery, they do not disappear completely. Topical tretinoin, 0.1% cream, has been shown to improve the appearance of striae, but can be very irritating to the skin.

HAIR AND NAIL CHANGES

Hirsutism – profuse growth of body hair – is seen in most pregnant women. It is more noticeable in women

18

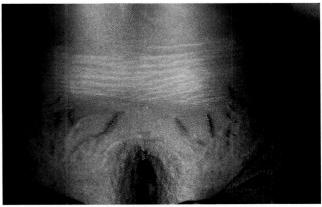

3.7 Striae distensae. Pigmentation of new striae that have developed during pregnancy; older striae remain pale.

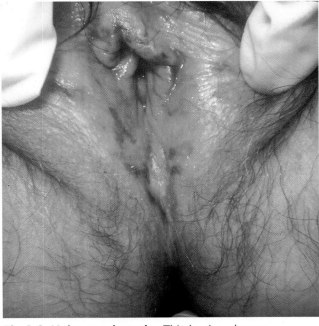

Fig 3.8 Vulvar melanosis. This benign change developed during pregnancy and did not require treatment.

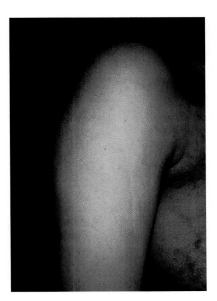

Fig 3.9 Pigmentary demarcation line. This can be seen on the upper arm. It has become more prominent during pregnancy.

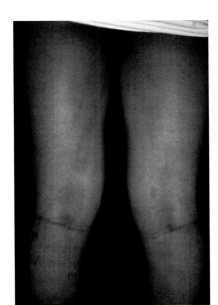

Fig 3.10 Pigmentary demarcation lines. These lines, also known as Voight or Futcher lines, can be seen on the posterior legs. They were not noticed by the patient until they darkened during pregnancy.

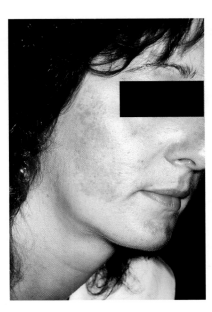

Fig 3.11 Melasma. The 'mask of pregnancy' in a typical distribution on the central face.

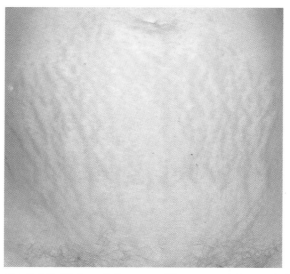

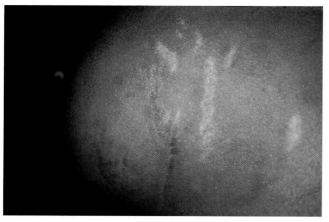

Fig 3.13 Striae distensae. Nonpigmented striae in an African American woman.

Fig 3.12 Striae distensae. These are striae, or 'stretch marks', over a fair-skinned abdomen.

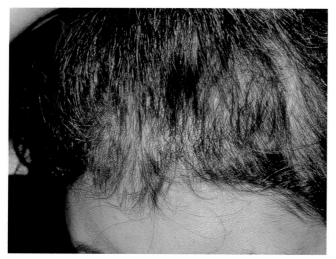

Fig 3.14 Telogen effluvium.

with dark and/or abundant body hair. The short lanugo hairs give the skin a 'furry' appearance; however, these disappear postpartum with the development of telogen effluvium.

Telogen effluvium results in the loss of terminal scalp hairs about 1–5 months postpartum; this hair loss can last for up to 1 year or more before regrowth occurs (3.14). The best explanation for this phenomenon is that pregnancy interrupts the normal hair-shedding cycle, thus allowing hairs to keep growing until delivery. Following delivery, the hair follicles rapidly resume their normal pattern of hair loss and regrowth, resulting in an apparently excessive loss of hair. However, patients can be reassured that baldness will not occur.

In rare cases, male-pattern baldness or diffuse thinning of scalp hairs may be seen late in pregnancy, but this also reverts to a normal pattern of hair growth postpartum.

Nail changes usually begin in the first trimester. Brittleness or softening may be seen, as can faster growth. Transverse grooving (Beau's line) has been noted after delivery, but this is a very nonspecific finding.

MUCOUS MEMBRANE CHANGES

Gingivitis of pregnancy is common, and occurs to a greater or lesser degree in most women. Hypertrophy of the gums increases gradually throughout pregnancy, and the mucosa become red and friable. Pyogenic granuloma (granuloma gravidarum) may be seen in this setting, but lesions usually regress after delivery and no treatment is required. They are thought to be caused by trauma to inflamed mucosa (3.15, 3.16).

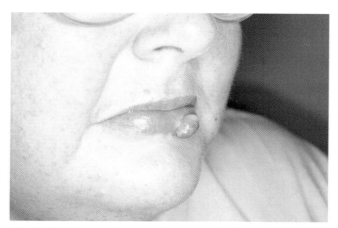

Fig 3.15 Pyogenic granuloma on the lip.

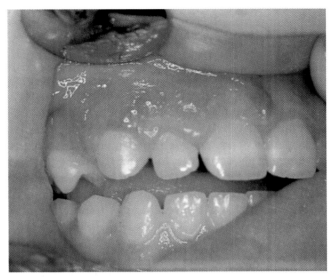

Fig 3.16 Pyogenic granuloma on the gingiva.

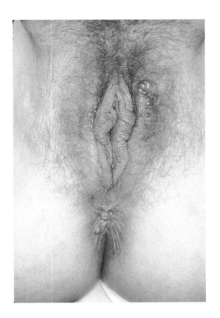

Fig 3.17 Hemorrhoids and vulvar varicosities developing during pregnancy.

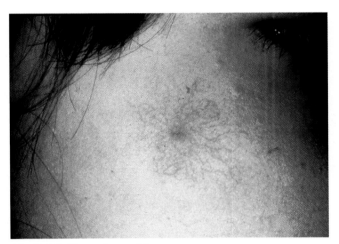

Fig 3.18 Vascular spider.

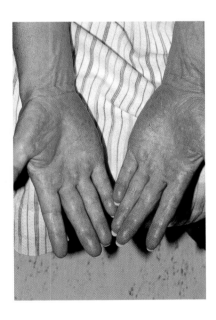

Fig 3.19 Palmar erythema.

VASCULAR AND HEMATOLOGIC CHANGES

Varicosities occur to some extent in almost half of all pregnancies (3.17), and are particularly bothersome around the anus (hemorrhoids) and on the legs. Leg and ankle edema is common and may also be accompanied by swelling of the hands and eyelids. For varicosities and swelling of the legs, supportive care with leg elevation and elastic stockings is recommended. Patients should avoid prolonged standing or sitting.

Spider angiomas (nevus araneus, spider nevus) usually develop in the first and second trimesters. Easily recognized by a central red punctum with radiating branches on the upper body, they may be seen in two-thirds of pregnant white women (3.18). Palmar erythema is also common in about the same number of patients (3.19). The etiology of both is unknown, but is thought to be associated with estrogen or angiogenic factors. These changes usually resolve postpartum.

FURTHER READING

Callen, J.P. Pregnancy's effects on the skin: common and uncommon changes. *Postgrad. Med.* 1984; **75**: 138–145.

Elson, M.L. Treatment of striae distensae with topical tretinoin. *J. Dermatol. Surg. Oncol.* 1990; **16**: 267–270.

James, W.D., Guill, M.A., Berger, T.G. *et al.* Pigmentary demarcation lines associated with pregnancy. *J. Am. Acad. Dermatol.* 1984; **11**: 438–440.

Martin, A.G. and Leal-Khouri, S. Physiologic skin changes associated with pregnancy. *Int. J. Dermatol.* 1992; **31**: 375–378.

Wade, T.R., Wade, S.L. and Jones, H.E. Skin changes and diseases associated with pregnancy. *Obstet. Gynecol.* 1978; **52**: 233–242.

Winton, G.B. and Lewis, C.W. Dermatoses of pregnancy. *J. Am. Acad. Dermatol.* 1982; **6**: 977–998.

Wong, R.C. and Ellis, C.N. Physiologic skin changes in pregnancy. *J. Am. Acad. Dermatol.* 1984; **10**: 929–940.

Wong, R.C. and Ellis, C.N. Physiologic skin changes in pregnancy. *Semin. Dermatol.* 1989; **8**: 7–11.

ACKNOWLEDGEMENTS

Figures **3.1** and **3.11** are reproduced from C.M. Lawrence and N.H. Cox *Color Atlas and Text of Physical Signs in Dermatology* (Figs 6.28 and 6.27), Wolfe, London, 1993.

Figure **3.12** is reproduced from G.M. Levene and C.D. Calnan *Color Atlas of Dermatology* (Fig. 464), Mosby–Wolfe, London, 1994.

Figure **3.16** is reproduced from W.R. Tyldesley *Color Atlas of Oral Medicine* (Fig. 146), Mosby–Wolfe, London, 1994.

4 A Systematic Approach to the Dermatoses of Pregnancy

Martin M. Black
Samantha Vaughan Jones

INTRODUCTION

Cutaneous symptoms and signs are not uncommon during pregnancy. The physiologic signs of pregnancy (*see also Chapter 3*) often involve the skin or mucous membranes, and can sometimes provide contributory evidence of pregnancy.

Although pruritus is the principal cutaneous symptom in pregnancy, itching in itself is not diagnostically helpful. Thus, a full clinical history and a thorough clinical examination are essential to confirm, or exclude, the possibility of any coexisting dermatosis or infestation. The clinical implications of pruritus in pregnancy are outlined in **Table 4.1**.

Chapter 8 describes the effect of pregnancy on other skin disorders. This chapter considers pruritus gravidarum and the difficult nomenclature of the specific dermatoses of pregnancy.

OBSTETRIC CHOLESTASIS

Obstetric cholestasis (OC) is manifested by pruritus in pregnancy, with or without laboratory evidence of cholestasis[1]. Although the condition is not accompanied by primary skin lesions, excoriations due to severe scratching are often present in more severe cases[2].

The disorder is a genetically linked, estrogen-dependent condition, which results in cholestasis, with or without jaundice. It usually begins in later pregnancy and resolves rapidly after delivery[1-4]. There is a positive family history in up to 50% of cases. OC is particularly prevalent in Scandinavia, northern Europe and Chile, and this has recently been linked to dietary factors[5]. A diagnosis of OC can be readily established or confirmed using the criteria given in **Table 4.2**.

PATHOGENESIS

No single biochemical abnormality has been found in OC. It has been postulated that the relative fall in hepatic blood flow during pregnancy leads to decreased clearance of toxins, and also estrogens[6]. Estrogens increase biliary cholesterol concentration and secretion, and also impair the capacity of the liver to transport anions, such as bilirubin and bile salts.

It has also been postulated that estrogens regulate actin molecules, which act intracellularly to mediate bile excretion[7].

Table 4.1 Clinical Implications of Pruritus in Pregnancy.

Normal skin (pruritus gravidarum)
Obstetric cholestasis
Associated skin rash
Pre-existing skin condition
Coincidentally acquired skin condition
Specific dermatosis of pregnancy

Table 4.2 Diagnostic Criteria of Obstetric Cholestasis.

Pruritus related to pregnancy, with no history of exposure to hepatitis or hepatotoxic drugs
Presence of generalized pruritus with or without jaundice
Absence of primary skin lesions
Localization of pruritus to palms and soles
Alteration of liver function consistent with cholestasis
Rapid disappearance of itching after delivery
Recurrence of itching in any subsequent pregnancy

CLINICAL AND LABORATORY FINDINGS

The disorder typically presents in the last trimester of an otherwise normal pregnancy, although initial presentation as early as 8 weeks' gestation has been reported. The incidence is increased in twin pregnancies[8]. Intense, generalized itching occurs, which is invariably worse at night, and persists throughout the duration of pregnancy. Pruritus is often localized, particularly to the palms and soles. The result of physical examination is usually normal, apart from the finding of widespread excoriations, and skin biopsies are unhelpful. Up to 50% of patients develop darker urine and light-colored stools, but only a few develop clinical jaundice, usually within 2–4 weeks of the onset of itching. Recurrences during subsequent pregnancies occur in about 70% of cases and follow a similar course. Oral contraceptives also provoke a recurrence of pruritus and cholestasis.

A typical biochemical finding is of markedly increased levels of total serum bile acids. Other laboratory findings may include moderately increased levels of serum-conjugated bilirubin, alkaline phosphatase, cholesterol, and lipids. Liver transaminases are usually only slightly raised; significantly higher levels of transaminases indicate that infectious hepatitis is the likely cause of the jaundice. Hepatic ultrasonographic findings are normal and liver biopsy is not indicated for typical OC but, if performed, shows centrilobular cholestasis and bile thrombi within dilated canaliculi[3].

JAUNDICE

The incidence of jaundice in pregnancy is about one in every 1500 pregnancies[6]. For comparison, viral hepatitis is a more common cause of jaundice in pregnancy. Meanwhile, OC accounts for about 20% of cases of obstetric jaundice. Since there is often a family history of obstetric jaundice, a possible genetic enzyme defect might be responsible.

FETAL RISKS

Obstetric cholestasis is associated with a high incidence of stillbirth, early delivery, and perinatal complications[9,10]. Serum abnormalities do not parallel fetal risk and are useful only to confirm the diagnosis. Postpartum and fetal intracranial hemorrhage are a particular risk, due to malabsorption of fat-soluble vitamin K. Intensive fetal surveillance is therefore recommended, including amniocentesis for meconium[9]. Induction at 38 weeks' gestation, or after demonstration of a mature lecithin: sphingomyelin ratio, may result in increased fetal survival[9,10].

MANAGEMENT

Treatment of the mother is largely symptomatic[1]. Cholestyramine or phenobarbital can be given, but there is no consensus about their efficacy. Phototherapy using ultraviolet B radiation may help relieve pruritus. Rest and a low fat diet have improved symptoms in some cases[3]. In prolonged OC, intramuscular administration of vitamin K may be necessary. Ursodeoxycholic acid (UDCA) is now used to treat this disorder, although patient consent is necessary as this drug is not yet licensed in pregnancy. The recommended dose is 15 mg/kg/day both to reduce symptoms and improve fetal outcome[5]. UDCA has been shown to reduce premature labor, fetal distress, and fetal deaths[5].

THE SPECIFIC DERMATOSES OF PREGNANCY

A group of inflammatory dermatoses closely related to pregnancy has caused great diagnostic confusion. Prior to 1982, the terminology became increasingly confused, with several names being used for similar clinical conditions (**Tables 4.3 and 4.4**). The author has extensively reviewed all the existing literature and has studied a large group of patients comprehensively, covering all the existing disease entities. Similar work was done by Holmes and Black before they published their proposals in 1982[21] and 1983[22] of a simplified clinical classification of the specific dermatoses of pregnancy. This classification basically subdivided the specific dermatoses of pregnancy into four groups:

- Pemphigoid (herpes) gestationis;
- Polymorphic eruption of pregnancy;
- Prurigo of pregnancy;
- Pruritic folliculitis of pregnancy.

Unfortunately, except for pemphigoid (herpes) gestationis, no reliable criteria exist to differentiate the specific dermatoses of pregnancy[23]. Nevertheless, the proposed, simplified, clinical classification appears gradually to have gained international acceptance[23]. For example, a recent prospective study of 3192 pregnant women with pruritus found that only seven cases could not be classified into a particular subgroup, according to the classification[24]. In a more recent study of 200 pregnancy dermatoses, 85 women had a specific dermatosis of pregnancy[25]. There are a number of other skin disorders that may present during pregnancy and may closely mimic the specific dermatoses of pregnancy (**Table 4.5**). These should always be considered in the differential diagnosis.

From time to time 'new' disease entities are reported in the literature, but to date they remain essentially anecdotal single case reports. Impetigo herpetiformis, for example, is now considered to be a variant of pustular

Table 4.3 Historical List of Specific Dermatoses of Pregnancy as Described by Various Authors.

Disorder	Reference	Year
Herpes gestationis	Milton[11]	1872
Herpes impetiginiformis (impetigo herpetiformis)	Hebra[12]	1872
Prurigo gestationis	Besnier et al.[13]	1904
Erythema multiforme	Gross[14]	1931
Prurigo annularis	Davis[15]	1941
Toxemic rash of pregnancy	Bourne[16]	1962
Papular dermatitis of pregnancy	Spangler et al.[17]	1962
Early and late-onset prurigo of pregnancy	Nurse[18]	1968
Pruritic urticarial papules and plaques of pregnancy	Lawley et al.[19]	1979
Pruritic folliculitis of pregnancy	Zoberman and Farmer[20]	1981

psoriasis (*see also Chapter 8*). Alcalay et al.[26] proposed the term linear IgM dermatosis of pregnancy, and described a single case of an intensely pruritic follicular papular eruption, which occurred in the third trimester. Linear deposition of IgM was noted at the dermoepidermal junction, but this disappeared after delivery. However, on clinical grounds, their case would have fitted well into the category of pruritic folliculitis of pregnancy.

CONCLUSION

It is clear that there is still much to be done in elucidating the pathogenesis of the specific dermatoses of pregnancy. Until this happens, the authors suggest that the above proposed simplified clinical classification should be used. The authors have designed an algorithm which provides a guide to the differential diagnosis, investigation, and treatment of the specific dermatoses of pregnancy (**4.1**). This will usually provide sufficient clinical diagnostic information to advise and manage the patient. The following chapters deal with each of the specific dermatoses of pregnancy in greater detail.

Table 4.4 Differential Diagnosis of Dermatoses of Pregnancy.

Diagnosis	Clinical Signs	Laboratory Findings	Risks/ Complications	Management
Pemphigoid (herpes) gestationis (See Chapter 5)	Erythema, wheals and blisters on abdomen (especially periumbilical), palms, soles, elsewhere	DIF positive (BMZ of skin and amnion)	Mother: discomfort and increased risk of other autoimmune diseases Fetus: blisters, increased risk of prematurity	Prednisone, plasmapheresis
Polymorphic eruption (pruritic urticarial papules and plaques) of pregnancy (See Chapter 6)	Papules, urticarial lesions on abdomen (common on striae distensae), thighs, buttocks; small vesicles may be present	DIF negative	None, other than mother's discomfort	Moderately potent topical corticosteroids
Prurigo of pregnancy (See Chapter 7)	Discrete erythematous papules on extremities, trunk	DIF negative	None, other than mother's discomfort	Moderately potent topical corticosteroids
Pruritic folliculitis of pregnancy (See Chapter 7)	Small red follicular papules and pustules on back, arms ('acne')	DIF negative	Mother: discomfort Fetus: none	5% benzoyl peroxide +1% hydrocortisone

DIF, direct immunofluorescence; BMZ, basement membrane zone.

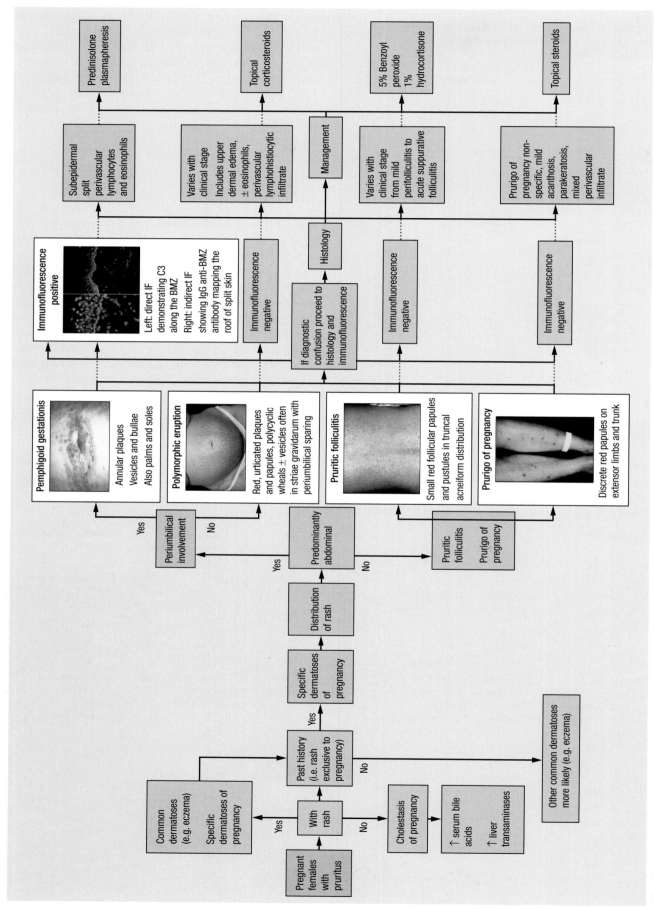

Fig. 4.1 An algorithmic approach to the pregnant woman presenting with pruritus.

Table 4.5 Common Skin Disorders that may Mimic Dermatoses of Pregnancy.

Disorder	Clinical Details
Allergic	
Urticaria (hives)	Does not blister, lesions transient
Drug reactions	Ingestion of medication
Contact dermatitis	Pattern, history of allergen
Common Skin Eruptions	
Atopic dermatitis or eczema	Family history of asthma, hay fever, rash on antecubital/popliteal folds, comes and goes with seasons, very itchy and chronic
Pityriasis rosea	Oval, slightly scaly plaques on trunk, 'herald patch' may precede rash by 1–2 weeks. May mimic secondary syphilis, consider serum test for syphilis
Erythema nodosum	Tender red nodules on shins and lower legs, occasionally seen with pregnancy
Miliaria	'Prickly heat', tiny vesicles on extremities or trunk in hot weather
Insect bites and scabies	Flea bites are most often on legs, sometimes blister in sensitive patient. Scabies has linear papules in fingerwebs, elbows, areolae

REFERENCES

1 Fagan, E. A. Intrahepatic cholestasis of pregnancy. *B.M.J.* 1994; **309**: 1242–1244.

2 Berg, B., Helm, G., Petersohn, L., *et al*. Cholestasis of pregnancy, clinical and laboratory studies. *Acta Obstet. Gynecol. Scand.* 1986; **65**: 107–113.

3 Reyes, H. The spectrum of liver and gastrointestinal disease seen in cholestasis of pregnancy. *Gastroenterol. Clin. North Am.* 1992; **21**: 905–921.

4 Shaw, D., Frohlich, J., Wittmann, B. A. K., *et al*. A prospective study of 18 patients with cholestasis of pregnancy. *Am. J. Obstet. Gynecol.* 1982; **142**: 621–625.

5 Reyes, H. Intrahepatic cholestasis. A puzzling disorder of pregnancy. *J. Gastroenterol. Hepatol.* 1997; **12**: 211–216.

6 Rustgi, V. K. Liver disease in pregnancy. *Med. Clin. North Am.* 1989; **73**: 1041–1047.

7 Reyes-Romero, M. A. Are changes in expression of actin genes involved in estrogen-induced cholestasis? *Med. Hypotheses* 1990; **32**: 39–43.

8 Gonzales, M. C., Reyes, H., Ribalta, J. *et al*. Intrahepatic cholestasis of pregnancy in twin pregnancies. *J. Hepatol.* 1989; **9**: 84–90.

9 Fisk, N. M. and Bruce Storey, G. N. Fetal outcome in obstetric cholestasis. *Br. J. Obstet. Gynaecol.* 1988; **95**: 1137–1143.

10 Fisk, N. M., Bye, W. B., and Bruce Storey G. N. Maternal features of obstetric cholestasis: 20 years' experience at King George V Hospital. *Aust. N. Z. J. Obstet. Gynaecol.* 1988; **28**: 172–176.

11 Milton, J. L. *The Pathology and Treatment of Disease of the Skin*. Robert Hardwicke, London, 1872, p. 205.

12 Hebra, F. Herpes impetiginiformis. *Lancet* 1872; i: 399–400.

13 Besnier, E., Brocq, L., and Jacquet, L. L. *La Pratique Dermatologique*. Masson et Cies, Paris, 1904, Vol. 1, p. 75.

14 Gross, P. Erythema multiforme gestationis. *Arch. Dermatol. Syph.* 1931; **23**: 567.

15 Davis, J. H. T. Prurigo annularis. *Br. J. Dermatol.* 1941; **53**: 143–145.

16 Bourne, G. Toxaemic rash of pregnancy. *Proc. R. Soc. Med.* 1962; **55**: 462–464.

17 Spangler, A. S., Reddy, W., Bardavil, W. A., *et al*. Papular dermatitis of pregnancy. *J.A.M.A.* 1962; **181**: 577–581.

18 Nurse, D. S. Prurigo of pregnancy. *Australas. J. Dermatol.* 1968; **9**: 258–267.

19 Lawley, T. J., Hertz, K. C., Wade, T. R., *et al*. Pruritic urticarial papules and plaques of pregnancy. *J.A.M.A.* 1979; **241**: 1696–1699.

20 Zoberman, E. and Farmer, E. R. Pruritic folliculitis of pregnancy. *Arch. Dermatol.* 1981; **117**: 20–22.

21 Holmes, R. C. and Black, M. M. The specific dermatoses of pregnancy: a reappraisal with special emphasis on a proposed simplified clinical classification. *Clin. Exp. Dermatol.* 1982; **7**: 65–73.

22 Holmes, R. C. and Black, M. M. The specific dermatoses of pregnancy. *J. Am. Acad. Dermatol.* 1983; **7**: 104–110.

23 Borradori, L. and Saurat, J. H. Specific dermatoses of pregnancy: towards a comprehensive view? *Arch. Dermatol.* 1994; **130**: 778–780.

24 Roger, D., Vaillant, L., Fignon, A., *et al*. Specific pruritic diseases of pregnancy: a prospective study of 3192 pregnant women. *Arch. Dermatol.* 1994; **130**: 734–739.

25 Vaughan Jones, S. A., Hern, S. Nelson-Piercy, C. *et al*. A prospective study of 200 women with dermatoses of pregnancy correlating the clinical findings with hormonal and immunopathological profiles. *Br. J. Dermatol.* 1999; **141**: 71–81.

26 Alcalay, J., Ingber, A., Hazaz, B., *et al*. Linear IgM dermatosis of pregnancy. *J. Am. Acad. Dermatol.* 1988; **18**: 412–415.

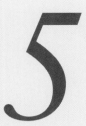

5 Pemphigoid (Herpes) Gestationis

Rachel E. Jenkins
Jeff Shornick

ETIOLOGY

Pemphigoid gestationis (PG) is a rare autoimmune bullous disease that occurs during pregnancy and the puerperium, being associated occasionally with trophoblastic tumors, hydatidiform mole, and choriocarcinoma[1]. Historically it has been known by many names, with Milton first applying the term herpes gestationis in 1872 (**Table 5.1**). Clinically and immunopathologically, PG is closely related to the pemphigoid group of bullous disorders and therefore the term pemphigoid gestationis is preferable to herpes gestationis, which may otherwise encourage confusion with virus-mediated disease. Despite a clinical resemblance to herpetic lesions, viral studies of PG have been consistently negative.

Table 5.1 Historical Terminology of Pemphigoid Gestationis.

Term	Original Citation
Pemphigus gravidarum	von Martius, 1829
Pemphigus pruriginosus	Chausit, 1852
Herpes circinatus bullosus	Wilson, 1867
Pemphigus hystericus	Hebra, 1868
Herpes gestationis	Milton, 1872
Dermatitis multiformis gestationis	Allen, 1889
Pemphigoid gestationis	Holmes and Black, 1982

CLINICAL FEATURES

Pemphigoid gestationis is estimated to complicate 1 in 40 000–60 000 pregnancies[1]. The disease has no racial predisposition, although there is evidence that the incidence may vary according to the incidence of human leucocyte antigen (HLA)-DR3 and DR4 in different populations[2].

ONSET OF DISEASE

Pemphigoid gestationis may develop at any time from 9 weeks' gestation to 1 week postpartum, but usually presents during the second and third trimesters. Approximately 18% present in the first trimester, 34% in the second trimester, and a further 34% in the third trimester[3]. Initial presentation postpartum may be 'explosive' and occurs in approximately 14% of women, but onset more than 3 days postpartum makes PG unlikely as the diagnosis[3]. The disease is likely to recur, usually with an earlier onset and more florid expression. When PG develops during the middle trimester there is often a period of relative remission in the last few weeks of pregnancy but this is frequently followed by abrupt relapse postpartum[1,3,4].

Occasionally, subsequent pregnancies are unaffected. Such 'skip pregnancies' have an incidence of approximately 8% but remain unpredictable on a prospective basis using available data[3]. What is clear, however, is that recurrence is not universal. Previous reports have suggested that such pregnancies may be more likely following a change in partner or when the mother and fetus are fully compatible at the HLA-D locus, but this is certainly not always the case[1].

RASH OF PEMPHIGOID GESTATIONIS

The disease typically presents with pruritic, erythematous, urticated papules and plaques which may become target-like, develop into annular wheals, or become polycyclic. Progression to clustered vesicobullous lesions on erythematous skin usually occurs within days to weeks of the initial onset of pruritus. Bullae may appear *de novo* on otherwise clinically uninvolved skin. Blisters are usually tense and contain serous fluid; however, pustules may be seen, albeit rarely. In 90% of patients the eruption is initially confined to the periumbilical area (5.1–5.3) with later spread to the abdomen (5.4–5.6), thighs (5.7), palms, and soles (5.8)[3]. The condition often becomes widespread but the face (5.9) and oral mucosa are usually spared. The blisters tend to resolve first with the plaques of erythema persisting longer. In the absence of secondary infection, resolution usually occurs without scarring.

NATURAL HISTORY

Occasionally there is spontaneous clearing of the disease during the latter part of pregnancy, only to flare at the time of delivery. Postpartum flares of disease are seen in 50–75% of patients, typically beginning within 24–48 hours of delivery. The duration of postpartum flares is variable but usually ranges from weeks to several months of involvement. Some patients have been reported with disease activity for as long as 11–12 years[5].

The duration of continued disease activity beyond delivery is variable and there is no correlation between disease activity and serum antibody titers. As the disease begins to resolve, recurrences associated with the menstrual cycle are common. Some women (20–50%) develop recurrences if treated with oral contraceptives (estrogens or progestogens).

HYDATIDIFORM MOLE AND CHORIOCARCINOMA

Pemphigoid gestationis is rarely associated with trophoblastic tumors such as hydatidiform mole and choriocarcinoma[1], which are most commonly produced by a diploid contribution of paternal chromosomes and have neither fetal tissue nor amnion[6]. Interestingly, there are no reports of PG-like disease in men with choriocarcinoma. This malignancy is relatively common and biochemically similar to normal pregnancy. Cytogenetic studies have demonstrated that the chromosomes in choriocarcinoma in men are also entirely of paternal origin[6]. It would, therefore, appear that placental tissue is required for the initial development of disease, not simply the presence of germinal tissue or the actual presence of fetus.

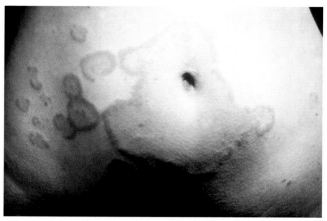

Fig 5.1 Early PG at 28 weeks' gestation. Pruritic polycyclic urticarial lesions have developed periumbilically.

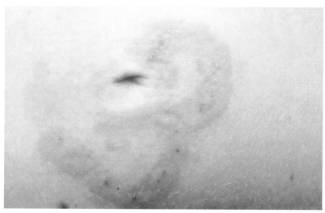

Fig 5.2 Early PG around the umbilicus. The urticarial lesions are beginning to develop vesicles.

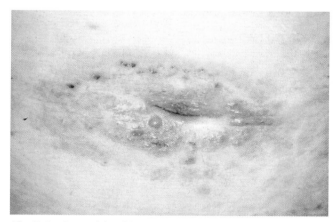

Fig 5.3 Pemphigoid gestationis. The periumbilical involvement is now clearly bullous.

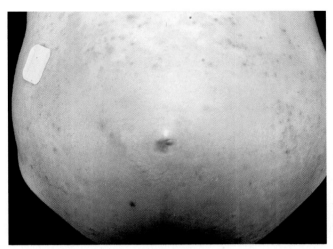

Fig 5.4   PG at 34 weeks' gestation. Pruritic urticarial lesions involve the entire abdomen.

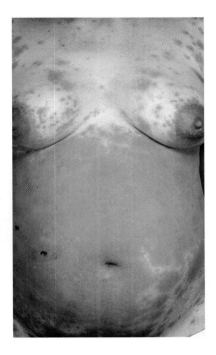

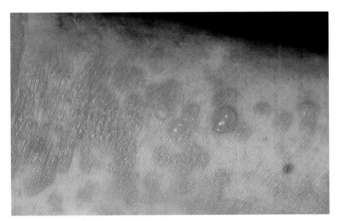

Fig 5.6   Pemphigoid gestationis. The same patient as in 5.5 Small bullae are developing within the areas of urticated erythema.

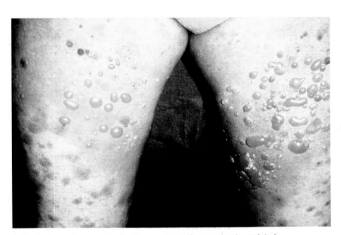

Fig 5.7   Severe PG, involving the anterior thighs.

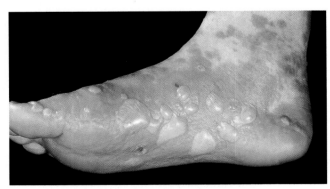

Fig 5.8   Pemphigoid gestationis. Large bullae developing on soles.

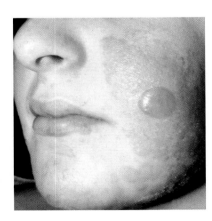

Fig 5.9 Severe PG, showing bulla and urticarial facial lesions.

FETAL AND NEONATAL DISEASE

Some 5–10% of infants born to mothers with PG have cutaneous lesions[1]. Transient urticarial or vesicular lesions are most common and resolve spontaneously within around 3 weeks, presumably as transferred maternal antibodies are catabolized (5.10). Long-term sequelae of disease have not been reported in children born to affected mothers, nor has an increased frequency of other autoimmune diseases.

Neonatal PG results from the passive transfer across the placenta of maternal immunoglobulin (Ig) G anti-basement membrane zone (BMZ) autoantibodies. These antibodies may be demonstrated in cord blood and neonatal skin. Subclinical disease is probably common since direct immunofluorescence (IF) of fetal skin is routinely positive despite a lack of clinically apparent disease. By the end of the first month of life, infants' skin biopsy specimens are normal and circulating IgG anti-BMZ autoantibodies can no longer be detected.

There has been controversy about whether or not PG is associated with an increase in fetal morbidity or mortality rate. In 1969 Kolodny remarked that there was no evidence of an increased incidence of stillbirth or spontaneous abortion associated with PG[7]. Lawley et al.[8] reviewed 41 cases of immunologically confirmed PG and, by contrast, reported increased fetal morbidity and mortality rates[8]. This review, however, relied extensively on published cases. A study of 50 pregnancies affected by PG demonstrated a slight increase in the frequency of infants that were small for dates and, because such infants have increased mortality and morbidity rates, these authors concluded that the fetal prognosis in PG was impaired[9]. A more recent large study found no evidence of an increased rate of spontaneous abortion or significant mortality but did demonstrate an increased incidence of both prematurity and small-for-dates babies with PG[10]. These observations would be consistent with low-grade placental dysfunction.

ASSOCIATED AUTOIMMUNE DISEASES

A few patients with PG have been reported to have additional autoimmune diseases (e.g. alopecia areata and Crohn's disease) but this is unusual. However, a recent study of 87 patients with PG reported that 13.8% also had Graves' disease[3] (5.11). Graves' disease is known to be associated with DR3, with a 0.4% female prevalence. This study also documented a slight increase in other autoantibodies in patients with PG, including antithyroid antibodies and platelet antibodies. In addition there is a 25% incidence of autoimmune diseases in the relatives of those with PG, particularly Graves' disease, Hashimoto thyroiditis and pernicious anemia[11].

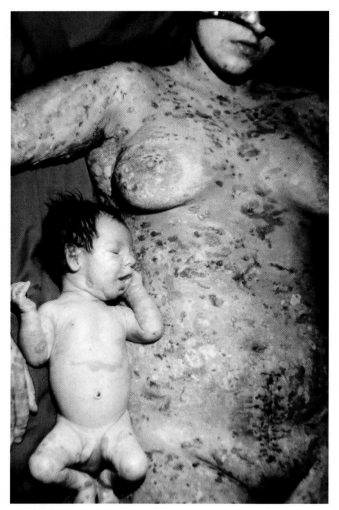

Fig 5.10 Mother to fetus transmission. The mother has severe PG, but only mild transient disease is present in the neonate.

PATHOLOGY

HISTOPATHOLOGY

The histopathology of PG classically shows subepidermal blistering, eosinophils within the blister fluid, and an edematous upper dermis that contains a mixed, perivascular, lymphohistiocytic infiltrate admixed with eosinophils, although these characteristic findings are seen only in a minority. More common findings include spongiotic vesicle formation or eosinophilic spongiosis. Eosinophils, neutrophils, or occasional lymphocytes may be seen to line up along the BMZ. The presence of eosinophils is the most constant feature in PG, being seen in nearly every case. Early urticarial lesions are characterized by epidermal and marked papillary dermal edema. Subepidermal separation results from basal cell necrosis leading to subepidermal bullae. Severe edema of the papillary dermis may result in bulbous, tear-drop-shaped dermal papillae.

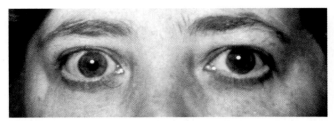

Fig 5.11 Thyrotoxicosis (Graves' disease) in the same patient as in **5.9**. Thyrotoxicosis developed 10 years after the onset of severe PG.

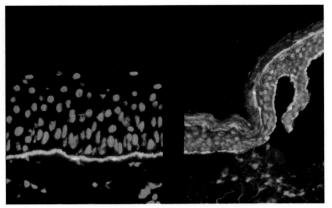

Fig 5.12 Direct immunofluorescence in PG. Bright linear deposition of C3 in the basement membrane zone and along the epidermal side of salt-split skin (pemphigoid pattern).

IMMUNOPATHOLOGY

The most characteristic finding in PG is linear deposition of C3, with or without IgG, along the BMZ of perilesional skin. Direct IF demonstrates C3 in the BMZ of clinically uninvolved skin in all patients with PG (5.12) and linear IgG deposition in about 25%. IgG deposition may be demonstrable in patients with negative routine IF with refined multistep techniques. For example, the use of split-skin specimens, chemically separated through the lamina lucida, demonstrates IgG deposits in the lamina lucida even when conventional direct IF is negative. There appears to be no difference in disease expression in patients who have deposition of complement alone compared with those who have IgG in addition to complement.

The herpes gestationis factor, now known as PG factor, is an IgG1 autoantibody directed against a normal cell surface component of cutaneous BMZ[1]. By contrast, in bullous pemphigoid (BP) the predominant autoantibody is IgG4 subclass. Circulating anti-BMZ IgG is detected in about 25% of patients using an indirect IF technique and binding is to the epidermal side of sodium chloride split skin; titers tend not to correlate with disease severity.

There have been a few reports of atypical IF staining in patients with PG, the significance of which is yet to be established[12,13].

IMMUNOGENETICS

Pemphigoid gestationis has previously been shown to be associated with the HLA antigens DR3 and DR4: 61–80% of patients express DR3, 52–53% express DR4, and 43–50% express both, compared with 3% of normal controls[14]. Advances in molecular analytical techniques such as restriction fragment length polymorphism (RFLP) and sequence-specific oligonucleotide probing have allowed the identification of HLA alleles previously difficult to define by serologic assays. HLA-DRB1*0301 (DR3) and DRB1*0401/040X (DR4; the 'X' denoting the combined subtypes of DR4 other than 0401) have, for instance, been shown to be associated

with PG[15]. There is no obvious relationship between HLA type and clinical severity, onset, duration, or recurrence, nor is there any relationship between HLA type and the presence or absence of IgG along the BMZ by direct IF. A significant increase in the frequency of paternal HLA-DR2 antigens has also led to the conclusion that both paternal HLA type and maternal HLA antibodies are important in the development of PG. The major histocompatibility complex (MHC) class II genes (DR, DP, and DQ) are located immediately adjacent to the class III genes which encode the complement components C4, with the multiple isomers of C4A and C4B, factor B and C2. The nonfunctioning C4 null allele is always present in patients with PG[16]. The C4A rather than the C4B null allele is seen and may impair immune complex degradation. However, because the C4 locus is adjacent to the DR locus on chromosome 6, with strong linkage disequilibrium, it is extremely difficult to determine what is the primary genetic marker in PG – DRB1*0301, DRB1* 0401/040X, or a C4 null allele.

IMMUNOPATHOGENESIS

Studies using immunoelectron microscopy have demonstrated that anti-BMZ IgG is directed towards a component just below the hemidesmosome in the upper lamina lucida of the BMZ. Immunoprecipitation has previously demonstrated that the majority (more than 95%) of BP sera react with a 230 kDa epidermal polypeptide known as BPAg1[17], with about 50% also reacting with a second epidermal antigen of 180 kDa, known as BPAg2[18]. The majority of PG sera recognize BPAg2 and some react to both BPAg2 and BPAg1. Cloning and sequencing have demonstrated that the two antigens are distinct gene products of different chromosomal locations, *BPAG1* at locus 6p11–12[19] and

BPAG2 at locus 10q24.3[20]. *BPAG2* has recently also been identified as *COL171A1*[21]. PG and BP, therefore, appear to share antigenic determinants, but in PG antibodies directed against the 180 kDa antigen are prevalent whereas in BP antibodies to the 230 kDa antigen are more common.

Immunoelectron microscopy using immunogold techniques has shown that BPAg2 is a type II transmembrane constituent of the hemidesmosome with collagenous segments in its extracellular domain and, for this reason, is also known as type XVII collagen[22]. BPAg1, on the other hand, is an intracellular, cytoplasmic plaque component[23]. The actual target epitope in PG has been localized to the NC16A region of the BPAg2 extracellular domain, positioned immediately adjacent to the plasma membrane of hemidesmosomes[24]. This immunodominant epitope is recognized by more than 50% of BP sera and 70% of PG sera. It has been further mapped to a 16 amino acid peptide.

Since BPAg1 is restricted to the intracellular compartment of the basal keratinocyte, it is not directly accessible to circulating antibodies. Anti-BPAg1 autoantibodies would, therefore, be predicted to arise as a secondary event in response to an initial insult to the basal keratinocyte. In contrast, BPAg2 is a transmembrane protein and is recognized by both PG and BP autoantibodies. Therefore, anti-BPAg2 autoantibodies may play an initiator role in subepidermal blister formation in PG and BP. Circulating autoantibodies in both PG and BP are likely to access to this newly defined antigenic site on the surface of intact keratinocytes.

Circulating autoantibodies which bind to skin cross-react with the basement membranes of chorionic epithelium and amnion, and immune complexes are found to be deposited in the placenta during the course of most cases of PG (5.13). In addition there is aberrant expression of MHC class II antigens in the placenta on amniochorionic stromal cells and trophoblastic cells which are derived from paternal genes[25]. This is not so in the skin, where only complement components (with or without IgG) are seen along the BMZ. These placental cells may be exposed to the maternal immune system, as it is known that in some anchoring villi there are focal deficiencies in the syncytiotrophoblast[26]. The cross-reactivity may be explained by the common origin of skin and amnion from the ectodermal germ layer.

In PG there is a universal presence of anti-HLA antibodies, which are directed mainly against class I antigens[27]. The actual role of these anti-HLA antibodies in the primary pathogenesis of PG is unknown but their presence does imply that women with PG are more able than normal women to mount an allogeneic response against their partner's antigens, and this may be a clue to the etiology of the disease. Anti-HLA antibodies may develop as a consequence of a placental bleed, which may then result in the partial destruction of the placenta, thereby exposing cryptic antigens and leading to the production of IgG autoantibody.

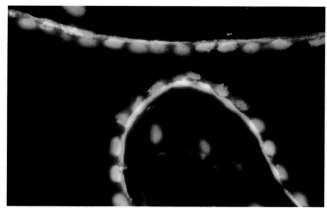

Fig 5.13 Placental immunology in PG. Linear binding of PG antibody to amniotic basement membrane.

DIFFERENTIAL DIAGNOSIS

Differentiation of PG from other cutaneous bullous eruptions is usually not difficult, especially once blisters have begun to develop (*see Chapters 4 and 6*). The vesicles and bullae found only in PG distinguish it from other pregnancy-related dermatoses such as papular dermatitis of pregnancy and prurigo of pregnancy. Nonclassical presentations could, however, easily be confused with polymorphic eruption of pregnancy (PEP) (**Table 5.2**) and other autoimmune bullous diseases (e.g. BP) (**Table 5.3**), dermatitis herpetiformis (DH), or linear IgA disease (LAD). Bullous systemic lupus erythematosus (SLE) also needs to be considered. Bullous pemphigoid is unusual in the childbearing age group; DH and LAD can be differentiated by routine histology or IF (**Table 5.4**). In most clinical settings the most important differential diagnosis is between pre-bullous PG and PEP. Although eosinophils are more commonly seen in PG, they may also be present in PEP, and the key to differentiating the two diseases is IF. Other diseases to be considered in the differential diagnosis include erythema multiforme, contact dermatitis, and bullous drug eruptions.

TREATMENT

The aim of therapy in patients with PG is to relieve pruritus, suppress blister formation, and prevent erosions, secondary infection, and scarring of lesional sites. In mild cases of PG careful but aggressive use of topical fluorinated corticosteroids combined with emollients and systemic antihistamines are adequate. Once bullae have developed, however, it is usually necessary to use systemic steroids[1,3,4]. A good response to prednisolone (e.g. 40 mg daily) is common, with control of pruritic symptoms, cessation of new vesicle formation and clearing within 10 days. Some patients receive greater symptomatic relief from divided doses of daily corticosteroids. Once these patients' disease is controlled, they can be converted to single morning

Table 5.2 Differences Between Polymorphic Eruption of Pregnancy and Pemphigoid Gestationis.

Feature	Polymorphic Eruption of Pregnancy	Pemphigoid Gestationis
Incidence	Common (1 : 150)	Very rare (1 : 50 000)
Primiparous	80%	50%
Multiple pregnancy	+	–
Morphology		
Erythematous papules	+	+
Target lesions	+	+
Vesicles	+	+
Bullae	–	+
Prominent striae	+	–
Periumbilical lesions	–	+
Fetal prognosis	Normal	Impaired
Recurrence in subsequent pregnancies	–	+
Direct IF for C3 at BMZ	–	100%
Indirect IF for C3 at BMZ	–	80%
HLA associations	–	DR3, DR4
Associated autoimmune conditions	–	+
Etiology	Unknown	Autoantibody to BMZ of skin and placenta

IF, immunofluorescence; C3, third component of complement; BMZ, basement membrane zone; HLA, human leucocyte antigen.

Table 5.3 Comparison of Bullous Pemphigoid and Pemphigoid Gestationis.

	Bullous Pemphigoid	Pemphigoid Gestationis
Similarities		
Clinical	Widespread pruritic bullous eruption	
Histopathology	Subepidermal bullae containing numerous eosinophils	
Direct IF	Deposition of C3 and IgG at the BMZ	
Indirect IF	Circulating complement fixing IgG1 autoantibody	
Immunogold electron microscopy	Deposition of the reaction product below hemidesmosome at *NC16A* domain of BPAg2 (180 kDa)	
Treatment	Invariable response to systemic corticosteroids	
Differences		
Sex	Male : female (1 : 1)	Female
Age	Over 60 years	15–45 years
Etiologic associations	Unknown	Pregnancy, hydatidiform mole, choriocarcinoma
Predilection for umbilicus	No	Yes
Hormonal modulation	No	Yes
HLA associations	?	DR3, DR4

IF, immunofluorescence; C3, third component of complement; BMZ, basement membrane zone; HLA, human leucocyte antigen.

35

Table 5.4 Immunofluorescence Findings for Differential Diagnosis of Pemphigoid Gestationis.

Diagnosis	Direct IF	Indirect IF
Pemphigoid gestationis	Linear IgG (25–30%) and C3 (100%) at BMZ	Circulating IgG (20%) against BMZ; PG factor in 25–50%
Bullous pemphigoid	Linear IgG (50–90%) and C3 (80–100%) at BMZ	Circulating IgG (70%) against BMZ
Dermatitis herpetiformis	Granular papillary deposition of IgA (100%)	No circulating IgA but 70% have anti-smooth muscle autoantibody
Linear IgA bullous dermatosis (adult and childhood)	Linear deposition of IgA at BMZ (90%)	Circulating IgA against BMZ (adult 50%, childhood 75%)
Pemphigus	Intercellular IgG	Circulating intercellular IgG

IF, immunofluorescence; C3, third component of complement; BMZ, basement membrane zone; PG, pemphigoid gestationis; Ig, immunoglobulin.

IMPLICATIONS FOR THE PREGNANT PATIENT

- Most patients with pemphigoid gestationis require treatment with moderate doses of systemic glucocorticosteroids for control of pruritus and lesion formation at some point in the course of their disease.
- All patients should be followed carefully and treated aggressively if postpartum flares of disease occur.
- Although lesions in infants are self-limiting, PG may be associated with an increased incidence of fetal risk. Patients with PG and their offspring should, therefore, be managed coordinately by dermatologists, obstetricians and neonatologists.
- Patients who require treatment postpartum should be advised about appropriate breastfeeding practices.
- Patients should be warned about the potential risk of PG flare up with oral contraceptive use.
- Patients must be warned about the significant risk of developing PG in a subsequent pregnancy.

doses of corticosteroids. If no new lesions develop 3 days after having commenced 40 mg prednisolone, the dose should be held constant for 1–2 weeks and then gradually decreased. If new lesions continue to develop after 3 days, the dose should be doubled and the guidelines as stated above followed. Some degree of disease activity (e.g. one or two new lesions developing every few days) is acceptable because much higher doses of prednisolone may be required to suppress all disease activity completely. Patients should, therefore, be tried on ever-lower doses of medication once the disease is controlled. The minimum effective dose of systemic corticosteroids should be used. It is important to remember that many patients actually improve during the latter part of pregnancy, only to have a recurrence at the time of delivery. Doses higher than 80 mg prednisolone are exceptional. The initial dose can often be reduced rapidly to maintenance levels (e.g. 10 mg daily). As postpartum exacerbations are frequent, it is usual to anticipate this by increasing the steroid dose temporarily immediately after delivery. Some patients may require reinstitution of their medication postpartum following quiescence of the disease during the latter part of the third trimester of pregnancy. Although systemic steroids do not appear to affect fetal prognosis, the mother must be carefully monitored as diabetes mellitus and hypertension may appear.

If PG should prove unresponsive to corticosteroids, or if these drugs are contraindicated in a particular patient, then plasmapheresis may be considered. It has been used with apparent success in a patient during pregnancy and also in a patient with PG persisting postpartum, thereby supporting claims for a circulating pathogenic factor in PG. There are no major technical difficulties in performing plasmapheresis during pregnancy, and in fact it has an established role in the treatment of rhesus disease for the removal of maternal rhesus antibodies. Other treatments have been tried in PG including pyridoxine[28], dapsone, and ritodrine[29]. Such approaches have not been entirely empiric. Dapsone is unhelpful and is now contraindicated during pregnancy as it can cause hemolytic disease of the newborn. In 1984 MacDonald and Raffle[29] reported a case of complete remission of severe PG when ritodrine, a β-sympathomimetic drug, was used for the treatment of premature labour.

Alternative drugs such as gold, methotrexate, and cyclophosphamide have been reported in the literature[30]. None is useful prior to term and the experience with each has been variable. Goserelin, a luteinizing hormone-releasing hormone (LHRH) analog, has been used in severe, long-standing PG with chemical oophorectomy leading to complete remission[31]. Intravenous IgG has been used with apparent success in a few isolated patients[32]. The use of second-line 'steroid-sparing' drugs during pregnancy is not advisable because of the possible teratogenic effects. Systemic corticosteroids, therefore, remain the mainstay of treatment.

Skin lesions in affected infants of patients with PG are transient and resolve as maternal autoantibodies are catabolized. Lesions in these infants usually require no specific therapy other than simple wound care. Infants of patients with PG who were treated with systemic steroids during pregnancy, however, should be assessed by a neonatologist for evidence of adrenal insufficiency.

REFERENCES

1 Jenkins, R. E., Shornick, J. K., and Black, M. M. Pemphigoid gestationis. *J. Eur. Acad. Dermatol. Venereol.* 1993; **2**: 163–173.

2 Garcia-Gonzalez, E., Castro-Llamas, J., Karchmer, S., *et al.* Class II major histocompatibility complex typing across the ethnic barrier in pemphigoid gestationis. A study in Mexicans. *Int. J. Dermatol.* 1999; **38**: 46–51.

3 Jenkins, R. E., Hern, S., and Black, M. M. Clinical features and management of 87 patients with pemphigoid gestationis. *Clin. Exp. Dermatol.* 1999; **24**: 255–259.

4 Engineer, L., Bhol, K., and Ahmed, A. R. Pemphigoid gestationis: a review. *Am. J. Obstet. Gynecol.* 2000; **183**: 483–491.

5 Jenkins, R. E., Vaughan Jones, S. M., and Black, M. M. Conversion of pemphigoid gestationis to bullous pemphigoid; two refractory cases highlighting this association. *Br. J. Dermatol.* 1996; **135**: 595–598.

6 Berkowitz, R. S., Goldstein, D. P., Chorionic tumors. *N. Engl. J. Med.* 1996; **335**: 1740–1748.

7 Kolodny, R. C., Herpes gestationis. A new assessment of incidence, diagnosis, and fetal prognosis. *Am. J. Obsetet. Gynecol.* 1969; **104**: 39–45.

8 Lawley, T. J., Stingl, G., and Katz S. I. Fetal and maternal risk factors in herpes gestationis. *Arch. Dermatol.* 1978; **114**: 552–555.

9 Holmes, R. C., and Black, M. M. The fetal prognosis in pemphigoid gestationis (herpes gestationis). *Br. J. Dermatol.* 1984; **110**: 67–72.

10 Shornick, J. K., and Black, M. M. Fetal risks in herpes gestationis. *J. Am. Acad. Dermatol.* 1992; **26**: 63–68.

11 Shornick, J. K., and Black, M. M. Secondary autoimmune diseases in herpes gestationis (pemphigoid gestationis). *J. Am. Acad. Dermatol.* 1992; **26**: 563–566.

12 Hashimoto, T., Amagai, M., Murakami, H., *et al.* Specific detection of anti-cell surface antibodies in herpes gestationis sera. *Exp. Dermatol.* 1996; **5**: 96–101.

13 Vaughan Jones, S. A., Bhogal, B. S., Black, M. M., *et al.* A typical case of pemphigoid gestationis with a unique pattern of intercellular immunofluorescence. *Br. J. Dermatol.* 1997; **136**: 245–248.

14 Shornick, J. K., Stastny, P., and Gilliam, J. N. High frequency of histocompatibility antigens HLA-DR3 and DR4 in herpes gestationis. *J. Clin. Invest.* 1981; **68**: 553–555.

15 Shornick, J. K., Jenkins, R. E., Artlett, C. M., *et al.* Class II MHC typing in pemphigoid gestationis. *Clin. Exp. Dermatol.* 1995; **20**: 123–126.

16 Shornick, J. K., Artlett, C. M., Jenkins, R. E., *et al.* Complement polymorphism in herpes gestationis: association with C4 null allele. *J. Am. Acad. Dermatol.* 1993; **29**: 545–549.

17 Stanley, J. R., Hawley-Nelson, P., Yuspa, S. H., *et al.* Characterization of bullous pemphigoid antigen: a unique basement membrane protein of stratified squamous epithelia. *Cell* 1981; **24**: 897–903.

18 Labib, R. S., Anhalt G. J., Patel, H. P., *et al.* Molecular heterogeneity of the bullous pemphigoid antigens as detected by immunoblotting. *J. Immunol.* 1986; **136**: 1231–1235.

19 Sawamura, D., Nomura, K., Sugita, Y., *et al.* Bullous pemphigoid antigen (BPAG1): cDNA cloning and mapping of the gene to the short arm of chromosome 6. *Genomics* 1990; **8**: 722–726.

20 Li K., Sawamura, D., Guidice, G. J., *et al.* Genomic organization of collagenous domains and chromosomal assignment of human 180-kDa bullous pemphigoid antigen-2, a novel collagen of stratified squamous epithelium. *J. Biol. Chem.* 1991; **266**: 24064–24069.

21 Li, K., Tamai, K., Tan, E. M. L., *et al.* Cloning of type XVII collagen. *J. Biol. Chem.* 1993; **268**: 8823–8834.

22 Guidice, G. J., Squiquera, H. L., Elias, P. M., *et al.* Identification of two collagen domains within the bullous pemphigoid auto-antigen, BP 180. *J. Clin. Invest.* 1991; **87**: 734–738.

23 Stanley, J. R., Tanaka, T., Muellers, S., *et al.* Isolation of complementary DNA for bullous pemphigoid antigen by use of patients' autoantibodies. *J. Clin. Invest.* 1988; **82**: 1864–1870.

24 Kitajima, Y., Adhesion molecules in the pathophysiology of bullous diseases. *Eur. J. Dermatol.* 1996; **6**: 399–405.

25 Kelly, S. E., Fleming, S., Bhogal, B. S., *et al.* Immunopathology of the placenta in pemphigoid gestationis and linear IgA disease. *Br. J. Dermatol.* 1989; **120**: 735–743.

26 Vince, G. S., and Johnson, P. M., Materno-fetal immunobiology in normal pregnancy and its possible failure in recurrent spontaneous abortion? *Hum. Reprod.* 1995; **10**: 107–113.

27 Shornick, J. K., Jenkins, R. E., Briggs, D. C., *et al.* Anti-HLA antibodies in pemphigoid gestationis (herpes gestationis). *Br. J. Dermatol.* 1993; **129**: 257–259.

28 Fosnaugh, R. P., Bryan, H. G., and Orders, R. L. Pyridoxine in the treatment of herpes gestationis. *Arch. Dermatol.* 1961; **84**: 90–95.

29 MacDonald, K. J. S., and Raffle, E. J. Ritodrine therapy associated with remission of pemphigoid gestationis. Br. J. Dermatol. 1984; **111**: 630.

30 Castle, S. P., Mather-Mondrey, M., Bennion, S., *et al.* Chronic herpes gestationis and antiphospholipid antibody syndrome successfully treated with cyclophosphamide. *J. Am. Acad. Dermatol.* 1996; **34**: 333–336.

31 Garvey, M. P., Handfield-Jones, S. E., and Black, M. M. Pemphigoid gestationis: response to chemical oophorectomy with goserelin. *Clin. Exp. Dermatol.* 1992; **17**: 443–445.

32 Hern, S., Harman, K., Bhogal, B. S., and Black, M. M. A severe persistent case of pemphigoid gestationis treated with intravenous immunoglobulins and cyclosporin. *Clin. Exp. Dermatol.* 1998; **23**: 185–188.

ACKNOWLEDGEMENT

Figure **5.10** has been reproduced by kind permission of Professor Ernesto Bonifazi, Bari, Italy.

6 Polymorphic Eruption of Pregnancy

Martin M. Black

INTRODUCTION

Polymorphic eruption of pregnancy (PEP), also known as pruritic urticarial papules and plaques of pregnancy (PUPPP), is probably the most common of the gestational dermatoses, affecting about one in 160 pregnancies. It is essentially a self-limiting, papular, urticarial eruption of late pregnancy and/or the puerperium. A few patients may develop vesicles or smaller bullae, target lesions, polycyclic wheals, and a widespread toxic erythema-like appearance.

HISTORICAL BACKGROUND

As PEP has a very variable clinical morphology[1], it is not surprising that various terms have been used to describe it. The disease was initially reported as 'toxemic rash of pregnancy'[2], but as the case was not associated with pre-eclampsia the term was little used. Since then other descriptive terms have been used, including prurigo of late pregnancy[3], toxic erythema of pregnancy[4], and PUPPP[5,6].

Although the term PUPPP is still widely used, particularly in the USA, it is generally agreed that PUPPP and PEP are identical dermatoses[7]. This discussion will refer to PEP, because it encapsulates the full range of clinical morphologic expressions, including papules, plaques, target lesions, polycyclic erythematous wheals, vesicles, and occasional bullae.

ETIOLOGY

Polymorphic eruption of pregnancy is an inflammatory dermatosis associated solely with pregnancy. No associations have been found with atopy, pre-eclampsia, or autoimmune phenomena[1], and the frequency of human leucocyte antigens (HLAs) in women with PEP is also normal[1,6]. The common clinical presentation of PEP in abdominal striae suggests that abdominal distension may be an important factor. A reaction to abdominal distension has also been implicated by the greater likelihood in PEP of higher maternal weight gain, higher neonatal birthweight, and increased incidence of twins[8,9] or multiple pregnancies[10]. A recent prospective study of 44 patients with PEP showed low serum cortisol levels compared with controls, suggesting a hormonal influence[10]. Furthermore, a male : female ratio of 2 : 1 was found in the offspring of affected women[10], although the relevance of this is currently not clear.

No evidence has been found to implicate autoimmune mechanisms[10–12], nor have circulating immune complexes been found[6]. A preliminary study of male DNA detection in PEP indicates that fetal cells can migrate to maternal skin during pregnancy[13]. Whether this initiates the inflammatory responses in PEP remains speculative. Although PEP is now a well-recognized entity, it is perhaps surprising that there is little substantial information about its etiology, and factors such as parity, multiple pregnancy, and paternity may well need further consideration[14].

CLINICAL FEATURES

The great majority of patients with PEP are primigravidas, and the development of PEP in a subsequent pregnancy is very likely to coexist with excessive maternal weight gain or multiple pregnancies[10,14,15]. The characteristic time of onset is between weeks 36 and 39 of gestation, but lesions may also develop in the immediate postpartum period. There is no particular maternal age at which PEP is likely to develop[6].

The mean duration of the eruption is 6 weeks, but the eruption is usually not severe for more than 1 week[1]. The eruption begins with pruritic urticarial papules, usually in association with striae distensae (6.1–6.4); however, these papules can develop on the abdomen without striae (6.5). Earlier reports of PEP indicated that the lesions consisted almost exclusively

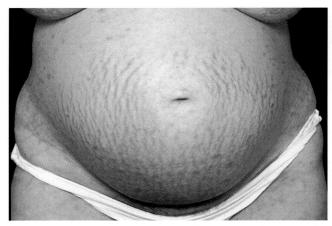

Fig 6.1   Early PEP at 38 weeks' gestation in an Asian primigravida. Pruritic urticaria in striae distensae. Note the periumbilical sparing.

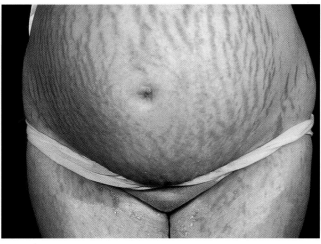

Fig 6.2   PEP at 37 weeks in a primigravida. Prominent pruritic urticarial lesions are present in striae distensae on the abdomen and thighs.

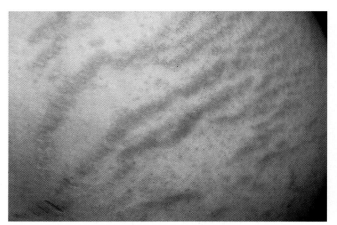

Fig 6.3   PEP in striae distensae. Close-up of **6.2**, showing confluent urticarial papules in striae distensae. Some papules occur adjacent to the striae.

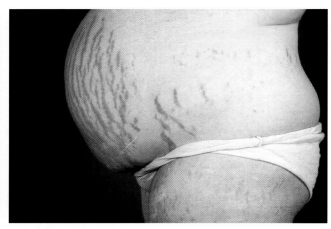

Fig 6.4   PEP in striae distensae. The pruritic eruption developed early (26 weeks) in a triplet pregnancy.

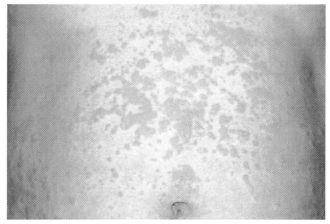

Fig 6.5   PEP at 36 weeks' gestation in a primigravida. Urticarial papules on the upper abdomen in the absence of striae distensae.

of urticarial papules and plaques[5]. However, the morphology of the eruption may vary greatly throughout its duration[1,10]. Some 40% of patients develop tiny vesicles (**6.6**), often on top of the papules overlying striae (**6.7**). Target-like lesions are present in 20% of cases (**6.8**) and annular or polycyclic wheals in 18% (**6.8**). In 70% of cases the lesions become confluent and widespread, resembling a toxic erythema (**6.9**). In a small number of cases, vesicles may coalesce to form smaller bullae[16]. The Koebner or isomorphic response in PEP is common[1], but facial involvement is very rare[17,18]. As the eruption slowly resolves, the great majority of cases exhibit fine scaling and crusting, reminiscent of eczema[1].

The eruption begins on the lower abdomen, but often spares the periumbilical area (**6.1, 6.2**). Other commonly affected sites include the thighs, back (**6.10**), buttocks (**6.11**), and the extensor surfaces of the arms (**6.12**). It is most unusual to see the hands and feet affected[19], but, if they are, the condition may resemble scabies (**6.13**) or pemphigoid (herpes) gestationis (PG).

Fig 6.6   PEP urticarial lesions and small vesicles on the abdomen, sparing striae distensae.

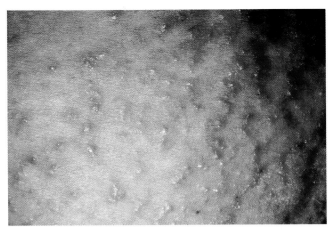

Fig 6.7   PEP morphology. 'Pinpoint-sized' vesicles are present, on top of the urticarial papules within striae distensae.

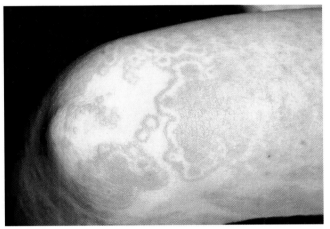

Fig 6.8   PEP morphology. Target-like and annular polycyclic lesions resembling erythema multiforme.

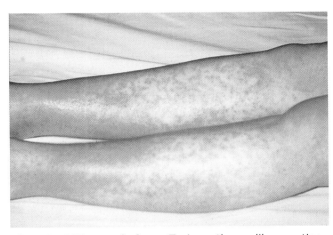

Fig 6.9   PEP morphology. Toxic erythema-like eruption on lower legs.

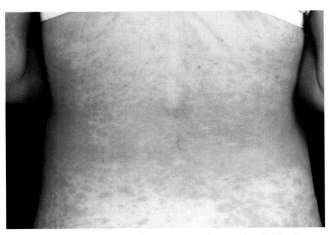

Fig 6.10   PEP morphology. Extensive urticarial lesions on the back.

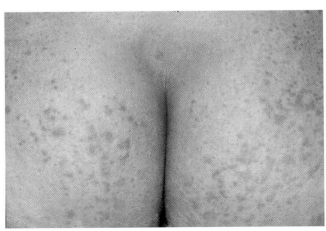

Fig 6.11   PEP morphology. Urticarial lesions on the buttocks.

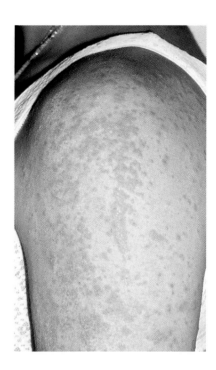

Fig 6.12 PEP morphology. Urticarial lesions on the upper arms.

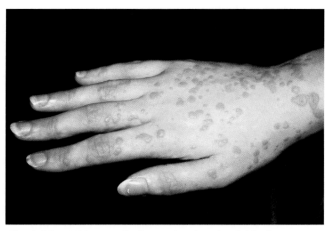

Fig 6.13 PEP morphology. Acral urticarial lesions resembling scabies.

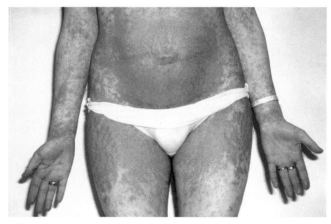

Fig 6.14 Severe PEP. The abdomen, thighs, and forearms are involved.

Mucosal lesions have not been described. In more severe PEP the erythema may confluently involve the entire abdomen, thighs, and even elsewhere (6.14). In view of the widespread clinical morphology in PEP, an attempt has been made to classify the clinical features. Aronson et al.[20] have categorized the clinical features into three types:

Type I	Mainly urticarial papules and plaques.
Type II	Nonurticarial erythema, papules or vesicles.
Type III	Combinations of the two forms.

HISTOPATHOLOGY AND IMMUNOFLUORESCENCE

Skin biopsy usually reveals a superficial and mid-dermal, perivascular, lymphohistiocytic infiltrate, with a variable number of eosinophils present. Spongiosis, parakeratosis, and marked papillary dermal edema may be present, leading to subepidermal vesicle formation[21]. These histopathologic changes in PEP may overlap with those seen in PG.

Direct immunofluorescence (DIF) is negative in the great majority of cases of PEP. However, some investigators have reported equivocal DIF findings in PEP, such as minimal C3 deposition along the basement membrane zone (BMZ), perivascular C3 and fibrin in the dermis[6,18,20], and in one case antiepidermal cell surface antibodies[22]. DIF can rarely show a speckled band of immunoglobulin (Ig) M deposition along the BMZ,

but indirect IMF is negative[10]. Saurat[23] has stressed the importance of performing DIF in patients with PEP, because some cases may be very similar clinically to PG.

DIFFERENTIAL DIAGNOSIS

As PEP may have a variable clinical morphology, it may be confused with several disorders, including drug eruptions, PG, scabies, and erythema multiforme. The following comparison may help to differentiate between PEP and PG:

- Examination of striae distensae is important because lesions overlying striae are found in 90% of patients with PEP but are seldom prominent in PG.
- Although vesicles are found in 40% of patients with PEP, they are unlikely to be larger than 2–3 mm in diameter. However, once vesicles occur in PG, they usually evolve rapidly into larger tense bullae.
- Involvement of periumbilical skin is a common finding (84%) in PG, but is observed in only 10% of patients with PEP[1].

Nevertheless, it is firmly recommended that DIF is performed for all patients with PEP to avoid any diagnostic confusion with PG.

PROGNOSIS

Apart from the discomfort of the pruritic urticarial eruption, the maternal prognosis is unaffected. However, the number of twin or multiple pregnancies in patients with PEP appears to be increased significantly[8-10]. Carruther's experience indicated that resolution of the eruption in PEP appeared to be unrelated to delivery of the infant[24], and it is generally agreed that fetal prognosis is normal[1,5,6,10,11,20,25]. Only one possible case of transient neonatal PEP involvement has been described[26].

MANAGEMENT

The disease is self-limiting without serious sequelae, and so only symptomatic treatment is usually required. Most patients can obtain relief with the use of moderately potent topical corticosteroid creams (e.g. clobetasone butyrate 0.05%, or hydrocortisone-17-butyrate 0.01%), either singly or combined with small doses of chlorpheniramine maleate (4 mg at night). However, the newer nonsedating antihistamines are not recommended in pregnancy[27]. More severe cases of PEP with a distressing degree of pruritus can be safely treated with oral prednisolone[9]. A tapering dose of prednisolone, 30 mg daily for 7–14 days, should be sufficient. A patient with severe PEP, unresponsive to therapy, was dramatically improved within 2 hours after delivery by cesarean section[28].

IMPLICATIONS FOR THE PREGNANT PATIENT

- Polymorphic eruption is the commonest gestational dermatosis, with an incidence of about one in 160 pregnancies. It is the commonest gestational dermatitis to be associated with multiple pregnancy.

- Onset is usually in the third trimester and in a primigravida.

- Lesions are commonly confined to striae distensae.

- Clinical morphology can be variable with urticarial papules, target-like lesions, polycyclic wheals, and vesicles often seen.

- Direct immunofluorescence is negative.

- Eruption is self-limiting, seldom severe, and lasts about 1–4 weeks.

REFERENCES

1 Charles-Holmes, R. Polymorphic eruption of pregnancy. *Semin. Dermatol.* 1989; 8: 18–22.

2 Bourne, G. Toxemic rash of pregnancy. *Proc. R. Soc. Med.* 1962; 55: 462–464.

3 Nurse, D. S. Prurigo of pregnancy. *Aust. J. Dermatol.* 1968; 9: 258–267.

4 Holmes, R. C., Black, M. M., Dann, J., *et al.* A comparative study of toxic erythema of pregnancy and herpes gestationis. *Br. J. Dermatol.* 1982; 106: 499–510.

5 Lawley, T. J., Hertz, K. C., Wade, T. R., *et al.* Pruritic urticarial papules and plaques of pregnancy. *J. Am. Med. Assoc.* 1979; 241: 1696–1699.

6 Yancey, K. B., Hall, R. P., and Lawley, T. J. Pruritic urticarial papules and plaques of pregnancy. *J. Am. Acad. Dermatol.* 1984; 10: 473–480.

7 Alcalay, J. and Wolf, J. E. Pruritic urticarial papules and plaques of pregnancy: the enigma and the confusion. *J. Am. Acad. Dermatol.* 1988; 19: 1115–1116.

8 Cohen, L. M., Capeless, E. L., Krusinski, P. A., *et al.* Pruritic urticarial papules and plaques of pregnancy and its relationship to maternal–fetal weight gain and twin pregnancy. *Arch. Dermatol.* 1989; 125: 1534–1536.

9 Bunker, C. B., Erskine, K., Rustin, M. H. A., *et al.* Severe polymorphic eruption of pregnancy occurring in twin pregnancies. *Clin. Exp. Dermatol.* 1990; 15: 228–231.

10 Vaughan-Jones, S. A., Hern, S. A., Nelson-Piercy C., *et al.* A prospective study of 200 women with dermatoses of pregnancy correlating clinical findings with hormonal and immunopathological profiles. *Br. J. Dermatol.* 1999; 141: 71–81.

11 Alcalay, J., Ingber, A., Kafri, B., *et al.* Hormonal evaluation and autoimmune background in pruritic urticarial papules and plaques of pregnancy. *Am. J. Obstet. Gynecol.* 1988; 158: 417–420.

12 Callen, J. P. and Hanno, R. Pruritic urticarial papules and plaques of pregnancy (PUPPP): a clinicopathologic study. *J. Am. Acad. Dermatol.* 1981; 5: 401–405.

13 Aractingi, S., Berkane, N., Bertheau, P., *et al.* Fetal DNA in skin of polymorphic eruptions of pregnancy. *Lancet* 1998; 352: 1898–1901.

14 Powell, F. C. Parity, polypregnancy, paternity and PUPPP. *Arch. Dermatol.* 1992; 128: 1551.

15 Beckett, M. A. and Goldberg, N. S. Pruritic urticarial plaques and papules of pregnancy and skin distension. *Arch. Dermatol.* 1991; 127: 125–126.

16 Holmes, R. C., McGibbon, D. H., and Black, M. M. Polymorphic eruption of pregnancy with subepidermal vesicles. *J. R. Soc. Med.* 1984; 77: 22–23.

17 Carruthers, A. Facial involvement in pruritic urticarial papules and plaques of pregnancy. *J. Am. Acad. Dermatol.* 1987; 17: 302.

18 Alcalay, J., David, M., and Sandbank, M. Facial involvement in pruritic urticarial papules and plaques of pregnancy. *J. Am. Acad. Dermatol.* 1986; **15**: 1048.

19 Vaughan Jones, S. A., Dunnill, M. G. S., and Black M. M. Pruritic urticarial papules and plaques of pregnancy. (polymorphic eruption of pregnancy): two unusual cases. *Br. J. Dermatol.* 1996; **135**: 102–105.

20 Aronson, I. K., Bond, S., Fielder, V. C., *et al.* Pruritic urticarial papules and plaques of pregnancy: clinical and immunopathologic observations in 57 patients. *J. Am. Aacad. Dermatol.* 1998; **39**: 933–939.

21 Holmes, R. C., Jureka, W., and Black, M. M. A comparative histopathological study of polymorphic eruption of pregnancy and herpes gestationis. *Clin. Exp. Dermatol.* 1983; **8**: 523–529.

22 Trattner, A., Ingber, A., and Sandbank, M. Antiepidermal cell surface antibodies in a patient with pruritic urticarial papules and plaques of pregnancy. *J. Am. Acad. Dermatol.* 1991; **24**: 306–308.

23 Saurat, J. H. Immunofluorescence biopsy for pruritic urticarial papules and plaques of pregnancy. *J. Am. Acad. Dermatol.* 1989; **20**: 711.

24 Carruthers, A. Pruritic urticarial papules and plaques of pregnancy. *J. Am. Acad. Dermatol.* 1993; **29**: 125.

25 Alcalay, J., Ingber, A., David, M., *et al.* Pruritic urticarial papules and plaques of pregnancy: a review of 21 cases. *J. Reprod. Med.* 1987; **32**: 315–316.

26 Uhlin, S. R. Pruritic urticarial papules and plaques of pregnancy. Involvement of the mother and infant. *Arch. Dermatol.* 1981; **117**: 238–239.

27 Jurecka, W. and Gebhart, W. Drug prescribing during pregnancy. *Semin. Dermatol.* 1989; **8**: 30–39.

28 Beltrani, V. P. and Beltrani, V. S. Pruritic urticarial papules and plaques of pregnancy: a severe case requiring early delivery for relief of symptoms. *J. Am. Acad. Dermatol.* 1992; **26**: 266–267.

7 The Papular and Pruritic Dermatoses of Pregnancy

Martin M. Black
Samantha Vaughan Jones

INTRODUCTION

The papular and pruritic dermatoses of pregnancy encompass three disease entities that are described in the same chapter because each of the terms applied are still quoted in the literature: prurigo of pregnancy, papular dermatitis of pregnancy, and pruritic folliculitis of pregnancy.

There may well be overlap between them and there is considerable doubt that they are all distinct clinical entities. Indeed, papular dermatitis of pregnancy is no longer regarded as a distinct condition (*see below*). In contrast to pemphigoid gestationis and polymorphic eruption of pregnancy, where the clinical features are quite distinct, the clinical features of these entities are characterized by discrete pruritic papules, which soon become excoriated. In general the intervening skin appears normal and the urticarial phase is absent. This chapter outlines the clinical and differentiating features of each entity.

PRURIGO OF PREGNANCY

HISTORICAL BACKGROUND

In 1904, Besnier first introduced the term 'prurigo gestationis' to include all patients with pregnancy-related dermatoses, other than those with herpes gestationis[1]. Costello, in 1941[2], estimated that 'prurigo gestationis of Besnier' occurred in 2% of pregnancies. In 1968, Nurse[3] outlined the clinical features of prurigo of pregnancy, but also included cases of polymorphic eruption of pregnancy under this term ('late-onset' prurigo of pregnancy).

CLINICAL FEATURES

Prurigo of pregnancy is not uncommon and affects about one in 300 pregnancies[3]. The onset is usually about 25–30 weeks' gestation, and it can persist for up to 3 months postpartum. The lesions are discrete erythematous or skin-colored papules, which are extremely pruritic, with the result that an excoriated surface soon develops over the papules. The papules tend to be small and are seldom larger than 0.5 cm in diameter. Usually, the lesions remain papular, and thus the surrounding skin does not develop features of eczema. Characteristically, the papules appear on the extensor surfaces of the extremities and trunk, and do not progress to vesicle formation[4] (7.1–7.4). There is little follow-up information on the reappearance of prurigo of pregnancy in subsequent pregnancies. Hayashi[4] believes it to be a rare occurrence.

The histologic features of prurigo of pregnancy have not been studied systematically, and consequently at present the diagnosis is made on clinical criteria alone. Where biopsies have been performed, the pathology usually shows mild acanthosis, parakeratosis, and surface excoriation. A mixed perivascular infiltrate is found, often containing eosinophils and some neutrophils[5]. Direct immunofluorescence (DIF) is negative[5].

PATHOGENESIS

Prurigo of pregnancy is perhaps the least studied of all the dermatoses of pregnancy. However, Holmes and Black[5] have postulated that prurigo of pregnancy might simply be the result of pruritus gravidarum occurring in atopic women. They based their argument on the

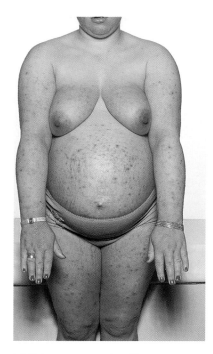

Fig 7.1 Prurigo of pregnancy. Diffuse prurigo papules scattered on the abdomen and extensor limb surfaces. The condition closely simulates 'papular dermatitis of pregnancy'.

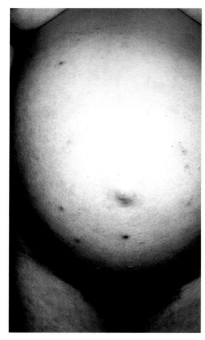

Fig 7.2 Prurigo of pregnancy. Discrete excoriated papules on the abdomen in late pregnancy.

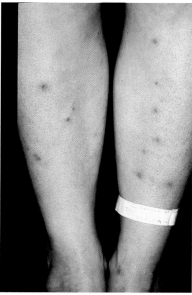

Fig 7.3 Prurigo of pregnancy. Same patient as in **7.2**, showing excoriated papules on the lower legs.

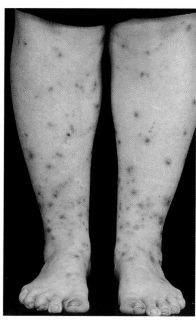

Fig 7.4 Prurigo of pregnancy. More extensive inflamed erythematous papules on lower legs.

finding that 18% of pregnancies are complicated by pruritus[6] and that 10% of the population displays atopy[7]. It might therefore be expected that both conditions would coincide in about 2% of pregnancies.

TREATMENT

Prurigo of pregnancy is a benign disorder, but the patient may find the persistent pruritus distressing. Symptomatic relief of pruritus usually can be achieved with moderately potent topical corticosteroid creams, such as class 4 or 5 clobetasone butyrate 0.05% cream or hydrocortisone-17-butyrate 0.1% cream, with oral chlorpheniramine maleate 4 mg at night. The use of

Cordran tape (translucent polythene adhesive film impregnated with flurandrenolone) can be effective in the management of a smaller number of discrete pruritic papules.

PAPULAR DERMATITIS OF PREGNANCY

Papular dermatitis of pregnancy was first described by Spangler *et al.*[8] in 1962. They identified a group of patients, whom they thought could be differentiated from patients with prurigo of pregnancy, both clinically and biochemically. They stressed the high fetal risk which they considered to be preventable by appropriate therapy. We have considerable doubt, however, that papular dermatitis of pregnancy is an entity separate from more widespread examples of prurigo of pregnancy. Nor is it likely that the disorder carries an appreciable fetal risk[9].

CLINICAL FEATURES

Spangler et al.[8] originally described 12 patients with papular dermatitis. The eruption occurred throughout pregnancy from 11 weeks' gestation to term. The condition was described as a generalized papular eruption over the trunk, arms, legs, and even the face. The papules were 3–5 mm in diameter and excoriated. Rahbari[10] later described 16 cases and noted that the papules could have an erythematous, urticated appearance, before excoriation.

Spangler et al.[8] estimated an incidence of about one in 2400 pregnancies and expressed concern about the high fetal mortality rate (27–37%). In recent years, very few new cases of papular dermatitis have been reported[11,12]. The similarity of the eruption to prurigo of pregnancy[9] (7.1) and pruritic folliculitis of pregnancy has been noted[12].

HISTOPATHOLOGY

The histopathologic findings in papular dermatitis have mainly been studied by Rahbari[10]. They clearly overlap with those of prurigo of pregnancy[5], with the following features occurring in both:

- Epidermal acanthosis
- Excoriation
- Perivascular accumulation of eosinophils and neutrophils

The few DIF observations made in papular dermatitis have been negative[12].

BIOCHEMISTRY

Spangler et al.[8,13] reported a raised chorionic gonadotrophin concentration, lowered plasma cortisol levels, and reduced urinary estriol levels in patients with papular dermatitis of pregnancy. These findings were also reported subsequently in individual case reports[11,12].

TREATMENT

Owing to the increased fetal mortality rate they found, Spangler et al.[8] recommended systemic administration of either prednisone (prednisolone), up to 200 mg daily, or diethystilbestrol 600–2500 mg daily. They claimed that these therapies cleared the dermatosis within a few days and reversed the potential fetal loss. However, subsequently, Rahbari[10] did not find a high fetal loss and recommended 'conservative treatment'. Individual case reports have reported on the beneficial use of tapering doses of prednisone[11,12].

REAPPRAISAL OF PAPULAR DERMATITIS

A comprehensive reappraisal of the startling claims of Spangler et al.[8,13] has cast considerable doubt on the nosology of papular dermatitis[5]. A recent study of 200 women with dermatoses of pregnancy found no cases that conformed to the diagnosis of papular dermatitis of pregnancy. In addition, hormonal investigation did not confirm Spangler's original findings, and fetal prognosis was found to be normal[14]. The present authors' view is that the cases of papular dermatitis described represent more widespread and severe cases of prurigo of pregnancy[9]. The main reason for the separate classification of papular dermatitis of pregnancy was based on the findings of raised urinary chorionic gonadotrophin, low urinary cortisol and low urinary estriol levels[8,13]. However, it is important to stress that similar biochemical studies were not performed in any other dermatoses of pregnancy.

Furthermore, the fetal mortality rate in the original report of Spangler et al.[8] was probably overestimated for the following reasons:

- The interpretation of fetal deaths that occurred in pregnancies preceding the development of papular dermatitis was not justified, and exaggerated the fetal risk.
- Their data included spontaneous abortions without reference to the period of gestation. This is important because spontaneous abortions in the first trimester are not uncommon in a normal population.

Now that a comprehensive prospective study of pruritic papular dermatoses with biochemical data has been published, the diagnosis of papular dermatitis of Spangler can be laid to rest[14].

PRURITIC FOLLICULITIS OF PREGNANCY

The term pruritic folliculitis of pregnancy was first introduced by Zoberman and Farmer in 1981[15]. They described six patients who had developed a pruritic, follicular, papular eruption between the fourth and ninth months of pregnancy, which then resolved within 2–3 weeks of delivery. The lesions were principally small, follicular, erythematous papules or pustules, distributed widely over the upper trunk. Histopathologic findings were interpreted as an acute folliculitis, but unfortunately no biochemical findings were presented. However, the clinical descriptions of pruritic folliculitis (PF) suggest that the eruption may mimic papular dermatitis[12].

The present authors have seen a number of patients with a similar widespread eruption consisting of small erythematous papules and pustules (7.5–7.7). Topical treatment with a cream containing 10% benzoyl peroxide and 1% hydrocortisone was beneficial. The authors' views are that the clinical appearance of PF of pregnancy is very similar to the monomorphic type of acne occurring after the administration of systemic corticosteroids or progestogens[5]. It is therefore possible that PF of pregnancy is a form of hormonally induced acne rather than a specific dermatosis of pregnancy. Wikinson *et al.*[16] recently reported a patient with PF in whom serum androgen levels were raised. However, a recent report of 12 patients with PF showed no significant increase in serum androgen concentration when compared with levels in matched normal pregnant controls[17].

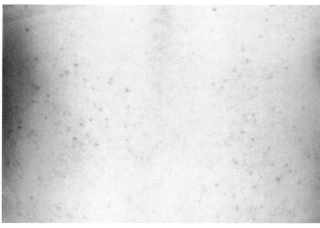

Fig 7.5 Pruritic folliculitis of pregnancy. Diffuse small monomorphic acneiform papules and pustules present on the patient's back.

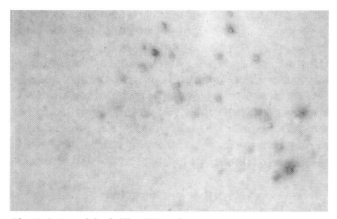

Fig 7.6 Pruritic folliculitis of pregnancy. A close-up of **7.5** shows small follicular papules and pustules.

IMPLICATIONS FOR THE PREGNANT PATIENT

- Prurigo and pruritic folliculitis can be managed with mild to moderately potent topical corticosteroids.
- Fetal prognosis is normal.
- Recurrence in future pregnancies is unlikely.
- Emollients are useful as an adjunct in topical therapy for relief of pruritus.
- Symptoms frequently disappear at the end of pregnancy or immediately postpartum.

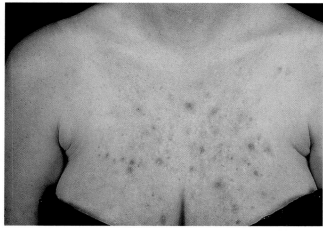

Fig 7.7 Acneiform eruption of pruritic folliculitis on the upper chest.

REFERENCES

1 Besnier, E., Brocq, L., and Jacquet, L. *La Pratique Dermatologique*, Vol. 1, p. 75. Masson et Cie, Paris, 1975.

2 Costello, M. J. Eruptions of pregnancy. *N. Y. State J. Med.* 1941; **41**: 849–855.

3 Nurse, D. S. Prurigo of pregnancy. *Australas. J. Dermatol.* 1968; **9**: 258–267.

4 Hayashi, R. H. Bullous dermatoses and prurigo of pregnancy. *Clin. Obstet. Gynecol.* 1990; **33**: 746–753.

5 Holmes, R. C. and Black, M. M. The specific dermatoses of pregnancy. *J. Am. Acad. Dermatol.* 1983; **8**: 405–412.

6 Kasdon, S. C. Abdominal pruritus in pregnancy. *Am. J. Obstet. Gynecol.* 1953; **65**: 320–324.

7 Rapaport, H. G., Appel, S. J., and Szanton V. L. Incidence of allergy in a pediatric population. *Am. J. Allergy* 1960; **18**: 45–49.

8 Spangler, A. S., Reddy, W., Bardawill, W. A., *et al.* Papular dermatitis of pregnancy. *J. Am. Med. Assoc.* 1962; **181**: 577–581.

9 Black, M. M. Prurigo of pregnancy, papular dermatitis of pregnancy and pruritic folliculitis of pregnancy. *Semin. Dermatol.* 1989; **8**: 23–25.

10 Rahbari, H. Pruritic papules of pregnancy. *J. Cutan. Pathol.* 1978; **5**: 347–352.

11 Michaund, R. M., Jacobson, D., and Dahl, M. V. Papular dermatitis of pregnancy. *Arch. Dermatol.* 1982; **118**: 1003–1005.

12 Nguyen, L. Q. and Sarmini, O. R. Papular dermatitis of pregnancy: a case report. *J. Am. Acad. Dermatol.* 1990; **22**: 690–691.

13 Spangler, A. S. and Emerson, K. Estrogen levels and estrogen therapy in papular dermatitis of pregnancy. *Am. J. Obstet. Gynecol.* 1971; **110**: 534–537.

14 Vaughan, Jones S. A., Hern, S., Nelson-Piercy, C., *et al.* A prospective study of 200 women with dermatoses of pregnancy correlating the clinical findings with hormonal and immunopathological profiles. *Br. J. Dermatol.* 1999; **141**: 71–81.

15 Zoberman, E. and Farmer, E. R. Pruritic folliculitis of pregnancy. *Arch. Dermatol.* 1981; **117**: 20–22.

16 Wilkinson, S. M., Buckler, H., Wilkinson, N., *et al.* Androgen levels in pruritic folliculitis of pregnancy. *Clin. Exp. Dermatol.* 1995; **20**: 234–236.

17 Vaughan Jones, S. A., Hern, S., and Black, M. M. Pruritic folliculitis and serum androgen levels. *Clin. Exp. Dermatol.* 1999; **24**: 392–395.

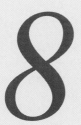

Effect of Pregnancy on Other Skin Disorders

Samantha Vaughan Jones
Martin M. Black

INTRODUCTION

Pregnancy causes immunologic, endocrine, metabolic, and vascular changes in the pregnant woman which modify her responses to skin diseases. Both the obstetrician and the dermatologist need to be aware of this potential if they are to provide optimal management during pregnancy. Particular attention should be given to any medication administered to a pregnant or nursing woman; the reader is advised to consult published guidelines and/or review articles[1-5].

PSORIASIS

Psoriasis affects 1.5–2% of the general population. It is an inflammatory disorder characterized by red scaly plaques on the skin. The nails are often involved and about 7% of patients have an associated seronegative inflammatory arthritis which may be debilitating. Local injuries to the skin, such as cuts, burns, or other skin infections, often lead to localized psoriasis at the site of injury (Koebner phenomenon).

TYPES OF PSORIASIS

In *plaque-type psoriasis*, the commonest form of psoriasis, there are well-demarcated erythematous plaques with adherent silver scales on the surface. The lesions are most common on the extensor surfaces of the elbows and knees, the sacral area (8.1), and the scalp (8.2). The groin may also be involved, as described in *Chapter 15*.

Guttate (drop-like) *psoriasis* is characterized by scattered pink papules, which are of uniform size and flare in crops mainly on the trunk (8.3) and proximal extremities. It often follows an upper respiratory infection, especially with streptococci. In *erythrodermic psoriasis*, the skin is red with a fine desquamative scale

Fig 8.1 Plaque-type psoriasis. Chronic, well-defined, slightly raised erythematous plaques, covered by a silver scale, are present, especially over the buttocks and extensor surfaces.

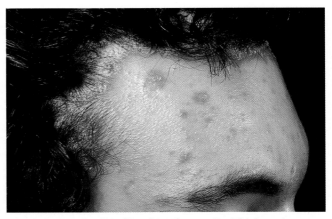

Fig 8.2 Psoriasis affecting the scalp. Thick scales are seen on the scalp and hairline, and smaller plaques on the forehead.

51

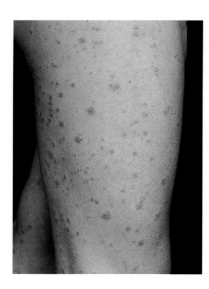

Fig 8.3 Guttate psoriasis. Small drop-like lesions occur in a shower-like distribution over the trunk and limbs, as shown here on the leg. The eruption occurs suddenly, often after a throat infection, and usually has a good prognosis.

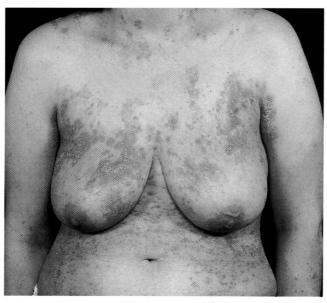

Fig 8.4 Generalized pustular psoriasis of von Zumbusch. The skin is red and sore with sheets of small sterile pustules erupting on the trunk.

present, often over its entire surface. There are several forms of *pustular psoriasis*, in which small sterile pustules appear either on pre-existing plaques or *de novo* on normal skin. Most patients with pustular psoriasis have had psoriasis previously. *Generalized pustular psoriasis* (von Zumbusch) may be life threatening, and treatment is urgently required (8.4). Pustular psoriasis exacerbated by pregnancy and controlled by cyclosporin A has recently been described[6]. Fever, arthralgia and leucocytosis often accompany the eruption. Pustular psoriasis of the palms and soles (*palmoplantar pustulosis*) consists of sterile itchy pustules on an erythematosquamous background.

MANAGEMENT

The treatment of psoriasis ranges from the application of mild tar products to the use of immunosuppressive agents. The location of lesions is important in selecting appropriate and effective therapy.

Drugs with direct therapeutic effects are used together with emollients, which will soften scaling, and keratolytics, such as salicylic acid, which help to remove the scale. Dithranol is the standard topical treatment for most cases of plaque psoriasis. However, it should be used with caution as it can irritate the skin and stain clothing. It is therefore essential to start with a low concentration and increase the dose gradually. Patients with fair skin do not tolerate dithranol as well as darker-skinned patients.

Coal tar ointment in concentrations up to 20% is often used, but as it is messy to apply and has a strong odor it is not very popular with patients. Topical calcipotriol, a vitamin D_3 metabolite, may be used for mild to moderately severe plaque psoriasis, but the total topical application should be less than 100 g weekly to minimize possible hypercalcemia. Topical corticosteroids may be required in some forms of psoriasis, such as guttate psoriasis. Side effects may arise with long-term treatment, and a rapid relapse may occur on withdrawal (rebound phenomenon). Ultraviolet B and PUVA may be given as adjuncts to topical therapy, with special considerations for the pregnant patient (*see below*).

PREGNANCY

Dithranol, tar, calcipotriol, and topical corticosteroids can all be used safely in pregnancy.

ULTRAVIOLET B AND PUVA

Ultraviolet B irradiation is safe in pregnancy, but the patient should be aware that UVB can increase the size and number of benign pigmented nevi. The use of PUVA (psoralen and ultraviolet A) may carry a risk of mutagenesis and teratogenesis, and neither sytemic nor topical (bath) PUVA should be used as a first-line treatment in pregnancy. However, a large study by Gunnarskog *et al.*[4] found no increased risk of spontaneous or induced abortions, nor an increased risk of congenital malformation or infant death, including pregnancies conceived following PUVA treatment.

The study, however, found an increased number of low birthweight infants in pregnancies begun following PUVA treatment. It therefore seems possible that PUVA treatment may cause germ cell mutations, resulting in chromosome anomalies or point mutations. Prenatal diagnosis should therefore be offered to women who become pregnant after PUVA treatment. Topical PUVA (bath PUVA) is safe to use in pregnancy.

SYSTEMIC DRUGS

Systemic drugs are sometimes required to treat psoriasis. Retinoic acid (acitretin) is highly teratogenic and should be used with caution (*see below*). Several cytotoxic drugs have been used for psoriasis, including methotrexate, hydroxyurea, and azathioprine. Methotrexate and hydroxyurea are known teratogens and must therefore be avoided in pregnancy, and azathioprine may be teratogenic. Cyclosporin A should be used with caution in pregnancy and during breastfeeding[7]. A recent paper reported the first British case of the successful use of cyclosporin to control pustular psoriasis in pregnancy from 25 weeks' gestation[6].

COURSE OF DISEASE

The hormonal changes in pregnancy do appear to influence the severity of psoriasis[8]. About 75% of women notice a significant change in their psoriasis during pregnancy, with 60% showing improvement and 15% an exacerbation; 80% of these will experience a postpartum flare of their diseases, usually within 4 months of delivery[9]. Pregnancy may also be a risk factor for psoriatic arthritis[10]. It is likely that the general downregulation of the immune system by the pregnancy hormones contributes to the improvement in psoriasis[9].

IMPETIGO HERPETIFORMIS

Impetigo herpetiformis is generally regarded as a very rare, acute, pustular form of psoriasis precipitated by pregnancy. It can affect pregnant women with no previous history of psoriasis. The onset is usually in the third trimester, and the disease tends to persist until delivery but may continue thereafter.

The eruption characteristically begins in the flexures with small sterile pustules on areas of acutely inflamed skin. These then extend centrifugally on to the trunk (8.5) and around the umbilicus (8.6) or form plaques with green-yellow pustules. The eruption may advance and become widespread, involving the tongue, buccal mucosa, and sometimes the esophagus. Constitutional symptoms are common, including fever, delirium, vomiting, diarrhea, and tetany due to hypocalcemia. Death may occur as a result of cardiac or renal failure.

The main obstetric problem in impetigo herpetiformis is placental insufficiency, with an increased risk of stillbirth, neonatal death, and fetal abnormalities[11]. The disease characteristically recurs with each pregnancy, with earlier onset and increased morbidity[11]. Between pregnancies, patients are free of the disorder and have no manifestations of psoriasis. The disease may also be exacerbated by oral contraceptives[12] and has recently been described in association with

Staphylococcus aureus lymphadenitis[13]. Corticosteroids are the treatment of choice for impetigo herpetiformis, but the results are generally unsatisfactory. In severe cases, termination of pregnancy is required; the impetigo herpetiformis usually resolves soon afterwards. Although the etiology of this condition is still unclear, a recent report showed extremely low levels of epidermal skin-derived antileucoproteinase/elafin in a patient with impetigo herpetiformis[14].

ACNE VULGARIS

Although acne may improve in pregnancy, it is occasionally exacerbated. This usually causes management problems, as most antiacne drugs are contraindicated during pregnancy. However, topical antiacne therapy, other than topical retinoic acid, does not seem to be teratogenic. Acne conglobata developing 10 days postpartum has recently been described[15]. Acne neonatorum has also been described with a family history of hyperandrogenism[16].

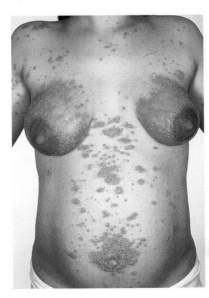

Fig 8.5 Impetigo herpetiformis. Sterile pustules develop on acutely inflamed skin and coalesce together on the trunk.

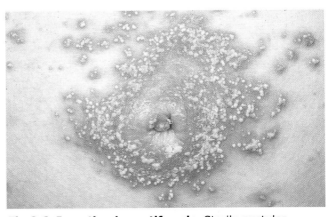

Fig 8.6 Impetigo herpetiformis. Sterile pustules around the umbilicus.

MANAGEMENT

The treatment of acne depends on the type of acne involved. If only comedones are present, a keratolytic agent such as benzoyl peroxide (2.5–10% cream, lotion, or gel) or azaleic acid cream 20% should be used to remove the surface keratin and unplug the follicular openings. These drugs are safe to use in pregnancy. Topical retinoic acid has been reported as causing multiple congenital defects in one patient[17] and ear deformities in another[18]. Ultraviolet light has an effect similar to that of topical keratolytics, but should be avoided in pregnancy.

ANTIBIOTICS

Long-term antibiotic therapy is usually required for inflammatory lesions with papules, pustules, or nodules. However, acne is slow to improve and beneficial effects are not usually seen for at least 2–3 months, with gradual improvement after 6–12 months of therapy. Maintenance treatment must be continued until the acne improves. Oral erythromycin is safe in pregnancy and is given at a dose of 250–500 mg twice daily.

Topical antibiotics are almost as effective as systemic antibiotics, but they may lead to the selection of resistant bacteria on the skin surface and to contact-allergic eczema. However, as there is negligible systemic absorption, this approach is safe in pregnancy. Examples include topical erythromycin (Stiemycin, Eryacne, Benzamycin, and Zineryt, which contains zinc in addition to erythromycin to help reduce bacterial resistance and make it more effective) and tetracycline (Topicycline, which is no longer available in the USA). The use of topical clindamycin during pregnancy has been associated with pseudomembranous colitis[19] and, in order to reduce systemic absorption, topical clindamycin phosphate is preferable to the hydrochloride salt. These topical preparations should be applied once or twice daily to the face and/or upper trunk.

SYSTEMIC DRUGS

Systemic antiandrogens and isotretinoin (Accutane, Roaccutane) are totally contraindicated in pregnancy. Vitamin A derivatives, such as oral isotretinoin etretinate, and the newer drug acitretin (Neotigason), are all potent teratogens and must not be used by those who are pregnant or who may become pregnant during the course of treatment. The most common teratogenic effects include nervous system anomalies, ear and eye deformities, cleft palate, renal and urogenital tract abnormalities, skeletal malformations, and toxic hepatocellular damage.

Although isotretinoin is rapidly cleared and is not stored in tissue, pregnancy should be avoided until 2 months after the drug has been discontinued.

However, etretinate and its metabolite acitretin (Neotigason) are a potential hazard for 2 years after therapy has been stopped because of their very slow elimination from the body.

HIDRADENITIS SUPPURATIVA

Hidradenitis suppurativa is a chronic cutaneous disease caused by the occlusion and rupture of follicular units, in which the resulting inflammatory response may secondarily involve the apocrine glands. Recurrent lesions develop in the axillae (8.7), groin, and perineal areas, with the formation of abscesses and with draining sinuses and progressive scarring.

In extreme cases, the entire vulva may be affected over many years, resulting in gross scarring and deformity, often associated with substantial psychosexual problems. The condition may remit during pregnancy as a result of reduced apocrine gland activity[20] but a recent review showed no consistent relationship between hidradenitis suppurativa and pregnancy in 38 women[21].

MANAGEMENT

Management often involves the use of long-term systemic antibiotics, such as erythromycin or tetracycline. However, tetracycline should be stopped before a

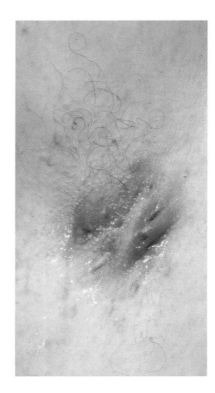

Fig 8.7 Hidradenitis suppurativa. Indolent painful pustules and nodules are present, with sinus and scar formation in the axilla.

planned pregnancy. If antibiotics are unsuccessful, alternatives include oral acitretin (which must also not be used in pregnancy) or surgery, where all the apocrine glands in the affected areas are excised. The carbon dioxide laser has been used to treat this condition, with considerable success[22]. Although repeat treatments may be necessary, the clearance rate and cosmetic results are excellent.

FOX–FORDYCE DISEASE

This is an uncommon chronic eruption of apocrine gland-bearing skin caused by the blockage and intraepidermal rupture of apocrine ducts. It mainly affects the axillary (8.8) and pubic regions, although other areas, such as the areolae, periumbilical region, and the perineum, are also sometimes involved. Itching can be intense and this may precede the formation of typical skin-colored follicular papules. Hormonal factors appear to influence this condition, as it usually improves in pregnancy[23].

ERYTHEMA NODOSUM

Erythema nodosum is a reactive inflammation of the subcutaneous fat, which is secondary to a wide variety of underlying conditions (Table 8.1). It can also occur *de novo* in pregnancy[24]. It presents with the sudden onset of ill-defined, tender, erythematous nodules or plaques, distributed symmetrically over the anterior legs (8.9). Lesions may also develop over the calves, arms, trunk, and face. Fever, malaise, and arthralgias may precede or accompany the eruption. Lesions usually resolve in 6–8 weeks.

MANAGEMENT

Treatment is supportive and includes bed-rest and mild analgesics such as acetaminophen (paracetamol). Nonsteroidal anti-inflammatory agents should not be used in pregnancy, especially in the third trimester. This is because they may constrict the ductus arteriosus

Table 8.1 Underlying Conditions of Erythema Nodosum.
Infections
Streptococcus spp.
Tuberculosis
Leprosy
Drug allergies
Sulfonamides
Oral contraceptives
Other disorders
Sarcoidosis
Inflammatory bowel disease

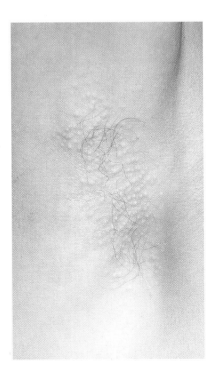

Fig 8.8 Fox–Fordyce disease. Flesh-colored papules in the axilla.

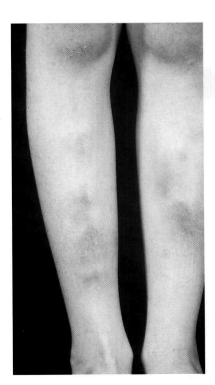

Fig 8.9 Erythema nodosum. Large, painful, shiny, erythematous plaques on the anterior aspect of the lower leg. The lesions are initially bright red in color and then become purple and fade like a bruise.

in utero, or inhibit or prolong labor by inhibiting prostaglandin synthetase. Systemic corticosteroids, if not contraindicated by an underlying infectious disease, are necessary in some cases. Treatment of the underlying disease or removal of the inciting drugs is essential.

BULLOUS DISORDERS

(See also Chapter 18)

PEMPHIGUS

Pemphigus is an uncommon autoimmune bullous dermatosis, which may develop or worsen during pregnancy and be transmitted to the fetus. In the literature there are at least 26 well-documented pregnancies in 22 women with immunopathologically confirmed pemphigus vulgaris. Eleven of these infants were healthy, seven had a transient pemphigus eruption, and eight were stillbirths or abortions[25]. It is therefore important that obstetricians and dermatologists maintain close antenatal and postnatal care of the mother and child. Pemphigus is caused by an autoantibody directed against epidermal antigens. Flaccid blisters of the skin (**8.10**) and mucous membranes develop, and are often widespread. The blisters rupture rapidly, leading to generalized erosions, crusting, and often secondary bacterial infections.

The presentation of pemphigus during pregnancy is extremely rare, although pregnancy has been reported to precipitate or aggravate the condition[26]. Exacerbations usually occur in the first or second trimester, and in most cases the disease continues chronically postpartum. It has been suggested that the improvement seen in pemphigus in the third trimester is due to a rising endogenous cortisol production and consequent immunosuppression. The clinical presentation

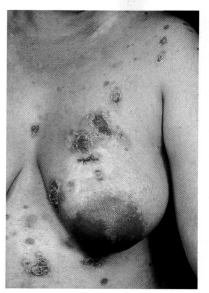

Fig 8.10 Pemphigus vulgaris. Superficial, flaccid blisters on the upper trunk rupture easily, leaving erosions. Blisters may become secondarily infected with bacteria and become crusted.

of pemphigus can be very similar to that of pemphigoid gestationis, and so skin biopsy with immunofluorescence studies is required for an accurate diagnosis[27].

MANAGEMENT

Pemphigus during pregnancy is usually treated with high doses of prednisone. Steroid doses as high as 100 mg prednisone daily may be required for initial control, with dose tapering thereafter. A potent topical corticosteroid cream, such as 0.05% clobetasol propionate, can be applied directly to lesions.

Immunosuppressants, such as cyclophosphamide, azathioprine, methotrexate, and gold, are best avoided. Azathioprine has not been associated with teratogenicity, but it could theoretically affect the immune system of the fetus or neonate. It is not recommended in breastfeeding mothers. Methotrexate is a potent teratogen, particularly if taken during the first trimester, causing multiple skeletal and neurologic defects and cleft palate. Although it is secreted in relatively low concentrations in breast milk, breastfeeding is usually not recommended. There are few data on the safety of cyclosporin A in pregnant patients with a skin condition. A study of pregnant women taking cyclosporin A following organ transplantation suggested a low risk of teratogenic effects. As cyclosporin A passes into breast milk, there is a potential risk of hypertension, nephrotoxicity, and malignancy in breastfed neonates. Cyclophosphamide is teratogenic, leading to skeletal defects and dysmorphic features.

Pemphigus antibody titers may help in assessing disease activity and planning effective treatment. If high antibody titers occur, transplacental transfer of pemphigus antibody and transient fetal pemphigus is probably more likely[27]. Plasmapheresis has been used but there is a risk of a rebound increase in circulating levels of pemphigus antibody. There appears to be, therefore, a need for continued plasmapheresis after delivery, with immunosuppressant adjunctive treatment (e.g. azathioprine) making this an option of last resort.

MATERNAL AND FETAL MORTALITY AND MORBIDITY

Severe cases of disseminated cutaneous disease have been associated with fetal death. Stillborn infants of mothers with pemphigus have been found to have skin lesions and immunofluorescence findings consistent with the disease[29,30]. Cases of well-controlled or mild disease are not usually associated with a significant risk of maternal and fetal morbidity or mortality. The mode of delivery needs careful consideration in each case. The trauma of vaginal delivery may result in the extension and worsening of erosions, while problems with wound healing in patients on long-term steroid therapy make cesarean section less attractive.

NEONATAL PEMPHIGUS

Neonatal pemphigus results from transplacental transmission of maternal pemphigus immunoglobulin (Ig) G autoantibody. Active pemphigus during pregnancy does not necessarily result in neonatal pemphigus. A recent report described a case in which the infant of a mother with purely oral disease was born with widespread cutaneous neonatal pemphigus[31]. Most neonates who develop blisters require no therapy, as the blisters usually heal spontaneously within 2–3 weeks[28]. Breastfeeding is not absolutely contraindicated, although local blister formation may occur with the potential risk of passive transfer of antibody to the infant.

DERMATITIS HERPETIFORMIS

Dermatitis herpetiformis is an autoimmune vesicular disorder characterized by grouped, intensely pruritic, vesicles, which are distributed symmetrically over the elbows, knees, buttocks, shoulders, and scalp (8.11). There is usually histologic and/or symptomatic evidence of gluten-sensitive enteropathy. The characteristic immunofluorescence feature of this disease is the presence of granular deposits of IgA in the upper papillary dermis.

MANAGEMENT

Dapsone administration – the treatment of choice – produces dramatic relief from pruritus within 24 hours and stops new lesion formation within 72 hours. Dapsone is probably safe in pregnancy[2,32]. Most patients respond to an initial dose of 100 mg daily. Those intolerant of dapsone should be tried on sulfapyridine 1–2 g daily. As dapsone may produce severe hemolysis in patients with glucose 6-phosphate

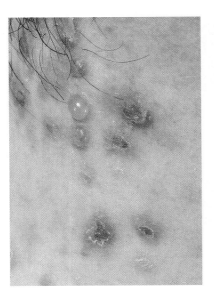

Fig 8.11 Dermatitis herpetiformis. Grouped, itchy, polymorphic lesions on the extremities, such as axillae, as shown here. Vesicles are excoriated, leaving urticarial papules.

dehydrogenase deficiency, patients should be screened before dapsone therapy is instituted.

Ideally, patients with dermatitis herpetiformis should adhere to a strict gluten-free diet, preferably for 6–12 months, before conception. This may obviate the need for dapsone during pregnancy. As dapsone is secreted in breast milk and produces hemolytic anemia in infants, patients taking dapsone should be discouraged from breastfeeding.

LINEAR IgA DISEASE

This is a rare, acquired, subepidermal blistering disorder. It has been defined on the basis of its unique immunopathologic finding of linear deposits of IgA along the cutaneous basement membrane. It resembles dermatitis herpetiformis clinically, but sometimes lesions similar to bullous pemphigoid develop on the trunk and limbs. Unlike dermatitis herpetiformis, there is no associated gluten-sensitive enteropathy.

Linear IgA disease may improve in pregnancy but a relapse may be seen postpartum[33]. The disease does not appear to affect fetal outcome adversely. Treatment is similar to that of dermatitis herpetiformis, with dapsone or sulfapyridine, but some patients may need a combination of dapsone and prednisone (*see also Chapter 18*).

PORPHYRIA CUTANEA TARDA

Porphyria cutanea tarda (PCT) is the most common type of porphyria and occurs in both autosomal dominant and acquired forms. The disorder is due to a defect in uroporphyrinogen decarboxylase activity. This results in a characteristic increase of uroporphyrin and 7-carboxyporphyrin in the urine, and increased isocoproporphyrin in the stool. Patients present with skin fragility, erosions, vesicles, bullae, and milia on sun-exposed areas, especially the dorsum of the hands (8.12) and forearms. Other cutaneous changes include facial hypertrichosis, periorbital hyperpigmentation, scarring alopecia, and dystrophic calcification with ulceration.

PREGNANCY

Although PCT is known to be affected adversely by estrogen, iron, and alcohol, there are conflicting reports about the effects of pregnancy. Case reports of patients whose illness was not exacerbated by pregnancy have led to speculation that endogenous estrogens may be less harmful than exogenous compounds[34]. However, other cases show findings of clinical and biochemical deterioration of disease, with increases in plasma and urine porphyrin levels during

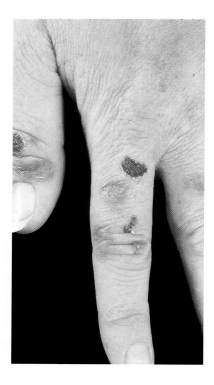

Fig 8.12 Porphyria cutanea tarda. Sun-exposed areas, such as the dorsum of the hand and fingers, are most severely affected. Minimal trauma results in erosions and blisters.

pregnancy[35,36]. In the nonpregnant individual, premenstrual exacerbation is a recognized feature of many of the porphyrias and the gonadotropin-releasing hormone analog, buserelin acetate, has been used successfully to treat hereditary coproporphyria by temporarily suppressing ovulation and menstruation[37]. However, this drug is contraindicated during pregnancy.

MANAGEMENT

The avoidance of sunlight and use of an opaque sun block, such as zinc oxide, are helpful. Venesection or phlebotomy, with careful monitoring of hematocrit, has been used successfully to treat PCT during pregnancy. In this procedure, 500 mL of blood is removed weekly or twice weekly until the hemoglobin level has fallen to 10–11 g/dL or serum iron concentration to 50–60 mg/dL.

Chloroquine is contraindicated in pregnancy because of its teratogenicity; it causes multiple defects in the fetus, including neurosensory hearing loss, intellectual impairment, and neonatal convulsions. Other less commonly applied therapies, such as cholestyramine, activated charcoal, and intravenous deferoxamine administration, are also contraindicated in pregnancy.

ERYTHEMA MULTIFORME

This disorder is characterized by acute, self-limiting, but often recurrent, episodes of erythematous maculopapular lesions, which may develop into classical target or iris lesions, or may blister. The lesions are typically distributed symmetrically on the extremities, especially the hands (8.13), and on the extensor aspects of the forearms and legs. The frequency of mucosal involvement varies widely, between 25% and 60%, with affected organs including the mouth, eyes, pharynx, esophagus, genitalia, and anus. Severe cases (Stevens–Johnson syndrome) may develop significant complications, such as visual impairment secondary to keratitis with conjunctival scarring (8.14).

There are several causes of erythema multiforme, such as herpes simplex or mycoplasmal infections, and sensitivity to drugs, especially to long-acting sulfonamides. Pregnancy may also cause erythema multiforme, and vaginal stenosis has been described in severe Stevens–Johnson syndrome in pregnancy[38]. Systemic corticosteroids, such as prednisone 30–40 mg daily, are sometimes required, particularly in Stevens–Johnson syndrome. The dose should be gradually reduced after a few days.

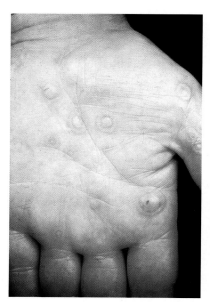

Fig 8.13 Erythema multiforme. Well circumscribed erythematous lesions occur on the hands, as shown here, and feet. The central area of the lesion is more involved than the periphery so it appears like a target. Blisters may develop in the center of the lesions.

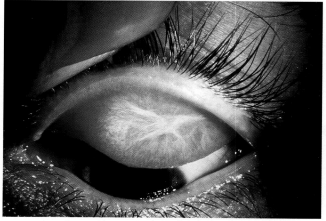

Fig 8.14 Stevens–Johnson syndrome. Severe blistering and ulceration of the conjunctiva results in corneal scarring.

NEOPLASIA

(See also Chapter 21)

Basal cell epithelioma and *squamous cell carcinoma* are both very rare in pregnancy, as they tend to be disorders of the elderly population. *Gorlin's syndrome* (basal cell nevus syndrome) is a rare autosomal dominant inherited condition, in which numerous basal cell carcinomas develop in a much younger age group; there are few reports in pregnant women. The disorder certainly does not appear to affect this group specifically.

BENIGN MELANOCYTIC NEVI

It is known that pre-existing benign pigmented nevi may darken temporarily during pregnancy owing to increased levels of melanocyte-stimulating hormone[39]. There is some debate as to whether benign melanocytic nevi increase in number and size during pregnancy (8.15). In one report 33% of women reported some enlargement or color change in their nevi during pregnancy[39]. Another recent study of 22 women found no significant change in measured size of their 129 nevi during pregnancy[40]. In addition, there is no evidence that pregnancy induces malignant transformation of pre-existing nevi.

MALIGNANT MELANOMA

The influence of pregnancy on the prognosis of malignant melanoma (8.16, 8.17) is controversial[41–43]. Many early observations suggested a link between hormones and malignant melanoma, but these have been disputed,

and the suspected adverse effect of pregnancy on malignant melanoma has not been confirmed. Mackie *et al.*[44] published a large study which suggests that malignant melanoma developing during pregnancy has a slightly worse prognosis. However, pregnancy following excision of a tumor does not appear to affect prognosis, which continues to be determined mainly by tumor thickness[41]. Grin *et al.*[45] recently reviewed the literature and concluded that pregnancy before, during, or after the diagnosis of melanoma does not appear to influence 5-year survival rates. Transplacental transmission of melanoma to the fetus is extremely rare, and maternal melanoma usually has no adverse effects on the fetus[42].

MANAGEMENT

Treatment for melanoma in pregnant women is no different to treatment in other patients. Surgical excision of primary lesions and clinically involved lymph nodes should be performed. Therapeutic termination in a

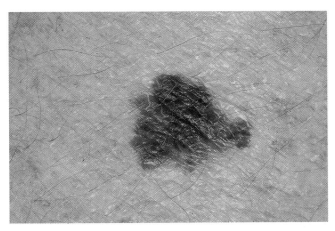

Fig 8.16 Superficial spreading malignant melanoma. The pigmented lesion is a slightly raised plaque with an irregular outline and irregular pigmentation.

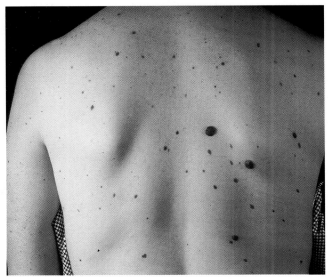

Fig 8.15 Benign melanocytic nevi. Multiple nevi on trunk have evenly distributed pigment and each nevus has a regular outline.

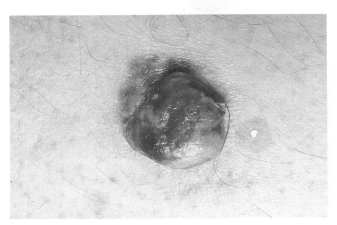

Fig 8.17 Nodular malignant melanoma. A nodule has developed in the center of an irregularly outlined pigmented lesion. The nodule itself appears to be relatively amelanotic.

woman who has a concurrent malignant melanoma and pregnancy has shown no benefit in inducing maternal tumor regression[41]. When melanoma occurs during pregnancy, a clinical and histologic examination of the placenta should be performed postpartum because the possibility of transmission of transplacental metastatic disease to the fetus does exist[27,42,46,47]. Chemotherapy may be indicated for rapidly progressive metastatic melanoma and is not necessarily associated with an adverse fetal prognosis[48,49].

TIMING OF PREGNANCY

Women from whom malignant melanomas have been excised should be counseled about future pregnancies. Mackie *et al.*[44] have observed that 83% of patients with metastatic disease present within 2 years after the initial diagnosis of primary malignant melanoma. Women should therefore be recommended to delay pregnancy by at least 2 years after diagnosis. Generally, women with melanoma should be advised about pregnancy on the basis of thickness and site of tumor and evidence of vascular spread, not hormonal status[44].

CUTANEOUS T-CELL LYMPHOMA

Cutaneous T-cell lymphoma (CTCL) or mycosis fungoides is a chronic, slowly evolving, T-cell lymphoma involving mainly the skin. The earliest lesions are flat, erythematous, slightly scaly patches, which gradually thicken to form plaques. Sometimes tumors may develop. Pregnancy may exacerbate the disease[50].

Early lesions may respond to potent topical steroids and ultraviolet B light, but PUVA should be avoided, if possible, because of the potential teratogenic effects of methoxypsoralen. Therapy with cytotoxic agents is generally contraindicated during pregnancy, especially in the first trimester.

MISCELLANEOUS CONDITIONS

SARCOIDOSIS

Sarcoidosis is a multisystem, granulomatous disorder of unknown etiology, which most commonly affects young adults in their reproductive years. Approximately 0.02–0.06% of pregnant women have sarcoidosis[51]. Both specific and nonspecific cutaneous lesions are associated with sarcoidosis. Specific lesions include papules, nodules (8.18), plaques (lupus pernio) (8.19), ichthyotic scaling, hypopigmentation, atrophy, ulcers, and scar infiltration. The nonspecific lesions are not actually granulomas, but skin changes that are characteristic associated with sarcoidosis, the most common of which is erythema nodosum.

PREGNANCY

Active sarcoidosis usually improves during pregnancy and relapses postpartum. In cases of already inactive disease, the condition remains inactive[52,53]. The positive effects of pregnancy on sarcoidosis may be due to an increased level of circulating free cortisol, and the postpartum relapse may represent a rebound phenomenon, as is usually seen after cessation of corticosteroid therapy. Improvement in some pregnant patients with sarcoidosis may be related to spontaneous resolution of the disease.

The frequency of abortions, obstetric complications, or congenital abnormalities is not increased by the presence of sarcoidosis[51]. Generally, the obstetric management of pregnancy, labor, and delivery does not differ from that for a normal patient. In some cases, however, such as those with advanced pulmonary disease or extrapulmonary lesions, exacerbations may occur and

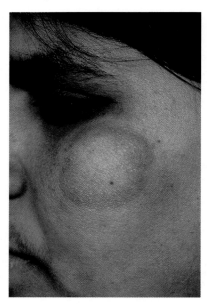

Fig 8.18 Sarcoidosis. Annular pigmented plaques on the face. Nasal infiltration may be extremely disfiguring and difficult to treat. In West Indians, red-brown nodules are especially common around the nose.

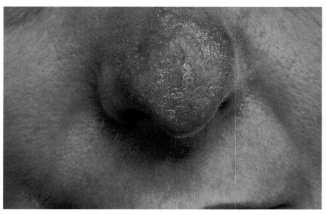

Fig 8.19 Lupus pernio. Thickened purple plaques occur on the nose and are caused by granulomatous involvement of the dermis and subcutaneous fat.

patients should be followed carefully. Disease activity should be carefully assessed soon after delivery in all patients who have, or have had, sarcoidosis[52,53].

PYODERMA GANGRENOSUM

There have been six reports of pyoderma gangrenosum in pregnancy to date associated with leukemia, lupus erythematosus, antiphospholipid syndrome, and three idiopathic cases. In one case this condition was a complication of cesarean section for delivery[54]. The patient described most recently developed marked pyoderma gangrenosum with pathergy but responded well to cyclosporin A[55].

ACRODERMATITIS ENTEROPATHICA

This is a rare autosomal recessive condition with reduced serum zinc levels. Acquired zinc deficiency can occur in patients with an inadequate intake of zinc, such as those receiving long-term parenteral nutrition without zinc supplementation, those who have zinc malabsorption, and those with increased losses of zinc. It is characterized by dermatitis, diarrhea, and alopecia. The dermatitis is vesiculobullous and eczematous, and develops on the acral areas of the extremities and periorificial sites, such as the mouth, anus, and genital areas. Paronychia and scalp alopecia are seen.

Acrodermatitis enteropathica flares during pregnancy, with a further decrease in serum zinc concentration[56]. This fall in zinc level is not entirely due to increased fetal demands, because zinc levels also decrease and the disease flares with oral contraceptive use[27]. Estrogens must therefore have an important primary role[27].

The skin eruption may resemble impetigo herpetiformis or pemphigoid gestationis. Having first appeared in childhood, the skin disease reappears early during pregnancy, progressively worsens until delivery, and then clears spontaneously postpartum.

Most pregnancies have produced normal offspring[27]. Zinc supplementation (e.g. zinc sulfate 200 mg three times daily) to maintain normal serum zinc levels seems to be effective in preventing adverse fetal effects.

NEUROFIBROMAS

Women with neurofibromatosis experience a higher than expected rate of first-trimester spontaneous abortion (21%), stillbirth (9%), and intrauterine growth retardation in pregnancy (13%)[57]. Genetic counseling is mandatory because of the disabilities that may be precipitated by pregnancy and because of the rare possible deformities associated with neurofibromatosis, an autosomal dominant disorder. Elective termination of pregnancy may be necessary in severely affected patients. During pregnancy, the skin lesions of neurofibromatosis may appear for the first time, or may increase in both size and number. Large, plexiform, neurofibromas may enlarge (8.20) and then hemorrhage into the core of the tumor. In most cases, the lesions regress postpartum. Of greater importance is the effect of pregnancy on the vascular system of patients with neurofibromatosis. Major blood vessels may rupture and hypertension may occur[58]. Patients with neurofibromatosis also have an increased risk of perinatal complications, so close monitoring of pregnancy is mandatory[59].

CONCLUSION

Obstetricians and dermatologists working together should be able to recognize and manage skin diseases in pregnant women. They should be aware of the often modified expression of disease in this special group of patients, and should also realize that therapeutic options are inevitably altered by the pregnant condition. It is important that patients with inherited disorders are counseled about the genetic nature of their condition, and if necessary the dermatologist and geneticist should offer counseling before conception.

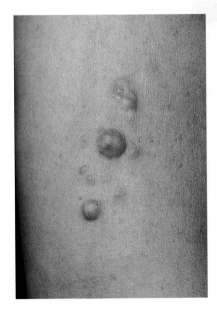

Fig 8.20 Neurofibromatosis. Large neurofibromas have developed on the upper arm.

REFERENCES

1 Reed, B. R. Pregnancy, drugs and the dermatologist. *Curr. Probl. Dermatol.* 1994; **VI**: 29–80.

2 Stockton, D. L. and Paller, A. S. Drug administration to the pregnant or lactating woman: a reference guide for dermatologists. *J. Am. Acad. Dermatol.* 1990; **23**: 87–103.

3 Jurecka, W. and Gebhart, W. Drug prescribing during pregnancy. *Semin. Dermatol.* 1989; **8**: 30–39.

4 Gunnarskog, J. G., Kallen, A. J. B., Lindelof, B. G., *et al.* Psoralen photochemotherapy (PUVA) and pregnancy. *Arch. Dermatol.* 1993; **129**: 320–323.

5 Cockburn, I., Krupp, P., and Monka, C. Present experience of Sandimmun in pregnancy. *Transplant. Proc.* 1989; **21**: 3730–3732.

6 Finch, T. M. and Tan, C. Y. Pustular psoriasis exacerbated by pregnancy and controlled by cyclosporin A. *Br. J. Dermatol.* 2000; **142**: 582–584.

7 Wright, S., Glover, H., and Baker, H. Psoriasis, cyclosporin, and pregnancy. *Arch. Dermatol.* 1991; **127**: 426.

8 Mowad, C. M., Margolis, D. J., and Halpern A. C. Hormonal influences on women with psoriasis. *Cutis* 1998; **61**: 257–260.

9 Boyd, A. S., Morris, L. F., and Phillips, C. M. Psoriasis and pregnancy: hormone and immune system interaction. *Int. J. Dermatol.* 1996; **35**: 169–172.

10 McHugh, N. J. and Laurent, M. R. The effect of pregnancy on the onset of psoriatic arthritis. *Br. J. Rheumatol.* 1989; **28**: 50–52.

11 Lotem, M., Katzenelson, V., Rotem, A., *et al.* Impetigo herpetiformis: a variant of pustular psoriasis or a separate entity? *J. Am. Acad. Dermatol.* 1989; **20**: 338–341.

12 Oumeish, O. Y., Farraj, S. E., and Bataineh, A. S. Some aspects of impetigo herpetiformis. *Arch. Dermatol.* 1982; **118**: 103–105.

13 Rackett, S. C. and Baughman, R. D. Impetigo herpetiformis and *Staphylococcus aureus* lymphadenitis in a pregnant adolescent. *Pediatr. Dermatol.* 1997; **14**: 387–390.

14 Kuijpers, A. L. A., Schalkwijk, J., Rulo H. F. C., *et al.* Extremely low levels of epidermal skin-derived antileucoproteinase/elafin in a patient with impetigo herpetiformis. *Br. J. Dermatol.* 1997; **137**: 123–129.

15 Van Pelt, H. P. A., and Juhlin, L. Acne conglobata after pregnancy. *Acta Derm. Venereol. (Stockh.)* 1999; **79**: 169.

16 Bekaert, C., Song, M., and Delvigne, A. Acne neonatorum and familial hyperandrogenism. *Dermatology* 1998; **196**: 453–454.

17 Lipson, A. H., Collins, F., and Webster, W. S. Multiple congenital defects associated with maternal use of topical tretinoin. *Lancet* 1993; **341**: 1352–1353.

18 Camera, G. and Pregliasco, P. Ear malformation in baby born to mother using tretinoin cream. *Lancet* 1992; **339**: 687.

19 Van Hoogdalem, E. J. Transdermal absorption of topical anti-acne agents in man: review of clinical pharmacokinetic data. *J. Eur. Acad. Dermatovenereol.* 1998; **11**: S13–19.

20 Graham–Brown, R. A. C. The ages of man and their dermatoses. In: Champion, R. H., Burton, J. L., Burns, D. A., and Breathnach, S. M. (eds) *Textbook of Dermatology*, pp. 3259–3287. Blackwell, Oxford, 1998.

21 Barth, J. H., Layton, A. M., and Cunliffe, W. J. Endocrine factors in pre- and postmenopausal women with hidradenitis suppurativa. *Br. J. Dermatol.* 1996; **134**: 1057–1059.

22 Dalyrumple, J. C. and Monaghan, J. M. Treatment of hidradenitis suppurativa with the carbon dioxide laser. *Br. J. Surg.* 1987; **74**: 420.

23 Shelly, W. B. and Levy, E. J. Apocrine sweat retention in man, II; Fox-Fordyce disease (apocrine miliaria). *Arch. Dermatol.* 1956; **73**: 38.

24 Bartelsmeyer, J. A. and Petrie, R. H. Erythema nodosum, estrogens, and pregnancy. *Clin. Obstet. Gynecol.* 1990; **33**: 777–781.

25 Yair, D., Shenhav, M., Botchan, A., *et al.* Pregnancy associated with pemphigus. *Br. J. Obstet. Gynaecol.* 1995; **102**: 667–669.

26 Honeyman, J. F., Eguiguren, G., Pinto, A., *et al.* Bullous dermatoses of pregnancy. *Arch. Dermatol.* 1981; **117**: 264–267.

27 Winton, G. B. Skin diseases aggravated by pregnancy. *J. Am. Acad. Dermatol.* 1989; **20**: 1–13.

28 Goldberg, N. S., DeFeo, C., and Kirshenbaum, N. Pemphigus vulgaris and pregnancy: risk factors and recommendations. *J. Am. Acad. Dermatol.* 1993; **28**: 877–879.

29 Terpestra, H. de Jong, M. C. J. M., and Klokke, A. H. *In vivo* bound pemphigus antibodies in a stillborn infant: passive intrauterine transfer of pemphigus vulgaris? *Arch. Dermatol.* 1979; **115**: 316–319.

30 Wasserstrum, N. and Lavros, R. K. Transplacental transmission of pemphigus. *J.A.M.A.* 1983; **249**: 1480–1482.

31 Hern, S., Vaughan Jones, S. A., Setterfield, J., *et al.* Pemphigus vulgaris in pregnancy with favourable fetal prognosis. *Clin. Exp. Dermatol.* 1998; **23**: 260–263.

32 Kahn, G. Dapsone is safe during pregnancy. *J. Am. Acad. Dermatol.* 1985; **13**: 838–839 (letter).

33 Collier, P. M., Kelly, S. E., and Wojnarowska, F. W. Linear IgA disease and pregnancy. *J. Am. Acad. Dermatol.* 1994; **30**: 407–411.

34 Marks, R. Porphyria cutanea tarda. *Arch. Dermatol.* 1982; **118**: 452.

35 Baxi, L. V., Rubeo, T. J., Katz, B., *et al.* Porphyria cutanea tarda and pregnancy. *Am. J. Obstet. Gynecol.* 1983; **146**: 333–334.

36 Rajka, G. Pregnancy and porphyria cutanea tarda. *Acta. Derm. Venereol. (Stockh.)* 1984; **64**: 444–445.

37 Yamamori, I., Asai, M., Tanaka, F., *et al* Prevention of premenstrual exacerbation of hereditary coproporphyria by gonadotropin-releasing hormone analogue. *Int. Med.* 1999; **38**: 365–368.

38 Graham–Brown, R. A. C., Cochrane, G. W., Swinhoe, J. R., *et al.* Vaginal stenosis due to bullous erythema multiforme (Stevens–Johnson syndrome). *Br. J. Obstet. Gynaecol.* 1981; **88**: 1156–1157.

39 Sanchez, J. L., Figueroa, L. D., and Rodriguez, E. Behaviour of melanocytic nevi during pregnancy. *Am. J. Dermatopathol.* 1984; **6**(suppl 1): 89–91.

40 Pennoyer, J. W., Grin, C. M., Driscoll, M. S., *et al.* Change in size of melanocytic nevi during pregnancy. *J. Am. Acad. Dermatol.* 1997; **36**: 378–382.

41 Colburn, D. S., Nathanson, L., and Belilos, E. Pregnancy and malignant melanoma. *Semin. Oncol.* 1989; **16**: 377–387.

42 McManamny, D. S., Moss, A. L. H., Briggs, J. C., *et al.* Melanoma and pregnancy: a long-term follow-up. *Br. J. Obstet. Gynaecol.* 1989; **96**: 1419–1423.

43 Driscoll, M. S., Grin-Jorgensen, C. M., and Grant-Kels, J. M. Does pregnancy influence the prognosis of malignant melanoma? *J. Am. Acad. Dermatol.* 1993; **29**: 619–630.

44 Mackie, R. M., Bufalino, R., Morabito, A., *et al.* Lack of effect of pregnancy on outcome of melanoma. *Lancet* 1991; **i**: 653–655.

45 Grin, C. M., Driscoll, M. S., and Grant-Kels, J. M. The relationship of pregnancy, hormones and melanoma. *Semin. Cutan. Med. Surg.* 1998; **17**: 167–171.

46 Ferreira, C. M. M., Maceira, J. M. P. M., and de Oliveira Coelho, J. M. C. Melanoma and pregnancy with placental metastases. *Am. J. Dermatopathol.* 1998; **20**: 403–407.

47 Baergen, R. N., Johnson, D., Moore, T., *et al.* Maternal melanoma metastatic to the placenta: a case report and review of the literature. *Arch. Pathol. Lab. Med.* 1997; **121**: 508–511.

48 Dipaola, R. S., Goodin, S., Ratzell, M., *et al.* Chemotherapy for metastatic melanoma during pregnancy. *Gynecol. Oncol.* 1997; **66**: 526–530.

49 Johnston, S. R. D., Broadley, K., Henson, G., *et al*. Management of metastatic melanoma during pregnancy – a difficult case. *B.M.J.* 1998; **316**: 848–851.

50 Vonderheid, E. C., Dellatorre, D. L., and van Scott, E. J. Prolonged remission of tumor-stage mycosis fungoides by topical immunotherapy. *Arch. Dermatol.* 1981; **117**: 586–589.

51 Abarquez, C., Pandya, K., and Sharma, O. P. Sarcoidosis and pregnancy. *Sarcoidosis J.* 1990; **7**: 63–66.

52 Selroos, O. Sarcoidosis and pregnancy: a review with results of a retrospective survey. *J. Intern. Med.* 1990; **227**: 221–224.

53 Chapelon, A. C., Ginsburg, C., Biousse, V., *et al*. Sarcoidosis and pregnancy. A retrospective study of 11 cases. *Rev. Med. Interne* 1998; **19**: 305–312.

54 Harland, C. C., Jaffe, W., Holden, C. A., and Ross, L. D. Pyoderma gangrenosum complicating cesarean section. *J. Obstet. Gynecol.* 1993; **13**: 115–116.

55 Sassolas, B., Le Ru, Y., Plantin, P., *et al*. Pyoderma gangrenosum with pathergic phenomenon in pregnancy. *Br. J. Dermatol.* 2000; **142**: 827–828.

56 Bronson, D. M., Barsky, R., and Barsky, S. Acrodermatitis enteropathica. *J. Am. Acad. Dermatol.* 1983; **9**: 140–144.

57 Weissman, A., Jakobi, P., Zaidise, I., *et al*. Neurofibromatosis and pregnancy. An update. *J. Reprod. Med.* 1993; **38**: 890–896.

58 Braude, P. B. and Bolan, J. C. Neurofibromatosis and spontaneous hemothorax in pregnancy: two case reports. *Obstet. Gynecol.* 1984; **63**(Suppl): 35–38.

59 Segal, D., Holcberg, G., Sapir, O., *et al*. Neurofibromatosis in pregnancy. *Eur. J. Obstet. Gynecol. Reprod. Biol.* 1999; **84**: 59–61.

ACKNOWLEDGEMENTS

Figure **8.3** is reproduced by kind permission of Dr I. R. White, St John's Institute of Dermatology, St Thomas' Hospital, London, UK. Figures **8.8** and **8.9** are reproduced by kind permission of Dr. A. C. Pembroke, King's College Hospital, London, UK. Figure **8.14** is reproduced by kind permission of Dr A. D. M. Bryceson, Hospital for Tropical Diseases, London, UK

Connective Tissue Diseases in Pregnancy

Catherine Nelson-Piercy

INTRODUCTION

The connective tissue diseases are multisystem disorders characterized by circulating nonorgan-specific autoantibodies. Many of them are more prevalent in women of childbearing age, so are not uncommonly encountered in pregnancy. Pregnancy is associated with suppressed cell-mediated immunity. Thus connective tissue diseases in general may remit or improve during pregnancy. However, this is not universal; for example, systemic lupus erythematosus (SLE) may flare or present in pregnancy, with disastrous consequences.

RHEUMATOID ARTHRITIS

Up to 75% of women with rheumatoid arthritis experience improvement of both joint and extra-articular features during pregnancy[1], although less than 20% are in complete remission[2]. Improvement usually begins

> ### IMPLICATIONS FOR THE PREGNANT PATIENT
>
> **Rheumatoid Arthritis**
>
> - Usually improves in pregnancy
> - Often deteriorates postpartum
> - Use corticosteroids rather than nonsteroidal antiinflammatory drugs

during the first trimester, and rheumatoid nodules may disappear. However, 90% of those who experience remission suffer postpartum exacerbations, and there is an increased incidence of rheumatoid arthritis onset in the postpartum period. Infants of women who have anti-Ro antibodies are at risk of neonatal lupus (see below). The relative safety of drugs used to treat connective tissue disease in pregnancy[3] is shown in **Table 9.1**.

Table 9.1 Drug Treatment of Connective Tissue Disease in Pregnancy[3].

Drug	Relative Safety
Prednisone	High (especially in doses of 20 mg daily or less)
Sulfasalazine	High
Aspirin (low doses)	High (doses above 150 mg/day should be discontinued before 32 weeks' gestation)
Nonsteroidal antiinflammatory drugs	Low (use steroids in preference and stop before 32 weeks if essential)
Heparin	High (although osteoporosis is a risk with prolonged high doses)
Gold	Caution (best avoided)
Azathioprine	Medium (probably safe)
Hydroxychloroquine	Medium (probably safe at the lower doses now used, e.g. 200 mg daily)
Penicillamine	Low
Methotrexate	Contraindicated in pregnancy
Cyclophosphamide	Low (avoid if possible)
Warfarin	Low (avoid during weeks 6–12)

SYSTEMIC LUPUS ERYTHEMATOSUS

The prevalence of SLE is approximately 1 per 1000 women, but may be increasing. SLE flares may be difficult to diagnose during pregnancy because many features, such as hairfall, edema, facial erythema, fatigue, anemia, raised erythrocyte sedimentation rate (ESR), and musculoskeletal pain, also occur in normal pregnancy[4]. About 60% of women with SLE have a flare during pregnancy or the puerperium, compared with about 40% of nonpregnant women over the same time period[5]. Cutaneous flares are the most common (9.1–9.3), followed by joint symptoms. Disease flares must be managed actively. Corticosteroids are the drug of choice[3], but do not prevent flares. They should not be prescribed prophylactically, nor the dose increased for that purpose[5]. Pregnancy does not seem to jeopardize

renal function in the long term for women with lupus nephritis, although SLE nephropathy may manifest for the first time in pregnancy. There is a greater risk of deterioration in patients with a higher baseline serum creatinine level. A renal flare may be difficult to distinguish from pre-eclampsia, as hypertension, proteinuria, thrombocytopenia, and renal impairment are all features of both (**Table 9.2**).

SLE is associated with an increased risk of spontaneous abortion, fetal death, pre-eclampsia, preterm delivery, and intrauterine growth restriction (IUGR)[6]. These adverse outcomes are associated with the presence of anticardiolipin antibodies (aCLs) or lupus anticoagulant (LA) (antiphospholipid antibodies; aPLs), lupus nephritis or hypertension, and either active disease at the time of conception or first presentation of SLE during pregnancy. In the absence of these features, the risk of adverse outcome is not increased.

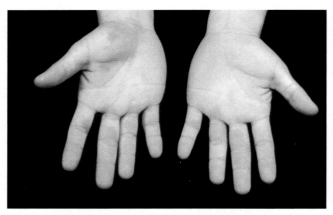

Fig 9.1 Florid erythema of the palms. Pregnancy-related palmar erythema may confuse the diagnosis of lupus vasculitis.

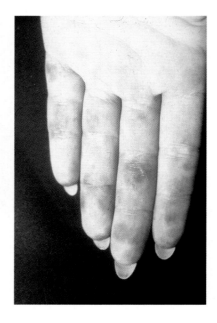

Fig 9.2 Peripheral lupus vasculitis. Vasculitic eruptions in lupus in pregnancy commonly affect the peripheries, especially the tips of the fingers and toes.

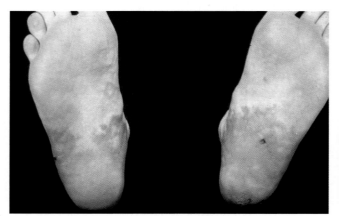

Fig 9.3 Lupus vasculitis of the soles. This young woman had marked lupus vasculitis of the soles of the feet, which had been confused with a fungal dermatosis by her family physician.

Table 9.2 Features that Distinguish Renal Flare in Lupus Pregnancy from Pre-eclampsia.
Evidence of clinical lupus activity in other systems
Rising titer of anti-DNA antibodies
Evidence of alternate pathway of complement activation (i.e. $\downarrow C_3$ or $\downarrow C_4$)
Presence of cellular casts on urine microscopy
Absence of other features of pre-eclampsia (e.g. IUGR, abnormal liver function test results, hyperuricemia)

NEONATAL LUPUS SYNDROMES

About 30% of patients with SLE have anti-Ro antibodies. They are most common in mothers with predominantly cutaneous lupus and with Sjögren's syndrome. These antibodies cross the placenta and may cause immune damage in the fetus.

The commonest manifestation (5% risk if anti-Ro positive) is cutaneous neonatal lupus. The eruption (9.4) usually appears in the first 2 weeks of life. The typical lesions tend to be geographical, annular, erythematous, and scaly, and occur over the face, scalp, or other light-exposed skin. The rash disappears spontaneously within 6 months and scarring is unusual.

The risk of congenital heart block is less (2–3% risk if anti-Ro positive), and is usually detected *in utero* at around 18–20 weeks. The perinatal mortality rate is increased, with 20% of affected children dying in the early neonatal period. Most infants who survive this period do well[7], although 50–60%[8] require a pacemaker. The risk of a second child being born with heart block is 25%, rising to 50% after two or more affected babies[7].

ANTIPHOSPHOLIPID SYNDROME

The combination of either aCLs or LA with one or more of the characteristic clinical features (**Table 9.3**) is known as the antiphospholipid syndrome (APS)[9]. Livedo reticularis (9.5) is the typical skin lesion but is

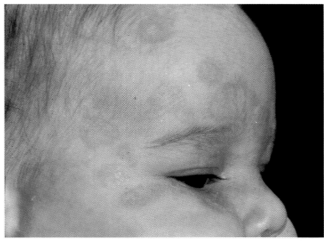

Fig 9.4 Cutaneous neonatal lupus. This baby shows the classic appearance of neonatal lupus.

not invariably present. Indolent cutaneous ulcers (9.6) are a rare feature. APS may complicate SLE, but many patients have primary APS with no features of SLE. Patients with primary APS should not be labeled as having 'lupus', but the antibodies should be regarded as markers for a high-risk pregnancy. Previous poor obstetric history is an important predictor of fetal loss. Many of the adverse outcomes described (early-onset pre-eclampsia, IUGR, placental abruption, stillbirth) are the end result of abnormal placentation, supporting the hypothesis that placental failure is the mechanism by which aPLs are associated with late loss[10].

The risk of recurrent thrombosis in patients with APS may reach 70%[11]. Management of pregnancy in women with APS includes low-dose aspirin (75 mg) and low molecular weight heparin[10], which reduce fetal mortality. Thromboprophylaxis with heparin is essential for those with previous thrombosis.

Table 9.3 Clinical Criteria for Antiphospholipid Syndrome[9].
Diagnostic criteria One or more of:
Thrombosis (venous or arterial)
Recurrent pregnancy loss (fetal death > 10 weeks, three or more miscarriages at < 10 weeks)
Premature birth before 34 weeks due to pre-eclampsia or IUGR
Additional Clinical Features
Thrombocytopenia and hemolytic anemia
Livedo reticularis
Cerebral involvement (particularly epilepsy, cerebral infarction, chorea and migraine)
Heart valve disease (particularly mitral valve)
Hypertension
Pulmonary hypertension
Leg ulcers

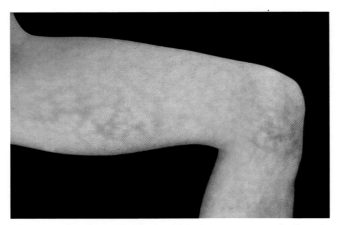

Fig 9.5 Livedo reticularis. This is a cutaneous hallmark of antiphospholipid antibodies. As well as miscarriage and thrombosis, these antibodies may be associated with cardiac murmurs due to valvular vegetations.

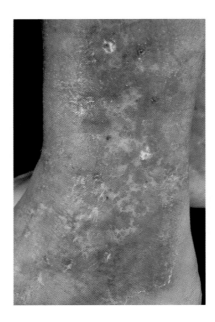

**Fig 9.6
Cutaneous ulcers
and atrophie
blanche.**
Cutaneous ulcers, especially on the lower legs, which are notoriously persistent, are a less usual manifestation of antiphospholipid syndrome.

Pregnancy complicated by SLE or APS requires expert care and a team approach by obstetricians, physicians, and hematologists. Close monitoring of both mother and fetus is essential[10].

SCLERODERMA

It is hypothesized that fetal antimaternal graft-versus-host reactions may be involved in the pathogenesis of scleroderma, which has clinical similarities to chronic graft-versus-host disease since persistent fetal microchimerism is more common in women with scleroderma than control women[12]. Pregnancy may have an etiological role in scleroderma[13].

Successful pregnancy is now reported to occur in 70–80% of patients[14]. The risks of adverse outcome are highest for women with early diffuse disease. Progressive cutaneous disease is unusual during or immediately after pregnancy. Raynaud's phenomenon usually improves as a result of vasodilation and increased blood flow. Reflux esophagitis often worsens, related to the decreased lower esophageal tone. Arthralgia usually worsens[15]. There is no evidence that pregnancy worsens cardiac or respiratory disease, although those with severe pulmonary fibrosis and pulmonary hypertension are at extremely high risk of postpartum deterioration[16], as with pulmonary hypertension from any cause.

DERMATOMYOSITIS AND POLYMYOSITIS

Dermatomyositis and polymyositis are rare in pregnancy. Dermatomyositis is a subacute systemic weakness of the proximal limb and trunk muscles associated with skin lesions (9.7, 9.8). There may be increased rash activity, proximal muscle weakness[17] or subcutaneous calcification in polymyositis during pregnancy (9.9, 9.10). Pre-existing dermatomyositis or polymyositis probably presents no increased risk to either mother or fetus, but the fetal mortality rate is increased when onset or relapse occur during pregnancy[18]. A significant improvement can usually be expected in the puerperium[19].

Pregnancy should be planned at a time of remission, and the patient should be monitored closely throughout the pregnancy for clinical and laboratory signs of disease exacerbation. Prednisone, administered in a minimally effective dosage, is the mainstay of treatment for dermatomyositis and polymyositis.

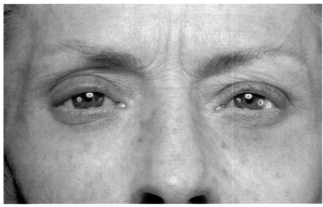

Fig 9.7 Dermatomyositis. Periorbital violescent (heliotrope) rash with associated edema.

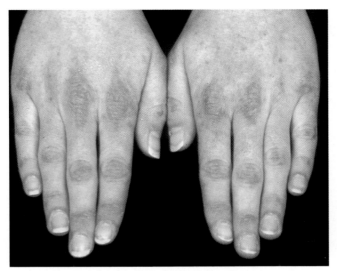

Fig 9.8 Dermatomyositis (Gottron papules).
Erythematous purple papules on the dorsal aspects of the metacarpophalangeal and interphalangeal joints.

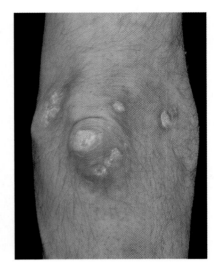

Fig 9.9 Polmyositis. Acceleration of subcutaneous calcification, shown here at the elbow, was noted by this young woman with polymyositis during pregnancy. The disease remained inactive in other respects.

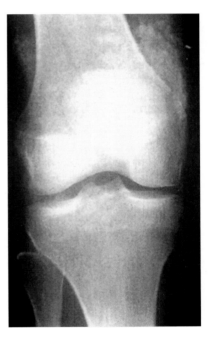

Fig 9.10 Polymyositis. Radiograph of the knee of the patient in **9.9**, showing calcification of subcutaneous tissue in the lower thigh.

EHLERS–DANLOS SYNDROME

Although Ehlers–Danlos syndrome and pseudoxanthoma elasticum are not regarded as 'connective tissue' diseases in the sense described above, they are included in this chapter for convenience. Ehlers–Danlos syndromes I–X are a group of inherited disorders of collagen metabolism, characterized by fragile skin and blood vessels, easy bruising, skin hyperelasticity, and joint hypermobility.

Obstetric problems include postpartum bleeding, poor wound healing and dehiscence, vaginal and perineal lacerations, bladder and uterine prolapse, and abdominal hernia[20–22]. There is an increased risk of premature rupture of the membranes, and perineal delivery has been described[23]. A favorable outcome for pregnancy has been reported for type II (mitis) and type X (fibronectin abnormality), and possibly mild forms of the disease[20]. Women with Ehlers–Danlos types I (classic or gravis) and IV (ecchymotic or arterial) are particularly likely to develop complications during pregnancy. Rupture and dissection of major blood vessels, including the aorta and pulmonary artery, and rupture of the bowel or uterus, especially with type IV disease, explain the increased maternal mortality rate[21]. Avoidance or early termination of pregnancy should be recommended in type IV disease, for which the reported maternal mortality rate (albeit probably an overestimate due to reporting bias) is 20–25%[21,22]. It is thus important to categorize the patient's condition accurately to enable accurate counselling regarding pregnancy.

IMPLICATIONS FOR THE PREGNANT PATIENT

Ehlers–Danlos Syndrome

- Women with Ehlers–Danlos types I (classic or gravis) and IV (ecchymotic or arterial) are particularly likely to develop dangerous complications during pregnancy.

- Catastrophic complications in patients with type I or IV disease are most likely to occur during labor, delivery, or in the first few days postpartum[21]. Cesarean section may not result in fewer complications than vaginal delivery[21].

PSEUDOXANTHOMA ELASTICUM

Pseudoxanthoma elasticum is an inherited disease characterized by widespread degeneration of elastic tissue involving the skin (**9.11**), eye (angioid streaks and loss of central vision), gastrointestinal tract, and blood vessels. Patients have premature vascular disease, and pseudoxanthoma elasticum is a model for accelerated aging[24].

IMPLICATIONS FOR THE PREGNANT PATIENT

Pseudoxanthoma elasticum

- The main complication during pregnancy is gastrointestinal (particularly gastric) bleeding with massive hematemesis[25,26].

- Hypertension should be treated aggressively in view of the risks related to cerebral and cardiovascular disease[27].

- Careful control of blood pressure may help to reduce the risk of hemorrhage.

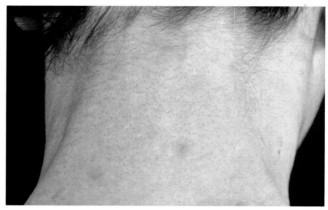

Fig 9.11 Pseudoxanthoma elasticum. The skin is loose and thickened, like that of a plucked chicken. This is a rather subtle clinical change. The sides of the neck are characteristic sites.

REFERENCES

1 Nelson, J.L. and Ostensen, M. Pregnancy and rheumatoid arthritis. *Rheum. Dis. Clin. North Am.* 1997; **23**: 195–212.

2 Barrett, J.H., Brennan, P., Fiddler, M. and Silman, A. Does rheumatoid arthritis remit during pregnancy and relapse postpartum? Results from a nationwide study in the United Kingdom performed prospectively from late pregnancy. *Arthritis Rheum.* 1999; **42**: 1219–1227.

3 Ostenson, M. and Ramsey-Golman, R. Treatment of inflammatory rheumatic disorders in pregnancy. *Drug Safety* 1998; **19**: 389–410.

4 Khamashta, M.A. and Hughes, G.R.V. Pregnancy in systemic lupus erythematosus. *Curr. Opin. Rheumatol.* 1997; **8**: 424–429.

5 Khamashta, M.A., Ruiz-Irastoza, G. and Hughes, G.R.V. Systemic lupus erythematosus flares during pregnancy. *Rheum. Dis. Clin. North Am.* 1997; **23**: 15–30.

6 Lima, F., Buchanan, N.M.M., Khamastha, M.A., Kerslake, S. and Hughes, G.R.V. Obstetric outcome in systemic lupus erythematosus. *Semin. Arthritis Rheum.* 1995; **25**: 184–192.

7 McCune, A.B., Weston, W.L. and Lee L.A. Maternal and fetal outcome in neonatal lupus erythematosus. *Ann. Intern. Med.* 1987; **106**: 518–523.

8 Waltuck, J. and Buyon, J.P. Autoantibody-associated congenital heart block: outcome in mothers and children. *Ann. Intern. Med.* 1994; **120**: 544–551.

9 Wilson, W.A., Gharavi, A.E., Koike, T. *et al.* International consensus statement on preliminary classification criteria for definite antiphospholipid syndrome: report of an international workshop. *Arthritis Rheum.* 1999; **42**: 1309–1311.

10 Langford, K. and Nelson-Piercy, C. Antiphospholipid syndrome in pregnancy. *Contemp. Rev. Obstet. Gynaecol.* 1999; **June:** 93–98.

11 Khamashta, M.A., Cuadrado, M.J., Mujic, F., Taub N.A., Hunt, B.J. and Hughes G.R. The management of thrombosis in the antiphospholipid-antibody syndrome. *N. Engl. J. Med.* 1995; **332**: 993–997.

12 Artlett, C.M., Smith, B. and Jimenez, S.A. Identification of fetal DNA and cells in skin lesions from women with systemic sclerosis. *N. Engl. J. Med.* 1998; **338**: 1186–1191.

13 Black, C.M. Systemic sclerosis and pregnancy. *Baillieres Clin. Rheumatol.* 1990; **4**: 105–124.

14 Steen, V.D. Pregnancy in systemic sclerosis. *Scand. J. Rheumatol.* 1998; **27**(Suppl 107): 72–75.

15 Steen, V.D. Scleroderma and pregnancy. *Rheum. Dis. Clin. North Am.* 1997; **23**: 133–147.

16 Scully, R.E., Mark, E.J., McNeely, W.F. and Ebeling, S.H. Case records of Massachusetts General Hospital. *N. Engl. J. Med.* 1999; **340**: 455–464.

17 Gutierrez, G., Dagnino, R. and Mintz, G. Polymyositis/dermatomyositis and pregnancy. *Arthritis Rheum.* 1984; **27**: 291–294.

18 Ishii, N., Ono, H., Kawaguchi, T. *et al.* Dermatomyositis and pregnancy. Case report and review of the literature. *Dermatologica* 1991; **183**: 146–149.

19 Ohno, T., Imai, A. and Tamaya, T. Successful outcomes of pregnancy complicated with dermatomyositis. Case reports. *Gynecol. Obstet. Invest.* 1992; **33**: 187–189.

20 Winton, G.B. Skin diseases aggravated by pregnancy. *J. Am. Acad. Dermatol.* 1989; **20**: 1–13.

21 Rudd, N.L., Nimrod, C., Holbrook, K.A. *et al.* Pregnancy complications in type IV Ehlers–Danlos syndrome. *Lancet* 1983; **i**: 50–53.

22 Lurie, S., Manor, M. and Hagay, Z.J. The threat of type IV Ehlers–Danlos syndrome on maternal well-being during pregnancy: early delivery may make the difference. *J. Obstet. Gynaecol.* 1988; **18**: 245–248.

23 Georgy, M.S., Anwar, K., Oates, S.E. and Redford, D.H.A. Perineal delivery in Ehlers–Danlos syndrome. *Br. J. Obstet. Gynaecol.* 1997; **104**: 505–506.

24 Yoles, A., Phelps, R. and Lebwohl M. Pseudoxanthoma elasticum and pregnancy. *Cutis* 1996; **58**: 161–164.

25 Berde, C., Willis, D.C. and Sandberg, E.C. Pregnancy in women with pseudoxanthoma elasticum. *Obstet. Gynecol. Surv.* 1983; **38**: 339–344.

26 Lao, T.T., Walters, B.N.J. and de Swiet, M. Pseudoxanthoma elasticum and pregnancy: two case reports. *Br. J. Obstet. Gynaecol.* 1984; **91**: 1049–1050.

27 Viljoen, D.L., Beatty, S. and Beighton, P. The obstetric and gynaecological implications of pseudoxanthoma elasticum. *Br. J. Obstet. Gynaecol.* 1987; **94**: 884–888.

ACKNOWLEDGEMENT

Figure **9.4** has been reproduced by kind permission of Dr D. J. Atherton, The Hospital for Sick Children, London, UK.

10

Eczema and Pregnancy

Samantha Vaughan Jones

INTRODUCTION

Atopic eczema is a chronic, relapsing, pruritic dermatitis, affecting 1–5% of the general population. The prevalence of this condition appears to be increasing, possibly because of environmental changes.[1-3] About 75–80% of patients with atopic eczema have a personal or family history of allergic disease. *Acute eczema* results in intensely pruritic, erythematous papules and vesicles, or extensive weeping areas covered with serous exudate. *Subacute eczema* is more organized and is most often associated with excoriated, scaling, and erythematous papules or plaques, grouped or scattered over erythematous skin. *Chronic eczema* is characterized by thickened, lichenified skin (10.1).

MANAGEMENT

A patient with eczema should try to avoid local heat and contact with irritants such as soap and detergents.

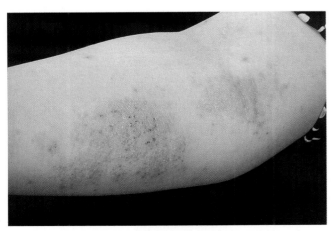

Fig 10.1 Eczema. Lichenified skin with excoriations in antecubital fossa and forearm in chronic atopic eczema.

The mainstay of treatment is keeping the skin moisturized with frequent use of topical emollients and bath oils. Topical emollients should also be applied during the day, between steroid applications. It is important to find an emollient that suits the individual patient. There are many available, ranging from white soft paraffin (petrolatum), which is very greasy, to aqueous cream, which is not greasy. Patients should also soak for 10–15 minutes daily in a lukewarm bath, and emulsifying ointment or aqueous cream should be used as a soap substitute. Emollient cream or ointment should be applied to the skin while still damp from the bath.

PREGNANCY

Several previous studies have shown an exacerbation of eczema during pregnancy. Kemmett and Tidman[4] noted that 50 of 150 atopic women reported a premenstrual exacerbation of the symptoms of atopic dermatitis. Similarly in 50 women with previous pregnancies, pregnancy had had an adverse effect in 52% of cases, usually in the first and second trimesters, although 24% of women had noticed an improvement during pregnancy[4]. The authors postulated that increased serum progesterone levels and other female sex hormones may influence skin sensitivity.

In a recent prospective study of 200 women with rashes in pregnancy, eczema was found to be the commonest pregnancy dermatosis[5]. Using the criteria recently modified by a UK Working Party for use in epidemiological studies[6], eczema accounted for 36% of the total number of cases[5]. Serum immunoglobulin (Ig) E levels were raised in only 18% of these, but the effect of pregnancy on serum IgE levels in normal pregnancy is not known (**Table 10.1**).

In the cases described, flares of dermatitis varied throughout all three trimesters. The clinical presentation was also variable and in 12% of cases there was a clear history of atopic eczema before the pregnancy, with an exacerbation during pregnancy. Three of these

Table 10.1 Eczema in Pregnancy.

Characteristics of Eczema	Proportion of Patients
Clinical features	36% of total cases
Classical eczematous lesions on trunk	
Flexural eczema on limbs	
Palmoplantar involvement in some cases	
Truncal follicular or discoid lesions	
Servere facial dermatitis (one case)	
Raised serum IgE level	18%
Past personal history of atopy	27%
Family history of atopy	50%
No antenatal history of atopy	23%
Fetal sex	Female 50%
	Male 50%
Infantile eczema in offspring	19%
Breastfed infants	13%

Source: Vaughan Jones et al.[5].

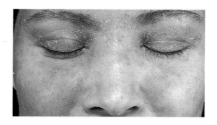

Fig 10.2 Florid facial eczema in a pregnant woman with no previous history of atopy. There is fine scaling, inflammation, and periorbital edema.

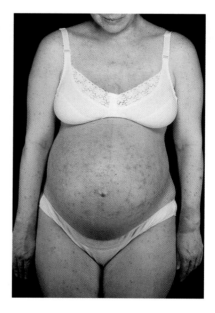

Fig 10.3 Same patient as 10.2 with widespread inflamed papules on the trunk and limbs. A patch of excoriated eczema on the left wrist at the watch strap site suggests underlying nickel allergy.

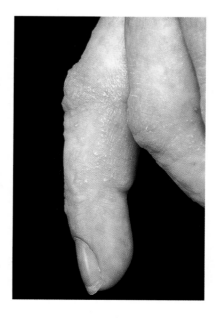

Fig 10.4 Pompholyx eczema affecting the fingers during pregnancy.

patients were multiparous and had developed a similar exacerbation in previous pregnancies. In a further 15% of cases there was a clear history of infantile atopic eczema.

Of the remaining patients, 50% gave a positive personal history of atopy or a family history of asthma, eczema, or hay fever in a first-degree relative. The other 23% of patients gave no such history and had therefore developed an eczematous eruption for the first time during the current pregnancy. Most patients presented with eczema on the limbs (10.1); in four patients the eruption began on the face, one of whom had a florid facial dermatitis (10.2) also spreading on to the abdomen and limbs (10.3). Other patients had palmoplantar pompholyx eczema (10.4), with secondary fissuring and excoriation, or truncal follicular and discoid lesions.

Four women flared in the immediate postpartum period, in three of whom there had been a history of eczema immediately before the onset of pregnancy. Subsequent follow-up found that 19% of the infants from these pregnancies had developed atopic eczema in the first 18 months of life, despite the fact that 13% had been breastfed for a variable period of time. Of the mothers affected by eczema during pregnancy, two women with severe atopic eczema developed a severe postpartum flare which settled within a few weeks, and six continued to have persistent pruritus and a rash consistent with eczema.

The influence of breastfeeding on atopic eczema is debated, and Kay et al.[7] showed that it had no influence on the development of atopic eczema. However, Chandra et al.[8] showed a significantly lower prevalence of eczema at 18 months of age in breastfed infants compared with nonbreastfed infants. It has been suggested that several other factors are important in determining an infant's relative risk of atopic eczema, including maternal diet, smoking, paternal or maternal atopy, and fetal sex. The first of these is maternal diet and some would recommend a reduction in dairy product consumption in the third trimester of pregnancy and during breastfeeding. However, a recent prospective study demonstrated no significant preventive effect of maternal diet[9]. Maternal smoking is now thought to be implicated in the development of atopic eczema during pregnancy and lactation, and should be avoided[10]. The prevalence of infant atopic eczema is the same regardless of whether the disease is inherited from father or mother[11]. One interesting finding in mothers with atopic asthma is that their symptoms appear to be worse when pregnant with a female fetus than with a male fetus, although this study has not been repeated with atopic eczema[12]. The key points of eczema in pregnancy are summarized in **Table 10.2**.

There are several reasons why eczema may appear to be more prevalent or to flare during pregnancy. Changes in the immune system during pregnancy appear to influence cytokine production, and the placenta is known to generate interleukin (IL) 4, a helper T cell type 2 (Th2) cytokine response to prevent fetal rejection[13]. IL-4 is known to be central to the induction of B lymphocyte synthesis of IgE, which might be relevant to atopic disease in pregnancy.[14] Howarth[13] postulated that the persistence of this placental Th2 drive may be a major factor in the increasing prevalence of allergic disease over the past 30–40 years.

Table 10.2 Eczema of Pregnancy: Key Points.

Clinical features identical to eczema in nonpregnant individuals

Personal or family history of atopy frequently present

Serum levels of IgE not necessarily raised in all cases

No adverse fetal outcome

Infant sex ratio equal

In cases of suspected contact dermatitis, delay patch testing until breastfeeding has stopped

---

TREATMENT IN PREGNANCY

The pregnant patient with atopic eczema should use only the weakest possible topical corticosteroid for routine maintenance, but in acute exacerbations high-potency class 1 or 2 corticosteroids may be applied for a few days, with a slow return to a low-potency steroid. Ointments rather than creams should be used to prevent loss of water from the skin. The adverse effects of topical corticosteroids include skin atrophy, depigmentation, acneiform papules, and, rarely, systemic effects. Tar-containing preparations, such as crude coal tar, are useful in treating eczema and are safe to use in pregnancy.

Occasionally, systemic corticosteroids, such as prednisone (prednisolone), are required for a short period in acute eczema. Prednisone, 30 mg daily, may be required initially, with the dose tapered over 1 week. Although fetal cleft palate has been reported in animal studies, prednisone is safe to use in pregnancy. A recent study by Nelson-Piercy and de Swiet[15] described the usefulness of corticosteroids in treating hyperemesis gravidarum. However, fetal or neonatal adrenal suppression may occur with continuous therapy with a prednisone dosage greater than 103 mg daily. Small amounts of corticosteroids also pass into the breast milk, although low doses of prednisone (e.g. 5 mg daily) are unlikely to have an adverse effect on the infant. The patient should be closely monitored for side effects, particularly maternal hypertension and gestational diabetes mellitus.

Systemic antibiotics are often necessary because of secondary bacterial infections, especially with *Staphylococcus aureus*. Penicillin and erythromycin are safe to use in pregnancy; penicillinase-resistant penicillins are recommended for skin infections. Topical antibiotics, such as bacitracin or neomycin, are sometimes used, but may cause skin sensitization. Mupirocin seems to be less sensitizing, but is more expensive. Systemic antihistamines, such as hydroxyzine, diphenhydramine, chlorpheniramine, and promethazine, are often required for pruritus, and are also safe when used in pregnancy. However, newer antihistamines, such as terfenadine and cetirizine, should be avoided[16].

Both ultraviolet B (UVB) irradiation and photochemotherapy using psoralens with long-wave ultraviolet irradiation (PUVA) may be useful adjuncts in treating chronic atopic eczema. However, PUVA should not be used as a first-line treatment because of its potential adverse effects on the fetus. Occasionally, immunosuppressive agents, such as azathioprine and cyclosporin A, are required for severe eczema. These drugs should be used only with great caution during pregnancy. There is a tendency for atopic dermatitis to improve in pregnancy, although in some patients it may be exacerbated.[4]

NIPPLE ECZEMA

Breastfeeding can sometimes be a problem because of nipple eczema (10.5). Painful fissures may develop and become secondarily infected with bacteria, particularly *S. aureus*. Anatomic features, such as relatively flat nipples, contribute to the development of this problem. Nipple eczema is treated with frequent application of moisturizers and a topical corticosteroid of mild potency, such as hydrocortisone. A topical corticosteroid combined with a topical antibiotic is useful for eczema that has become infected by bacteria. A systemic antibiotic, such as erythromycin, may then be required.

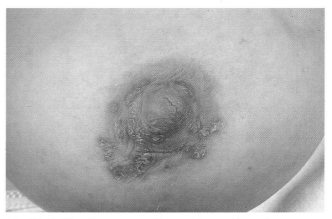

Fig 10.5 Nipple eczema. Dry, scaly, erythematous areas on the nipple, with painful fissures.

HAND ECZEMA

Hand eczema may be exacerbated during the puerperium because of the constant exposure to irritants used in providing care for young children (10.6). Once the skin barrier has been broken, only minor re-exposure to the irritant is needed to keep the eczema active. Treatment is prophylactic and aimed at protecting the hands from all skin irritants by using rubber gloves.

Topical corticosteroids of moderate potency (class 4 or 5), such as betamethasone valerate 0.1% cream, are needed, and emollients should be applied frequently. Hand eczema may appear for the first time in women not previously affected; atopic patients are particularly susceptible. Contact dermatitis should be suspected in patients who fail to improve with standard treatment, but patch testing should be delayed until breastfeeding has stopped.

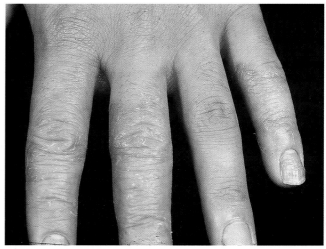

Fig 10.6 Hand eczema. Erythematous scaly areas on the dorsal and lateral aspects of the fingers. Painful fissures develop which may become secondarily infected with bacteria. There is horizontal ridging of involved nails.

IMPLICATIONS FOR THE PREGNANT PATIENT

- Eczema is common in pregnancy, particularly if a positive personal or family history of atopy is present.
- Maternal smoking during pregnancy and lactation increases the risk for atopic eczema in the offspring and should therefore be avoided[8].
- Nipple and hand eczema are both common postpartum.
- Breastfeeding reduces the risk of infant atopy[10].
- Topical ointments are preferable to creams.
- Emollients and bath additives are helpful in management and in the reduction of pruritus.

REFERENCES

1 Williams, H. C. Is the prevalence of atopic dermatitis increasing? *Clin. Exp. Dermatol.* 1992; **17**: 385–391.

2 Charman, C. Atopic eczema. *B.M.J.* 1999; **318**: 1600–1604.

3 Butland, B. K., Strachan, D. P., Lewis, S., *et al.* Investigation into the increase in hay fever and eczema at age 16 observed between 1958 and 1970 British birth cohorts. *B.M.J.* 1997; **315**: 717–721.

4 Kemmett, D., and Tidman, M. J. The influence of the menstrual cycle and pregnancy on atopic dermatitis. *Br. J. Dermatol.* 1991; **125**: 59–61.

5 Vaughan Jones, S. A., Hern, S., Nelson-Piercy, C., *et al.* A prospective study of 200 women with dermatoses of pregnancy correlating the clinical findings with hormonal and immunopathological profiles. *Br. J. Dermatol.* 1999; **141**: 71–81.

6 Williams H. C., Burney P. G. J., Hay R. J., *et al.* The UK Working Party's diagnostic criteria for atopic dermatitis. I. Derivation of a minimum set of discriminators for atopic dermatitis. *Br. J. Dermatol.* 1994; **131**: 102–105.

7 Kay J., Gawkrodger D. J., Mortimer M. J., *et al.* The prevalence of childhood atopic eczema in a general population. *J. Am. Acad. Dermatol.* 1994; **30**: 35–39.

8 Chandra, R. K., Shakuntla, P., and Hamed, A. Influence of maternal diet during lactation and use of formula feeds on development of atopic eczema in high risk infants. *B.M.J.* 1989; **299**: 228–230.

9 Herrmann, M. E., Dannermann, A., Gruters, A., *et al.* Prospective study on the atopy preventive effect of maternal avoidance of milk and eggs during pregnancy and lactation. *Eur. J. Pediatr.* 1996; **155**: 770–774.

10 Schafer T. Dirschedl P, Kunz B., *et al.* Maternal smoking during pregnancy and lactation increases the risk for atopic eczema in the offspring. *J. Am. Acad. Dermatol.* 1997; **36**: 550–556.

11 Uehara, M., Sugiura, H., and Omoto, M. Paternal and maternal atopic dermatitis have the same influence on development of the disease in children. *Acta Derm. Venereol. (Stockh.)* 1999; **79**: 235.

12 Beecroft, N., Cochrane, G. M., and Milburn, H. J. Effect of sex of fetus on asthma during pregnancy: blind prospective study. *B.M.J.* 1998; **317**: 856–857.

13 Howarth, P. H. ABC of allergies. Pathogenic mechanisms: a rational basis for treatment. *B.M.J.* 1998; **316**: 758–761.

14 Coleman, R., Trembath, R. C., and Harper, J. I. Genetic studies of atopy and atopic dermatitis. *Br. J. Dermatol.* 1997; **136**: 1–5.

15 Nelson-Piercy, C., and de Swiet, M. Corticosteroids for the treatment of hyperemesis gravidarum. *Br. J. Obstet. Gynaecol.* 1994; **101**: 1013–1015.

16 Jurecka, W., and Gebhart: W. Drug prescribing during pregnancy. *Semin. Dermatol.* 1989; **8**: 30–39.

ACKNOWLEDGEMENT

Figure **10.6** has been reproduced by kind permission of Dr I. R. White, St John's Institute of Dermatology, St Thomas' Hospital, London, UK.

11 Infectious Diseases in Pregnancy

Eithne MacMahon,
Annemiek de Ruiter,
Diana Lockwood

This chapter focuses on those acute and chronic infections that may have adverse consequences for the fetus or neonate, or warrant special attention and/or management during the course of pregnancy. The viral exanthems will be considered first, followed by notes on the dermatological manifestations of HIV. The viral vulvar infections (herpes simplex virus and human papilloma virus) are considered next and leprosy is discussed in the concluding section.

VIRAL EXANTHEMS AND PREGNANCY

INTRODUCTION

The viral exanthems, which cause mild disease in childhood, may be asymptomatic or give rise to severe disease in the expectant mother. Dermatologic manifestations generally take the form of a vesicular or maculopapular type rash (**Table 11.1**). Primary maternal infection during pregnancy may have potentially serious consequences for the fetus or newborn (**Table 11.2**). The fetus may be infected *in utero*, giving rise to congenital infection, or acquire infection perinatally, with presentation in the neonatal period. The major risk period for exposure of the fetus or neonate depends on the viral etiology and the timing of maternal infection[1]. **Table 11.2** summarizes measures to minimize maternal and fetal sequelae following exposure or infection. Practical points noted below supplement the tabular information.

VARICELLA-ZOSTER VIRUS (VZV)

Primary infection with varicella-zoster virus (VZV) causes chickenpox (varicella) (**11.1**) and induces VZV-specific immunoglobulin (Ig) G, which persists for life[2]. Reactivation, typically occurring decades later, results in shingles (zoster). In temperate climes, where approximately 90% adults are VZV-seropositive, varicella is uncommon during pregnancy and may be further reduced by VZV vaccination policies. In contrast, primary infection is delayed in subtropical and tropical climates, where about 50% of women may be susceptible[2]. Primary VZV infection may be severe in adults, and associated with greater morbidity and mortality during pregnancy[1] (**Table 11.1**). Although aciclovir (acyclovir) is not licensed for use in pregnancy, it has been used extensively without adverse effects and should be considered in confirmed cases[2] (**Table 11.2**).

In contrast to primary infection with VZV, there is no evidence that shingles/zoster in pregnancy presents any risk to the fetus or neonate[3]. The possibility of underlying human immunodeficiency virus (HIV) infection should, however, be considered in prospective mothers who suffer a recurrent attack, or cutaneous or visceral dissemination of shingles.

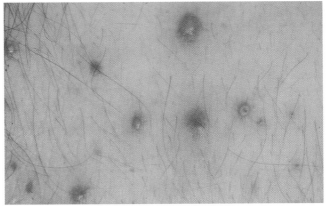

Fig 11.1 Varicella (chickenpox). Multiple, discrete, vesiculopustular, and maculopapular lesions on day 5 of rash.

Table 11.1 Viral Exanthems in Pregnancy – 1 Maternal Infection.

Primary Viral Infection	Incubation Period to Rash	Clinical Features in Mother	Dermatological Manifestations	Laboratory Diagnosis in Mother
Varicella-zoster virus	7–23 days[2]	Varicella Increased risk of complications including pneumonitis[2] Increased mortality rate in pregnancy?	Vesicular rash[2] Lesions progress rapidly (maculopapular → vesicles → pustules → crusting) Itchy Centripetal distribution Scalp lesions Oral ulceration	Lesion scrapings[2]: electron microscopy Tzanck smear antigen detection culture polymerase chain reaction (PCR)
Rubella	13–20 days[5]	Fever Rash Lymphadenopathy Arthropathy (finger joints, wrists, knees, ankles) Up to 25% of cases asymptomatic	Maculopapular rash[5]: pinpoint → confluent exanthem	Specific IgM[5]
Parvovirus B19 Fifth disease Erythema infectiosum Slapped cheek syndrome	18 days[6] (8d to non-specific symptoms)	Rash Acute symmetric arthropathy: finger joints (metacarpophalangeal, proximal interphalangeal joints), wrists, ankles, knees, elbows, axial spine, hips Aplastic crisis in patients with hemoglobinopathy Up to 50% asymptomatic	Maculopapular rash[6]: discrete → confluent → central clearing → 'lacy'/reticular pattern	Specific IgM[6]
Enterovirus infection	2–40 days[10]	Majority asymptomatic[10]	Maculopapular or vesicular[10]	Stool[10]: culture PCR

Table 11.2 Viral Exanthems in Pregnancy – 2 Consequences for the Fetus/Neonate.

Primary Viral Infection	Stages of Pregnancy at which Maternal Infection may Harm Fetus or Neonate	Manifestations in Fetus or Neonate	Specific Prevention or Management
Varicella-zoster virus	0–20 weeks	Congenital varicella (1–2%)[3] Manifestations ranging from skin scarring or limb hypoplasia to severe multisystem involvement	VZIG administration to seronegative mother within 72 hours postexposure may prevent or ameliorate maternal infection[3] Treat confirmed maternal varicella early with aciclovir[a] p.o. or i.v. for pneumonitis or other complications[2]
	13–40 weeks	Shingles in infancy (1–2%)[3]	
	-7 to +7 days from delivery	Neonatal varicella	VZIG prophylaxis to neonate if mother develops varicella rash within the period of 7 days before to 7 days after delivery, or infant of seronegative mother has maternal or other VZV contact before 28 days[4] Treat neonatal varicella with i.v. aciclovir
Rubella	0–8 weeks	Spontaneous abortion (<20%)[5]	HNIG may be offered to seronegative pregnant contacts of rubella for whom termination is unacceptable
	0–12 weeks	Congenital rubella syndrome (85%)[5]: sensorineural deafness congenital heart defects retinopathy, cataract microphthalmia microcephaly psychomotor retardation	Therapeutic abortion[5]
	13–16 weeks	Congenital rubella[5]: sensorineural deafness retinopathy	
Parvovirus B19 (Fifth disease Erythema infectiosum Slapped cheek syndrome)	0–20 weeks	Mid-trimester abortion 4–6 weeks later (incidence increased by 9%)[8]	
	9–20 weeks	Hydrops fetalis after 2–12 weeks (3%)[8] Congenital red cell aplasia?[3]	Monitor for hydrops fetalis and consider intrauterine transfusion[9]
Enterovirus infection	Perinatal period	Neonatal infection; variable severity Asymptomatic → fulminant multisystem disease[10,11]: meningoencephalitis myocarditis pneumonitis hepatitis pancreatitis disseminated intravascular coagulation	Consider HNIG administration to neonates born within 5 days of maternal infection (efficacy unproven)[11] Infection control measures to prevent nosocomial spread from index case[10]

[a]Unlicensed in pregnancy. HNIG, human normal immunoglobulin; VZIG, varicella zoster immune globulin.

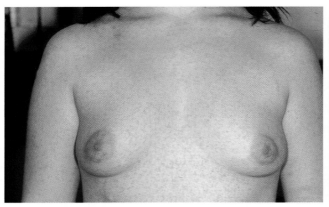

Fig 11.2 Rubella. Discrete and confluent erythematous maculopapular lesions are present.

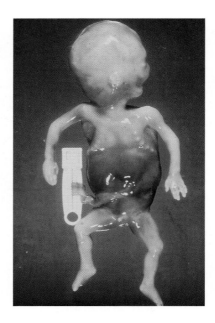

Fig 11.3 Parvovirus B19 infection. Hydropic fetus following primary infection during pregnancy.

MACULOPAPULAR RASHES

Rubella (11.2), parvovirus B19, and enterovirus infections may all present with red rashes, which in practice are clinically indistinguishable[5,6,10]. Neither a past history nor a current clinical diagnosis is reliable, and laboratory confirmation is required during pregnancy[1]. The arthropathy associated with both rubella and parvovirus B19 may persist for some weeks[5,6]. The possibility of HIV seroconversion should always be considered in the differential diagnosis of maculopapular rashes.

RUBELLA

Rubella (Table 11.1) is currently a rare disease in women in many countries as a result of successful vaccination programmes[5]. Congenital rubella syndrome (Table 11.2) continues to be a problem in developing countries, however, partly as a result of unsatisfactory vaccination strategies[7]. Where therapeutic abortion is considered following rubella in the first trimester, the diagnosis should be confirmed by testing a second blood sample for specific IgM and/or a rise in specific IgG. Congenital rubella is diagnosed by the detection of rubella-specific IgM in cord or infant blood[5].

Rubella reinfection has been described in seropositive individuals[5]. Reinfection in the first 16 weeks of pregnancy carries an 8% or lower risk of fetal infection, but fetal malformations are rare[5].

PARVOVIRUS B19

Primary parvovirus B19 infection is most common between 4 and 10 years of age. Whereas seropositivity is almost universal among adults in developing countries, about 40% of women in the developed world remain susceptible[6]. Parvovirus B19 infects red cells via the erythrocyte P antigen, classically causing a biphasic illness, the period of infectivity coinciding with the first phase of fever, mild anemia, and nonspecific symptoms[6]. In the second phase, coinciding with specific IgG and IgM production, rash and arthropathy are the main features (Table 11.1). One or other phase, or both phases, may be subclinical. Joint involvement occurs in 80% of women with rash, and arthropathy may be the sole feature. The rash may wax and wane for some weeks after onset[6]. Primary infection during pregnancy is associated with an excess fetal loss of 9% and with nonimmune *hydrops fetalis* (fetal anemia in the absence of hemolysis) in 3% of fetuses 2–12 weeks following maternal illness[8] (11.3). Intrauterine transfusion has been used to treat fetal hydrops[9] (Table 11.2).

ENTEROVIRUSES

Enteroviral infections occur frequently in healthy adults, usually without symptoms. Symptomatic infection may be associated with rubelliform or vesicular rashes[10] (Table 11.1). Some 1–2% of pregnant women may be excreting enteroviruses at term, with a high risk of transmission[10]. Neonatal infection presents at 3–7 days of age as an illness of wide-ranging severity. Coxsackie B viruses and echoviruses types 6, 7 and 11 have been associated with severe or fatal neonatal infection[10, 11] (Table 11.2).

HUMAN IMMUNODEFICIENCY VIRUS

HIV infection is frequently associated with dermatologic manifestations. These are not usually altered by pregnancy. The ability to recognize them, however, is crucial. Knowledge of a pregnant woman's HIV status allows her to take up recognized interventions to reduce mother-to-child transmission of HIV[12,13]. Although antenatal HIV testing should be recommended to all pregnant women, uptake is variable, and the diagnosis may not be made until the woman presents with symptoms and/or a history of associated manifestations.

IMPLICATIONS FOR THE PREGNANT PATIENT

- The use of antiretroviral therapy, elective cesarean section, and the avoidance of breastfeeding reduce the risk of mother to child transmission of HIV-1 from around 35% to less than 2%.

FOLLICULITIS

Several conditions may affect the hair follicle in HIV. Itchy, excoriated, follicular papules and pustules on the face, trunk, and upper arms are typical of eosinophilic folliculitis (11.4), which is almost diagnostic of HIV infection. Treatment includes systemic antibiotics, phototherapy and 13-*cis*-retinoic acid. Other causes of folliculitis include *Staphylococcus aureus* and *Pityrosporum ovale*. Postinflammatory pigmentation may occur in nonwhite skin[14,15].

KAPOSI SARCOMA

Kaposi sarcoma usually affects homosexual men but can affect women, particularly those from endemic areas. Human herpesvirus 8 is the causative agent. Lesions may appear as patients become more immunosuppressed, but can occur early. Cutaneous lesions are usually purple-brown macules, nodules, or plaques (11.5). Oral lesions may be visible, and pulmonary involvement carries a poor prognosis. Histologic examination confirms the diagnosis and differentiates the condition from bacillary angiomatosis, which it may resemble. Treatment includes radiotherapy, local or systemic chemotherapy, and Highly Active Antiretroviral Therapy (HAART)[14].

VARICELLA-ZOSTER VIRUS

HIV should be considered in patients with shingles. It may occur early in the course of HIV infection before

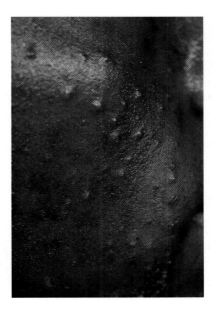

Fig 11.4 Eosinophilic folliculitis affecting the right cheek.

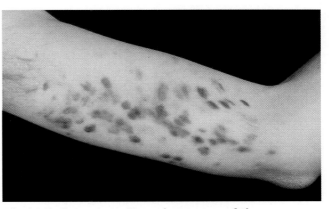

Fig 11.5 Cutaneous Kaposi sarcoma of the upper arm.

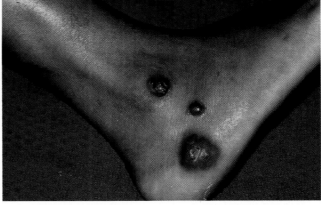

Fig 11.6 Verrucous lesions of varicella-zoster virus.

the onset of other signs or symptoms. Multidermatomal involvement occurs, usually associated with significant immunosuppression. Atypical presentations include verrucous lesions (11.6) and indolent ulcers. Prolonged suppressive aciclovir treatment may be required for persistent or recurrent disease[14].

GENITAL CONDITIONS

Genital warts may be associated with immunosuppression, and HIV should be considered in women with extensive recalcitrant genital warts and multifocal genital intraepithelial neoplasia. Similarly, frequent recurrent herpes simplex virus infection may be a presenting symptom. Lesions may be extensive with advanced immunosuppression[14].

OTHER CONDITIONS

Molluscum contagiosum, seborrheic dermatitis, ichthyosis, scabies, and psoriasis are frequently seen in patients with HIV infection. More rarely, cutaneous cryptococcosis or histoplasmosis occurs.

HERPES SIMPLEX VIRUS

Genital herpes simplex infection in the mother may have severe consequences for the neonate. Although this book is concerned with the presence of dermatologic manifestations, it must be emphasized that maternal genital herpes infection warrants consideration even in the absence of genital lesions, past or present. Furthermore, disseminated neonatal herpes infection and herpes encephalitis may present in the absence of mucocutaneous lesions.

Genital herpes can be caused by either herpes simplex virus type 2 (HSV-2) or type 1 (HSV-1)[16,17]. These closely related herpes viruses are characterized by lifelong persistence in the host following primary infection, the establishment of latency in neuronal ganglia, and intermittent reactivation. HSV-2 is predominantly sexually transmitted, first acquired in adolescence or early adulthood and associated with symptoms 'below the waist'. In contrast, HSV-1 is classically acquired in childhood and is associated with disease 'above the waist', with primary infection manifest as gingivostomatis and clinical reactivation as 'cold sores'. In practice there is considerable crossover, with up to 50% of initial presentations of genital herpes attributable to HSV-1[18].

GENITAL HERPES

EPIDEMIOLOGY

Serological testing, using assays that can discriminate between HSV-1 and HSV-2, has indicated that enumeration of clinical cases grossly underestimates the prevalence of genital herpes infection. Between 1988 and 1994, the seroprevalence of HSV-2 infection in persons aged 12 years or over in the United States was 21.9%, a 30% increase compared with the late 1970s[19]. Yet less than 10% of seropositive individuals reported a history of genital herpes infection[19]. Female sex, black race or Mexican-American ethnic background, older age, less education, poverty, cocaine use and a greater lifetime number of sexual partners were independent predictors of infection. The prevalence of HSV-2 infection in the UK is considerably less, with values ranging from 3% (male blood donors) to 23% (STD clinic patients)[17]. These figures necessarily underestimate the size of the problem as sexually acquired HSV-1 is not considered[18].

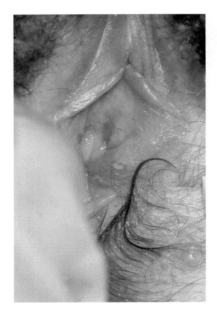

Fig 11.7 Genital herpes. Multiple discrete vulvar ulcers.

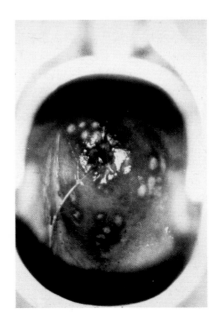

Fig 11.8 Genital herpes. Cervical lesions identified by speculum examination.

CLINICAL FEATURES

Primary genital herpes is defined as genital infection with either HSV-1 or HSV-2 in an individual without previous HSV-1 or HSV-2 infection[17,20]. It may pass unnoticed or present clinically after an incubation period of 2–12 days. *First-episode (initial) genital herpes* is the first recognized attack of genital herpes in an individual previously infected with HSV-1 or HSV-2[17,20]. Primary or first-episode genital herpes presents with multiple painful lesions on the external genitalia, buttocks, cervix, vagina, and/or rectum. The initial blisters soon rupture to form shallow ulcers with erythematous margins (11.7, 11.8). There is often dysuria and even urinary retention.

Symptomatic primary genital infection may be accompanied by constitutional symptoms of fever, malaise, myalgia, and lymphadenopathy. There are large quantities of replicating virus in the genital tract, and viral excretion continues for 3 weeks on average. HSV is not cleared, but persists in a latent state in the local sensory ganglion, reactivating periodically.

Acquisition of genital infection may be asymptomatic, but then present clinically for the first time months or years later. Previous HSV-1 infection does not reduce the rate of HSV-2 infection, but significantly increases the likelihood of asymptomatic seroconversion[18].

Recurrent genital herpes is the second or subsequent episode of clinical disease. Recurrent attacks generally become progressively less frequent and less severe over time. Symptomatic recurrences are fewer and less frequent with genital HSV-1 infection, so that HSV-2 accounts for 95% of recurrent cases[21]. Asymptomatic or unrecognized herpes reactivation is the rule, however, with viral shedding estimated to occur in 1% of HSV-2-seropositive subjects on any given day regardless of any history of genital herpes[22].

DIAGNOSIS AND TREATMENT

Table 11.3 lists the techniques available to detect viruses in patients with suspected herpes infection.

The oral antiviral agents aciclovir, valaciclovir (valacyclovir), and famciclovir (famcyclovir) are effective in reducing the severity and duration of symptoms during attacks and in suppressing clinical recurrences. Aciclovir has also been shown to suppress subclinical shedding and may therefore have a role in preventing transmission[23]. Herpetic skin lesions may be invasive and persistent in individuals with HIV-1 infection, who may ultimately develop resistance to antiviral agents[17]. Genital herpetic infection promotes transmission of HIV infection.

NEONATAL HERPES

Neonatal herpes occurs far less frequently than genital herpes infections in women of childbearing age. In the UK the incidence is 1 in 60 000 live births[17], compared with more than 1 in 5000 in the USA[16]. The variable incidence of neonatal herpes in different countries cannot be explained adequately by differences in the prevalence of HSV-2 infection, or underreporting of neonatal cases[16].

HSV infection in the neonate may result from intrauterine, perinatal, or postnatal transmission of HSV-1 or HSV-2. Postnatal transmission from staff or family members with active herpetic infections accounts for about 10% of cases. Some 85% are acquired perinatally by contact with infected maternal secretions during vaginal delivery. The incubation period of neonatal herpes is 5–21 days. Intrauterine transmission is implicated in the 5% of infants with neonatal herpes presenting on the day of birth following rupture of membranes for less than 24 hours or born by cesarean section initiated before membrane rupture[24,25].

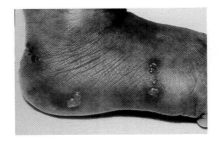

Fig 11.9 Neonatal herpes. Lesions on the foot of an infant with fatal disseminated infection.

Table 11.3 Techniques for Viral Detection in Material from Suspected Herpetic Lesions.

Electron microscopy
Immunofluorescence
Antigen detection
Virus culture
Nucleic acid amplification/detection techniques

Table 11.4 Clinical Presentation of Neonatal Herpes.

Localized to the skin, eye, and/or mouth
Encephalitis with or without skin, eye, and/or mouth involvement
Disseminated infection that involves multiple organs including central nervous system, lung, liver, adrenals, skin, eye, and/or mouth

CLINICAL FEATURES

Infection may be limited to the portals of viral entry (skin, eyes, mouth) or progress to involve the brain and/or other organs[16] (**Table 11.4**). In localized presentation, cutaneous lesions appear at sites of trauma (e.g. the presenting part, scalp electrode sites, etc). Lesions usually appear at 1–2 weeks but are sometimes present at birth[24,25]. Vesicular lesions are usually 1–2 mm in diameter, but may be larger and have an erythematous base with clear or slightly cloudy fluid (**11.9**). More pustular lesions have been confused with bullous impetigo or erythema toxicum. Prompt diagnosis and treatment is required as untreated neonates may develop encephalitis or disseminated infection. Survival is 100% when neonates with localized infection receive intravenous aciclovir therapy. The relative proportions of cases with localized versus disseminated disease may reflect early recognition and treatment of localized infection[26].

Disseminated infection presents during the first week of life with signs and symptoms suggestive of overwhelming bacterial infection, including liver dysfunction, bleeding diathesis, and respiratory distress[16]. The CNS subgroup accounts for about one third of cases[26] presenting in the third week of life with nonspecific symptoms of fever and irritability followed by seizures. Disseminated and CNS infection in the neonate frequently present in the absence of skin lesions. The initial nonspecific symptoms and signs, together with the lack of a maternal history of genital herpes, may contribute to diagnostic delay. Although aciclovir therapy reduces the mortality rate in both disseminated and CNS cases, a large proportion of survivors suffer substantial long-term sequelae[16].

RISKS OF VERTICAL TRANSMISSION

Both symptomatic and asymptomatic viral shedding can result in HSV transmission during vaginal birth. Despite the anxieties of mothers with a history of genital herpes, their risk of perinatal infection is very small. In two prospective studies of 64 such women with recurrent HSV-2 at labor (the majority asymptomatic), there was one case (less than 2%) of neonatal herpes[27,28]. The women at greatest risk of transmitting infection to their babies are those who first acquire genital HSV in pregnancy, most often without their knowledge. Asymptomatic first-episode maternal genital herpes is the source of infection in 60–70% of infected newborns[28]. In a prospective study of 7046 pregnant women seronegative for HSV-1 and/or HSV-2, 94 (1.3%) acquired genital HSV infection during pregnancy. When adjusted for a 40-week gestation, an estimated 2.1% seroconverted during pregnancy. Among the 64 HSV-2 and 30 HSV-1 infections, subclinical cases were of similar frequency: 64% overall[29]. Neonatal herpes infection occurred in four of nine infants born to women who had acquired genital HSV infection shortly before labor. In contrast, among a further 51 pregnancies (including nine earlier third-trimester infections) where the timing of maternal primary infection was known, there were no cases of neonatal or congenital infection[29]. Maternal seroconversion before labor is thought to account for these observations[29,30].

MANAGEMENT OF GENITAL HERPES IN PREGNANCY

DIAGNOSIS AND ANTIVIRAL THERAPY

Owing to the lack of evidence from randomized controlled trials, policies for the management of herpes in pregnancy are often based on the recommendations and opinions of expert committees[20,30]. Pregnant women with symptoms or lesions suggestive of genital herpes should have appropriate samples taken to confirm the diagnosis (**Table 11.3, 11.10**). First-episode genital herpes or recurrent attacks may warrant the use of oral or intravenous antiviral therapy. The oral antiviral agents aciclovir, valaciclovir, and famciclovir are all effective but are not licensed for use in pregnancy.

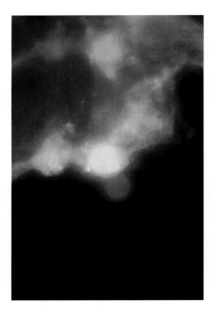

Fig 11.10 Laboratory diagnosis. Immunofluorescent detection of HSV in cellular material scraped from the base of a lesion.

Although as yet inconclusive, the available data suggest that aciclovir (and by inference its more bioavailable prodrug valaciclovir) is likely to be safe in pregnancy. Prospective registration of cases with the Aciclovir in Pregnancy Register since 1984 has so far failed to find any evidence that it is teratogenic[31]. Aciclovir crosses the placenta, concentrates in amniotic fluid and breast milk, and reaches therapeutic levels in the fetus[32]. There are no data to support the use of valaciclovir or famciclovir in pregnancy.

FIRST-EPISODE GENITAL HERPES DURING PREGNANCY

Cesarean section should be considered for all women who develop first-episode genital herpes in the third trimester of pregnancy[30]. This applies particularly to those whose symptoms first appear within 6 weeks of delivery as the risk of viral shedding in labor is very high[29,30]. If vaginal delivery is unavoidable, or the membranes have been ruptured for more than 4 hours before a cesarean section, administration of aciclovir to the mother and baby may be indicated[30]. Vaginal procedures such as application of scalp electrodes, fetal blood sampling, or instrumental delivery should be avoided, as damage to the baby's skin may be the portal of entry for infection[20,30]. Viral swabs from the oropharynx, eyes, and surface sites for HSV detection should be collected from babies born to mothers with first-episode genital herpes to allow early identification of infected babies. Consideration should be given to immediate commencement of intravenous aciclovir treatment pending test results, and the baby monitored closely for early signs of neonatal herpes: lethargy, poor feeding, fever, skin lesions.

First-episode genital herpes in the first and second trimesters presents a lesser risk of perinatal transmission[29] and, providing delivery does not ensue, it has been suggested that the pregnancy may be managed expectantly and vaginal delivery anticipated[30]. Continuous oral aciclovir in the last 4 weeks of pregnancy may prevent recurrence at term and hence the need for delivery by cesarean section[30,33].

HISTORY OF RECURRENT GENITAL HERPES PRIOR TO CURRENT PREGNANCY

Women with recurrent genital herpes can be reassured that the risk of transmission of infection to their babies is very small. Screening tests to detect asymptomatic shedding during late gestation and at term are not recommended[20,30]. Vaginal delivery is recommended in the absence of lesions[20,30] and prodromal symptoms[20] at delivery.

Cesarean delivery has been recommended for women with a history of recurrent infection who have genital lesions or prodromal symptoms at onset of labor[20]. The risk benefit ratio of this approach has been called into question[30], and cessation of this practice has not resulted in any increase in the number of cases[34]. In the absence of randomized controlled trial data to settle this issue, the mode of delivery may best be determined on an individual case basis by clinical assessment and discussion with the prospective mother[30].

In a study of suppressive aciclovir in late pregnancy, there was no significant reduction in the number of cesarean section deliveries but clinical recurrences were significantly reduced, although some asymptomatic shedding was detected in women receiving aciclovir[33]. Following vaginal delivery in the presence of active herpetic lesions, samples may be collected from the neonate to facilitate early identification of herpes simplex exposure, and parents advised to report any early signs of infection.

PREVENTION OF GENITAL HSV ACQUISITION DURING PREGNANCY

Routine antenatal type-specific HSV antibody testing has been advocated as a means of preventing neonatal herpes[35]. In a prospective study of 190 pregnant women, in which samples were also available from their partners, 18 (9.5%) were found to be at risk of contracting primary HSV-2 infection from their HSV-2-positive partners. The risk was unsuspected in over half these women as their partners had no history of genital herpes[36]. One woman seroconverted during pregnancy. The cost:benefit ratio of this approach is currently the subject of considerable debate[35,37].

In the meantime, pregnant women and their partners should be asked whether either has a history of genital herpes. Where a woman has no history but her partner does, the couple should be warned to avoid sexual intercourse at the time of any recurrences. The use of

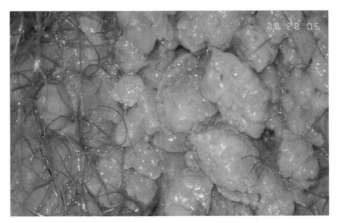

Fig 11.11 Genital warts. Florid condylomata acuminata occupying the perineum.

condoms throughout pregnancy should be advised to minimize the risk of infection[30]. Clear, tactful explanations about genital herpes, the risk of acquisition of infection, and possible consequent adverse outcome of pregnancy should be given.

HUMAN PAPILLOMA VIRUS

Human papilloma virus (HPV) is the cause of genital warts (condylomata acuminata) (**11.11**), and types 16, 18 and other high-risk types are linked etiologically with cervical carcinoma. There is no known association between HPV and any adverse outcome of pregnancy, but perinatal transmission of HPV types 6 and 11 has been implicated in juvenile laryngeal papillomatosis[38]. Given the rarity of this condition and the high prevalence of asymptomatic HPV infection, cesarean section has not been advocated in women with genital warts. While recent evidence suggests that high-risk types are often transmitted vertically, no adverse consequences have yet been observed[39].

Most genital HPV infection is asymptomatic but genital warts are said to grow more rapidly in pregnancy, when they may become florid or hemorrhagic. Rarely, they may cause obstruction sufficient to warrant delivery by cesarean section. A variety of approaches are currently available for the treatment of genital warts. With the exception of imiquimod, an immune response modifier that should not be used in pregnancy, all share tissue destruction as their mode of action. Podophyllin may be teratogenic and is contraindicated throughout pregnancy, but topical therapy with trichloroacetic acid (90%) may be used safely. Other approaches suitable for use in pregnancy include cryotherapy, laser, and other surgical methods. Recurrence of warts after treatment remains a problem. The antiviral agent cidofovir in topical formulation holds promise for the treatment of warts in the future.

PREGNANCY AND LEPROSY

There is a paucity of contemporary data on leprosy and pregnancy; Lockwood and Sinha[40] have recently reviewed all published data on leprosy and pregnancy. Most studies were done in pre-multidrug therapy days, with inappropriate controls, and are difficult to interpret. Pregnancy results in depression of cell-mediated immunity (CMI) by the fetoplacental unit; thus, theoretically, the pregnant patient with leprosy may be at risk of new disease, relapse, and reactions. An Ethiopian study[41] of 120 pregnancies in 154 patients suggested that reactivation of leprosy does occur during pregnancy, whereas a recent Venezuelan[42] study of 54 pregnancies did not find this, and data from large field studies do not show an excess of pregnant women amongst newly diagnosed patients.

REACTIONS

There is a clear temporal association between parturition and the development of type 1 reactions, when CMI returns to pre-pregnancy levels. In the Ethiopian study, 60% of type 1 reactions occurred during the postpartum and lactation phase, with 42% of pregnancies in patients with borderline lepromatous leprosy being complicated by a type 1 reaction[41]. In the same cohort, patients with lepromatous leprosy experienced erythema nodosum leprosum (ENL) reactions throughout pregnancy and lactation[42,43]. ENL in pregnancy is associated with early loss of nerve function, compared with nonpregnant individuals. Neuritis is an important complication of pregnancy and parturition, as significant numbers of women may develop nerve damage associated with pregnancy and lactation. Thus, pregnant and newly delivered women should have regular neurologic examination. Without appropriate treatment, the patient risks developing nerve damage and disability.

MANAGEMENT

Multidrug therapy of rifampin, dapsone, and clofazimine is safe during pregnancy. Clofazimine crosses the placenta, and babies may be born with mild clofazimine pigmentation. Leprosy reactions should be treated with prednisolone, 40–60 mg daily for 2 weeks, followed by a steady reduction in dose. Thalidomide is totally contraindicated in woman planning pregnancy, because it is teratogenic. Whenever possible, before they become pregnant, patients should be told that there is a significant risk that their condition will deteriorate after delivery. Ideally, pregnancies should be planned when leprosy is well controlled.

REFERENCES

1 Remington, J.S. and Klein, J.O. *Infectious Diseases of the Fetus and Newborn Infant*. 5th ed. W.B. Saunders, Philadelphia, 2001.

2 Breuer, J., Harper, D.R. and Kangro, H.O. Varicella Zoster. In: Zuckerman, A.J., Banatvala, J.E. and Pattison, J.R. (eds) *Principles and Practice of Clinical Virology*, 4th edn, pp. 47–77. John Wiley, Chichester, 2000.

3 Enders, G., Miller, E., Cradock-Watson, J., Bolley, I. and Ridehalgh, M. Consequences of varicella and herpes zoster in pregnancy: prospective study of 1739 cases. *Lancet* 1994; **343**: 1548–1551.

4 Miller, E., Cradock-Watson, J.E. and Ridehalgh, M.K.S. Outcome in newborn babies given anti-varicella-zoster immunoglobulin after perinatal maternal infection with varicella-zoster virus. *Lancet* 1989; **ii**: 371–373.

5 Best, J.M. and Banatvala, J.E. Rubella. In: Zuckerman, A.J., Banatvala, J.E. and Pattison, J.R. (eds) *Principles and Practice of Clinical Virology*, 4th edn, pp. 387–418. John Wiley, Chichester, 2000.

6 Pattison, J.R. Human parvoviruses. In: Zuckerman, A.J., Banatvala, J.E. and Pattison, J.R. (eds) *Principles and Practice of Clinical Virology*, 4th edn, pp. 645–658. John Wiley, Chichester, 2000.

7 Banatvala, J.E. Rubella – could do better? *Lancet* 1998; **351**: 849–850.

8 Miller, E., Fairley, C.K., Cohen, B.J. and Seng, C. Immediate and long term outcome of human parvovirus B19 infection in pregnancy. *Br. J. Obstet. Gynaecol.* 1998; **105**: 174–176.

9 Fairley, C.K., Smoleniec, J.S., Caul, O.E. and Miller, E. Observational study of effect of intrauterine transfusions on outcome of fetal hydrops after parvovirus B19 infection. *BMJ* 1995; **346**: 1335–1337.

10 Minor, P.D., Morgan-Capner, P. and Muir, P. Enteroviruses. In: Zuckerman, A.J., Banatvala, J.E. and Pattison, J.R. (eds) *Principles and Practice of Clinical Virology*, 4th edn, pp. 427–450. John Wiley, Chichester, 2000.

11 Modlin, J.F. Echovirus infections of newborn infants. *Pediatr. Infect. Dis. J.* 1988; **7**: 311–312.

12 de Ruiter, A. and Brocklehurst, P. HIV infection and pregnancy. *Int. J. STD AIDS* 1998; **9**: 647–655.

13 European Mode of Delivery Collaboration. Elective caesarean-section versus vaginal delivery in prevention of vertical HIV-1 transmission: a randomised clinical trial. *Lancet* 1999; **353**: 1035–1039.

14 Aftergut, K. and Cockerell, C.J. Update on the cutaneous manifestations of HIV infection. *Dermatol. Clin.* 1999; **17**(3): 445–471.

15 Simpson-Dent, S., Fearfield, L.A. and Staughton, R.C. HIV associated eosinophilic folliculitis – differential diagnosis and management. *Sex. Transm. Infect.* 1999; **75**(5): 291–293.

16 Whitley, R.J. and Arvin, A.M. Herpes simplex virus infections. In: Remington, J.S. and Klein, J.O. (eds) *Infectious Diseases of the Fetus and Newborn Infant*, 4th edn, pp. 354–376. W.B. Saunders, Philadelphia, 1995.

17 Drake, S., Taylor, S., Brown, D. and Pillay, D. Improving the care of patients with genital herpes. *BMJ* 2000; **321**: 619–623.

18 Langenberg, A.G.M., Corey, L., Ashley, R.L. *et al*. A prospective study of new infections with herpes simplex virus type 1 and type 2. *N. Engl. J. Med.* 1999; **341**: 1432–1438.

19 Fleming, D.T., McQuillan, G.M., Johnson, R.E. *et al*. Herpes simplex virus type 2 in the United States, 1976 to 1994. *N. Engl. J. Med.* 1997; **337**: 1105–1111.

20 American College of Obstetricians and Gynecologists. Management of herpes in pregnancy. Clinical management guidelines for obstetrician–gynecologists. *Int. J. Gynaecol. Obstet.* 2000; **68**: 165–173.

21 Benedetti, J., Corey, L. and Ashley, R. Recurrence rates in genital herpes after symptomatic first-episode infection. *Ann. Intern. Med.* 1994; **121**: 847–854.

22 Wald, A., Zeh, J., Selke, S. *et al*. Reactivation of genital herpes simplex virus type 2 infection in asymptomatic seropositive persons. *N. Engl. J. Med.* 2000; **342**: 844–850.

23 Wald, A., Zeh, J., Barnum, G. *et al*. Suppression of subclinical shedding of herpes simplex virus type 2 with acyclovir. *Ann. Intern. Med.* 1996; **124**: 8–15.

24 Stone, K.M., Brooks, C.A., Guinan, M.E. and Alexander, E.R. National surveillance for neonatal herpes simplex virus infections. *Sex. Transm. Dis.* 1989; **16**: 152–156.

25 Koskiniemi, M., Happonen, J.-M., Järvenpää, A.-L. *et al*. Neonatal herpes simplex virus infection: a report of 43 patients. *Pediatr. Infect. Dis. J.* 1989; **8**: 30–35.

26 Whitley, R.J., Corey, L., Arvin, A. *et al*. Changing presentation of herpes simplex virus infection in neonates. *J. Infect. Dis.* 1988; **158**: 109–116.

27 Prober, C.G., Sullender, W.M., Yasukawa, L.L. *et al*. Low risk of herpes simplex virus infections in neonates exposed to the virus at the time of vaginal delivery to mothers with recurrent genital herpes simplex virus infections. *N. Engl. J. Med.* 1987; **316**: 240–244.

28 Brown, Z.A., Benedetti, J., Ashley, R. *et al*. Neonatal herpes simplex virus infection in relation to asymptomatic maternal infection at the time of labor. *N. Engl. J. Med.* 1991; **324**: 1247–1252.

29 Brown, Z.A., Selke, S., Zeh, J. *et al*. The acquisition of herpes simplex virus during pregnancy. *N. Engl. J. Med.* 1997; **337**: 509–515.

30 Smith, J.R., Cowan, F.M. and Munday, P. on behalf of the Pregnancy Subgroup of the Herpes Simplex Advisory Panel. The management of herpes simplex virus infection in pregnancy. *Br. J. Obstet. Gynaecol.* 1998; **105**: 255–260.

31 Centers for Disease Control. Pregnancy outcomes following systemic prenatal acyclovir exposure – June 1, 1984-June 30, 1993. MMWR. *Morb. Mortal. Wkly. Rep.* 1993; **42**: 806–809.

32 Frenkel, L.M., Brown, Z.A., Bryson, Y.J. *et al*. Pharmacokinetics of acyclovir in the term human pregnancy and neonate. *Am. J. Obstet. Gynecol.* 1991; **164**: 569–576.

33 Brocklehurst, P., Kinghorn, G., Carney, O. *et al*. A randomised placebo controlled trial of suppressive acyclovir in late pregnancy in women with recurrent genital herpes infection. *Br. J. Obstet. Gynaecol.* 1998; **105**: 275–280.

34 Van Everdingen, J.J., Peeters, M.F. and ten Have, P. Neonatal herpes policy in The Netherlands. Five years after a consensus conference. *J. Perinat. Med.* 1993; **21**: 371–375.

35 Brown, Z.A. HSV-2 specific serology should be offered routinely to antenatal patients. *Rev. Med. Virol.* 2000; **10**: 141–144.

36 Kulhanjian, J.A., Soroush, V., Au, D.S. *et al*. Identification of women at unsuspected risk of primary infection with herpes simplex virus type 2 during pregnancy. *N. Engl. J. Med.* 1992; **326**: 916–920.

37 Wilkinson, D., Barton, S. and Cowan, F. HSV-2 specific serology should *not* be offered routinely to antenatal patients. *Rev. Med. Virol.* 2000; **10**: 145–153.

38 Arvin, A.M. and Maldonado, Y.A. Other viral infections of the fetus and newborn (human papillomavirus (condyloma acuminatum), Epstein–Barr virus, human herpesvirus 6, influenza A and B, respiratory syncytial virus, lymphocytic choriomeningitis virus, molluscum contagiosum, rabies virus). In: Remington, J.S. and Klein, J.O. (eds) *Infectious Diseases of the Fetus and Newborn Infant*, 4th edn, pp. 745–756. W.B. Saunders, Philadelphia, 1995.

39 Mant, C., Cason, J., Rice, P. and Best, J.M. Non-sexual transmission of cervical cancer-associated papillomaviruses: an update. *Papillomavirus Rep.* 2000; **11**: 1–5.

40 Lockwood, D.N.J. and Sinha, H.H. Pregnancy and leprosy: a comprehensive literature review. *Int. J. Lepr.* 1999; **67**: 6–12.

41 Duncan, M.E. *et al.* The association of pregnancy and leprosy I; new cases, relapse of cured patients and deterioration in patients on treatment during pregnancy and lactation – results of a prospective study of 154 pregnancies in 147 Ethiopian women. *Lepr. Rev.* 1981; **52**: 245.

42 Ulrich, M., Zulueta, A.M., Caceres-Dittmar, G. *et al.* Leprosy in women: characteristics and repercussions. *Soc. Sci. Med.* 1993; **37**(4): 445–456.

43 Duncan, M.E. and Pearson, J.M.H. The association of pregnancy and leprosy III, erythema nodosum leprosum. *Lepr. Rev.* 1984; **55**: 129.

ACKNOWLEDGEMENT

Figure **11.3** has been reproduced from the slide collection of the late Dr James C. Booth, St George's Hospital Medical School, London, UK.

12 Infectious Vulvovaginitis: Candidiasis, Trichomoniasis, and Bacterial Vaginosis

Marilynne McKay

INTRODUCTION

Vulvovaginal symptoms represent one of the most common reasons for a woman to consult her doctor, a genitourinary medicine clinic, or an emergency room. Although a majority of patients may be treated for infection, infectious vaginitis is not always the cause of vaginal discharge or vulvar discomfort. With the exception of candida, most vaginal infections do not involve the vulvar skin. Diagnostic testing should be performed to ensure proper management, as overtreatment with antibiotics can disrupt the normal physiologic and microbiologic vaginal environment. Patients with chronic undiagnosed vulvovaginitis are at risk of psychological and psychosexual problems, and may require specialized counseling. A detailed discussion of vaginal and cervical disorders and sexually transmitted diseases is beyond the scope of this chapter, but the three most common infectious causes of chronic and/or recurrent vulvovaginitis will be discussed, especially as they might present in the context of a vulvar clinic. (*See Appendix C for vaginal examination technique and evaluation of the vaginal smear.*)

NORMAL VAGINAL DISCHARGE

The quantity of vaginal discharge accepted as 'normal' will vary from woman, and complaints occur with changes in volume or the consistency of discharge. During the reproductive years, the fluid is white and fairly thick, diluted during sexual excitement by a transudate of serious fluid from the vaginal wall. Under the microscope, normal vaginal discharge contains a large proportion of superficial squamous cells with small pyknotic nuclei that stain pink with Papanicolaou reagents. Lactobacilli are common, and there may be a variety of other bacteria. In mid-cycle, leucocytes are rare, but increase in number immediately before the start of or after the end of the menstrual cycle.

Vaginal discharge increases shortly after birth in response to high maternal estrogen levels. In the prepubertal and postmenopausal years, the volume of discharge tends to be less, and postmenopausal dryness is often a complaint. The predominant cells seen under the microscope are parabasal and intermediate in type, with proportionately larger nuclei that stain blue with Papanicolaou reagents. Leucocytes may be common, and a variety of microorganisms are seen on staining.

In pregnancy, intermediate 'navicular cells' predominate. Exogenous hormones tend to modify the cellular pattern. For example, unopposed estrogen given after hysterectomy tends to result in mature cells, whereas progesterone-dominated oral contraceptives tend to produce a pattern of intermediate-type cells.

Vaginal acidity (pH) varies with age and hormonal changes. During the reproductive years, the vagina is acid (pH 4.0–4.5) due to the metabolism of glycogen in the cells of the vaginal walls. Before puberty and after the menopause, the pH level is greater than 4.5 (**Table 12.1**)

Table 12.1 Causes of Raised Vaginal pH (> 4.5).
Physiologic
Hypoestrogenism
Menses
Heavy cervical mucus (i.e. ovulation)
Recent intercourse with ejaculation
Pregnancy with rupture of membranes
Infectious
Trichomoniasis
Bacterial vaginosis
Foreign body with secondary infection
Streptococcal vaginitis (group A) (rare)
Desquamative inflammatory vaginitis (rare)

CERVICAL CONDITIONS CAUSING VAGINAL DISCHARGE

Lesions or changes on the uterine cervix may cause a vaginal discharge. As the squamocolumnar junction may be on the vagina rather than the vaginal portion of the cervix, the vagina may be included in these changes. Before reaching any conclusion about the cause and nature of vaginal disease, the uterine cervix must be seen clearly in a good light. The result of a current or recent cervical smear must be available at the time of treatment or soon afterwards. Any suspicious appearance of the cervix should be investigated by colposcopy and biopsy, as cytological examination alone may not detect cervical carcinoma. Blood and necrotic debris may obscure the diagnostic features of malignant change in such slides.

COLUMNAR CELL ECTOPY

Columnar cell ectopy, sometimes misnamed 'cervical erosion', is the presence of visible columnar epithelium on the vaginal portion of the uterine cervix. In its exaggerated form, it extends out onto the upper portion of the vagina, and is then referred to as vaginal adenosis. Use of the bivalve speculum increases the impression of cervical ectopy by forcing open the canal of the parous cervix; if the blades are allowed to close slightly after opening fully, the area of change will decrease to its proper size.

Columnar cell ectopy is a normal feature on the uterine cervix. It is prominent at birth and increases again at the menarche when hormones cause the lips of the cervix to evert. Columnar epithelium subjected to the vaginal environment (especially low acidity) undergoes the process of squamous metaplasia, in which it is replaced by metaplastic squamous epithelium. Such change may be delayed by hormones (especially oral contraception) and by pregnancy.

Columnar epithelium is prone to nonspecific infection, which may cause excessive discharge. Rarely, if this cannot be controlled by local or systemic treatment, the area of ectopy may be destroyed with cryotherapy or diathermy. Healing usually results in the development of squamous epithelium, especially if an acid environment is maintained during healing.

MICROBIOLOGY

The normal vagina contains a high density of a large variety of microorganisms. With very few exceptions, such as *Treponema pallidum*, *Neisseria gonorrhoeae*, *Chlamydia trachomatis*, and possibly *Trichomonas vaginalis*, almost any microorganism may be found in the healthy vagina. Pathogenic organisms such as group B streptococci, *Mycoplasma hominis*, *Ureaplasma urealyticum*, *Gardnerella vaginalis*, and *Candida albicans* are each present in approximately 20% of healthy asymptomatic women, with wide variations depending on the patient population[1]. For this reason, routine bacterial cultures are strongly discouraged because the results may be misleading. Moreover 'normal' vaginal flora must be defined according to the age, estrogenic state, and sexual experience of the woman concerned (**Table 12.2**).

Before puberty the vagina is thinned and hypoestrogenic. Culture shows a variety of organisms, including skin flora (e.g. *Staphylococcus epidermidis* or *Corynebacterium*), fecal flora (e.g. *Escherichia coli* or *Enterococcus* spp.), and vaginal flora (e.g. *Lactobacillus* spp.). With estrogenization at puberty, lactobacilli become the dominant flora and the vaginal pH decreases to less than 4.5. It is now thought that the production of hydrogen peroxide by lactobacilli is extremely important in protecting the vagina from infection[2]. While the presence of lactobacillus-dominant flora is associated with a decreased risk for bacterial vaginosis, it does not seem to decrease the incidence of symptomatic candida vaginitis[3].

Before the menarche, vulvovaginitis is not usually infectious or necessarily related to poor hygiene, specific irritants, or sexual abuse, although any of these can present with genital irritation[4]. Patients with a demonstrable infectious cause tend to have visible discharge and moderate to severe inflammation of the genital area. Diagnostic testing with a swab and smear for Gram staining should be reserved for patients with these symptoms, and a pinworm test should also be considered if there is severe itching. Antibiotics should be used only if the relevant pathogen is identified. Candida is an unlikely pathogen in toilet-trained prepubertal girls. Initial treatment should be simple and symptomatic (gentle bathing with salt water or dilute vinegar baths) and irritants should be avoided. (See also Chapter 16, Pediatric Vulvar Disorders.)

A recent study of postmenopausal women who had never received estrogen replacement therapy (mean age 67 years) showed a significant decrease in the concentration of *Lactobacillus* compared with women of childbearing age (**Table 12.2**)[5]. None of them had bacterial vaginosis. Some of the other organisms that were recovered, including *G. vaginalis* (27% of the women), *U. urealyticum* (13%), *C. albicans* (1%), and *Prevotella bivia* (33%), were isolated less frequently from postmenopausal women than from women of reproductive age, whereas coliforms (41%) were recovered at a higher frequency. The postmenopausal decrease in lactobacilli, yeasts, and bacterial vaginosis-associated bacteria may explain the decrease in the incidence of bacterial vaginosis and yeast vaginitis in this age group.

Table 12.2 Comparison of the Vaginal Microflora of Prepubertal Girls, Women of Child-bearing Age, and Postmenopausal Women.

	Percentage of Women with Indicated Isolate		
Isolate	Prepubertal (*n* = 19)	Pregnant (*n* = 132)	Postmenopausal (*n* = 73)
Mycoplasma hominis	0	23	0
Yeasts	0	26	1
Group B streptococcus	0	16	23
Gardnerella vaginalis	0	58	27
Provotella bivia	11	61	44
Facultative lactobacilli	11	92	49
Ureaplasma urealyticum	20	82	13
Fusobacterium spp	26	12	7
Actinomyces	32	8	15
Enterococci	32	33	38
Coliforms	32	16	41
Coryneforms	42	78	58
Viridans streptococci	42	59	74
Staphylococci	68	86	59
Peptostreptococcus	89	92	88
Anaerobic Gram-negative rods	89	90	89

Pregnant women with bacterial vaginosis were excluded.
Source: Hillier and Lau[5].

SYMPTOMS OF VAGINAL INFECTION

The symptoms of vaginal infection are often associated and/or confused with symptoms related to associated areas. The commonest presenting symptoms are an increase in vaginal discharge, vaginal soreness, and vaginal odor, with or without discharge (**Table 12.3**).

VAGINAL DISCHARGE

Discharge may be due to a vaginal condition, but blood-stained fluid is more likely to relate to the cervix or uterus. The following characteristics should be noted:

- Color – clear, yellow, green, bloodstained, brown, or black
- Quantity – assessed by the need to use sanitary pads or other protection
- Smell – offensive or nonoffensive
- Irritancy – present or not

LOCATION OF SYMPTOMS

Vulva, introitus, or deep vagina.

VAGINAL SORENESS

This may be a symptom by itself or may be related to tampon use or sexual intercourse. Soreness on intercourse (dyspareunia) may be superficial (at the start of penetration) or deep (related to deep penetration only). Deep dyspareunia tends to be related to pelvic conditions other than vaginitis. Dysuria may also be a presenting symptom of vaginitis.

VAGINAL ODOR, WITH OR WITHOUT DISCHARGE

This may be more noticeable or unpleasant during particular times, such as menstruation, and may be further exacerbated by sexual intercourse. The complaint of odor alone does not necessarily imply a problem, as patients may complain of a 'terrible odor' that is indistinguishable to several examiners. Careful questioning

Table 12.3 Differential Diagnosis of Vaginitis.

Diagnosis	Symptoms	Vulvar Signs	Vaginal Signs	pH	Amine Test	Saline Microscopy	10% Potassium Hydroxide	Culture	Treatment of Patient (or Partner)	Complications
Normal	None or mild	–	–	4.0–4.5	Negative	PMN : EC ratio < 1 rods dominate	Negative	–		
Vulvovaginal candidiasis (VVC), yeast, thrush, moniliasis	Itching, soreness, dyspareunia, discharge	Vulvar erythema, edema, fissuring	Erythema, often a thick white discharge	4.0–4.5	Negative	PMN : EC ratio < 1, rods dominate; pseudohyphae (~40%)	Pseudohyphae (~70%)	Culture if microscopy negative (*Candida albicans, C.parapsilosis, C.crusei, C.glabrata*)	Antifungal creams, tablets, suppositories; oral fluconazole or ketoconazole if resistant	Possible HIV transmission
Bacterial vaginosis	Malodorous discharge, no dyspareunia	Minimal	None or white, thin, adherent; fishy odor typical, especially postcoital	> 4.5	Positive (~70–80%)	PMN : EC ratio < 1, loss of rods, clue cells > 90%	Negative	Culture of little value (*Gardnerella, Prevotella bivia, Mycoplasma hominis*)	Metronidazole or clindamycin, topical or oral (none for partner)	Pelvic infections resulting in greater infertility and tubal (ectopic) pregnancy, increased risk of GC and HIV
Trichomoniasis 'Trich'	Malodorous purulent discharge, dyspareunia	Erythema, irritation	Purulent discharge	5.0–6.0	Often positive	PMNs ++++, mixedflora: motile trichomonads (60%)	Negative	Culture if microscopy negative	Single-dose metronidazole for patient (and partner)	
Atrophic vaginitis	Dyspareunia, vaginal dryness	Vestibular thinning, urethral caruncle	Vaginal thinning	> 6.0	Negative	PMN + to ++, loss of rods, parabasal cells, coliforms	Negative		Consider estrogen replacement therapy, topical or systemic	

PMN, polymorphonuclear leucocytes; EC, vaginal epithelial cells; HIV, human immunodeficiency virus; GC, gonococcus.

in these cases often reveals anxiety related to an offhand comment by a partner or friend. Frank discussion and reassurance may be all that is required to resolve the problem.

SPECIFIC CONDITIONS

PHYSIOLOGIC DISCHARGE

The complaint of 'excessive discharge' is not unusual; in most cases, it is not associated with odor, itching, or pain. The patient, usually young, insists that her vaginal secretions have increased significantly beyond what has been 'normal' for her in the past. She may be wearing a sanitary pad or panty shield to prevent 'soaking' of underwear. Examination is completely normal and the discharge, if present, is clear and inoffensive.

A careful history may reveal that the patient has undergone some hormonal change – starting or discontinuing oral contraceptives, for example, or has just delivered her first baby. Some adolescents become alarmed at puberty as they notice an increase in vaginal secretions, particularly at different times of the menstrual cycle. Patients often describe a discharge 'coming down' when they are on the toilet, because they notice secretions on toilet paper.

Cervicitis should be ruled out by examination, but vaginal culture is not required. In most cases, an explanation of the changing viscosity of vaginal secretions during a normal menstrual cycle is all that is necessary, especially for adolescent patients. It is not unusual for secretions to pool at the hymenal ring, where pressure from a tissue may reveal their presence. Amounts of 'normal' secretions may vary before, during, and after menses and pregnancy as well as puberty. Despite reassurance and explanation of normal function, some patients remain fixated on physiologic discharge. Douching is not recommended, as patients tend to overuse this modality; in fact, patients who are already douching regularly may report similar symptoms.

VULVOVAGINAL CANDIDIASIS (VVC, THRUSH, MONILIASIS, CANDIDOSIS)

(See also Chapter 15)

Although only 20–25% of all cases of infectious vaginitis are caused by candida, it is so notorious for producing symptomatic inflammatory vulvitis that candida infection is the presumptive diagnosis in a majority of patients presenting with vulvitis. Patients with culture-positive candida infection typically complain of vulvar and vaginal itching, with or without discharge. If a discharge is present, it is typically yellow-white and has a thick, cheesy consistency. The condition develops most commonly in the week preceding menstruation, and symptoms are worse when the genital area is both warm and confined, for example in bed at night or when wearing tights, denim trousers, or clothes made from synthetic materials. Patients may complain of burning or irritation from vaginal creams due to candida-induced local inflammation of the skin. Dyspareunia and dysuria are common for the same reason. There is usually no complaint of odor.

On clinical examination, the vulva and vestibule are obviously inflamed. Typically there will be redness and edema, often with fissuring and erosions due to scratching. Speculum examination of the vagina shows thick plaques of curdy discharge on the vaginal walls and cervix. The vaginal pH is less than 4.5. Microscopic examination of a wet preparation or a Gram-stained film reveals budding yeast cells, and hyphal forms may be seen. Culture can be performed using selective media, and a specific latex agglutination test is available for the identification of *C. albicans*.

CAUSATIVE ORGANISMS

It has been estimated that *C. albicans* is responsible for 80–94% of episodes of VVC worldwide[6], but recent studies suggest that there may be a shift to non-albicans species, especially *Candida glabrata* (previously known as *Torulopsis glabrata*)[7]. Symptomatic disease has been attributed to *C. tropicalis* and *C. parapsilosis*, as well as other species, and there have also been reports of vaginal infection with *Saccharomyces cerevisiae*, transmitted from yeast used in baking.[8]

PATHOGENESIS

C. albicans is found in the mouth and the intestinal tract of a substantial proportion of the normal population. It should probably also be regarded as a normal inhabitant of the female genital tract, occurring in the vagina in up to 10% of nonpregnant women and up to 30% of pregnant women. It may be argued that the development of the disease process represents a failure of the host's defence mechanisms, although allergy is thought to be an important factor in some cases, and some strains are more virulent than others.

PREDISPOSING FACTORS

Although many factors are claimed to be precipitating factors for VVC, definitive evidence is hard to find. In a recent multivariant analysis of 774 women with vaginal symptoms at an urban genitourinary medicine clinic, risk factors for positive *C. albicans* culture included condom use, presentation after day 14 of the menstrual cycle, sexual intercourse more than four times per month, recent antibiotic use, young age, past gonococcal infection, and absence of current gonorrhea or bacterial vaginosis.[9] Sexual intercourse with the use of a diaphragm or spermicide in the preceding 3 days is associated with a marked increase in the rate of candida colonization, and vaginal sponges and intrauterine devices also increase the risk of VVC. There is an increased risk of VVC with oral contraceptive use[10], especially pills containing a high dosage of estrogen. Probably in response to the changed immune status, VVC appears to be more common in pregnancy, with a reported incidence of up to 30%. Women with diabetes, ongoing antibiotic therapy, and any immunodepressed state are more likely to develop VVC.

TREATMENT

Today the azoles are the first-line options for treatment of VVC: clotrimazole, miconazole, econazole, and isoconazole are all available as single-application treatments. The first three may also be used for longer courses, and topical clotrimazole and micronazole are safe to use in pregnancy. There have been no significant differences in efficacy among topical and systemic azoles, and both offer a greater than 80% chance for cure in uncomplicated cases[11]. Oral medication (ketoconazole, itraconazole, and fluconazole) is best regarded as a second-line treatment for VVC. Ketoconazole may be hepatotoxic, and *C. tropicalis* is resistant to fluconazole; all are expensive. Single-dose fluconazole therapy provides therapeutic concentrations of drug in vaginal secretions and vaginal tissue for at least 72 hours. (Note that vaginal creams containing mineral or vegetable oil may compromise the integrity of condoms.)

Non-albicans candida species such as *C. glabrata* and *S. cerevisiae* are less susceptible to azoles and may require boric acid suppository therapy (600 mg/day intravaginally for 14 days)[12]. Nystatin, a polyene antifungal agent, is normally given as vaginal tablets (pessaries). However, patient compliance is often poor, as nystatin has the disadvantage that it must be used for 14 consecutive nights. It also stains underclothes. In severe pruritus, a mixture of an antifungal agent and a weak hydrocortisone cream is soothing when applied to the vulva.

RECURRENT VULVOVAGINAL CANDIDIASIS (RVVC)

RVVC is defined as four or more episodes of infection over a period of 12 months. Although many patients may carry this diagnosis, culture-positive confirmation of infection is estimated at less than 5% in healthy women[13]. In contrast to subjects with human immunodeficiency virus infection or mucocutaneous candidiasis, women with RVVC do not seem to be susceptible to oropharyngeal candidiasis, which suggests a vaginal site-specific predisposition. Current views regarding pathogenesis of idiopathic RVVC suggest that local vaginal immune mechanisms may be responsible for the frequent relapses[14]. In such cases, it is vital to confirm the diagnosis by microbiologic culture and to exclude other causes of the symptoms and signs. Evidence for an underlying immune deficiency should also be sought if there are predisposing risk factors. The role of sexual transmission in RVVC is debatable. While most authorities would not consider investigating and treating a sexual partner at the first attack, this should be considered if the condition is recurrent[15].

For patients in whom no cause of recurrence can be found, relief may be provided by intermittent prophylactic treatment. Several controlled long-term studies have confirmed the value of maintenance suppressive therapy for 6 months after an initial full treatment course successfully makes the vagina culture-negative for candida[16]. Regimens that have proven effective include ketoconazole (100 mg daily), itraconazole (50–100 mg daily), fluconazole (100 mg weekly), or clotrimazole vaginal suppositories (500 mg) inserted once a week.

TRICHOMONIASIS

Some 15–20% of all cases of infectious vaginitis seen in gynecology clinics are caused by *Trichomonas vaginalis*. It is considered to be a sexually transmitted disease, and organisms can be identified in 30–40% of the male sexual partners of infected women[11]. The incubation period has been estimated to range from 3 to 28 days. Symptoms often appear during or immediately after menstruation.

Clinically, trichomonal infection ranges from an asymptomatic carrier state to severe acute inflammatory disease. A malodorous discharge is reported by 50–75% of women diagnosed with trichomoniasis, and itching occurs in 25–50%. Patients also complain of soreness, dysuria, and dyspareunia, but less than 10% report lower abdominal pain. Vulvar findings are often absent, with severe cases demonstrating only diffuse vulvar erythema and edema, along with a copious discharge. The vaginal pH is greater than 4.5, usually 5.5–6.0. On colposcopic examination, the vaginal walls have a typical punctate appearance, the so-called 'strawberry' vagina. (It should be noted, however, that this description was coined before the recognition of bacterial vaginosis as a clinical entity, and a similar appearance also occurs with this condition. Trichomonal vaginosis and bacterial vaginosis commonly coexist in florid clinical presentations.) 'Pure' trichomonal vaginitis is often a much milder condition.

CAUSATIVE ORGANISM

The causative organism is *T. vaginalis*, a large, single-celled flagellate. It has a very distinctive appearance, especially when moving. The diagnosis can almost always be made microscopically in the clinic on viewing typical mobile organisms of *T. vaginalis* in a film of discharge emulsified in normal saline. There will be numerous polymorphonuclear leucocytes as well. Routine Papanicolaou cytology staining has a sensitivity of only 60–70%, compared with saline preparation microscopy. If symptoms and signs are not present, and the diagnosis has not been confirmed by another method, cytologic diagnoses should be regarded as unproven. Trichomonad organisms can be confirmed by culture in selective media, and rapid diagnostic kits using DNA probes and monoclonal antibodies are now available with high sensitivity and specificity.

TREATMENT

The group of 5-nitroimidazole drugs – metronidazole, tinidazole, and ornidazole – remain the basis for therapy, and all have similar efficacy[17]. Oral therapy is preferred to topical vaginal therapy because of the frequency of infection of the urethra and periurethral glands, where reinfection can arise if inadequately treated. Treatment is with oral metronidazole, 500 mg twice daily for 7 days, with a cure rate of 85–95%. Comparable results (82–88% cure rate) have been obtained with a single oral dose of 2 g metronidazole. This cure rate increases to more than 90% when sexual partners are treated simultaneously. Single-dose therapy is preferred because of better patient compliance, lower total dose, shorter period of alcohol abstinence, and possibly decreased subsequent candidal vaginitis; a disadvantage is the need to insist on simultaneous treatment of sexual partners. Side effects of metronidazole include metallic taste, nausea (10%), transient neutropenia (7.5%), disulfiram-like effect with alcohol ingestion, interaction with warfarin, and peripheral neuropathy. Metronidazole should not be used in pregnancy.

Relative resistance to metronidazole has been reported in a small number of cases, but treatment failure is more likely to be due to poor compliance, malabsorption, or reinfection. In a few cases, the male is a long-term reservoir of infection, which sometimes causes urethritis. Thus, if the woman fails to respond to standard treatment, her partner(s) should be examined and treated. In most such cases, retreatment with a 7-day course at double dosage, or the use of rectal or parenteral preparations of the same drug, should suffice. Topical povidone–iodine may be used as a support measure for treatment with metronidazole, and is available as vaginal pessary, vaginal gel, or vaginal douche.

BACTERIAL VAGINOSIS

Bacterial vaginosis is the most common cause of vaginitis in women of childbearing age, although symptoms of vulvitis are rare in affected patients. It typically affects young, sexually active, women but may also occur in the absence of sexual intercourse. This term is used to describe a syndrome characterized by a malodorous vaginal discharge and raised vaginal pH. A typical complaint is a vaginal discharge that is excessive, stains clothes green or yellow, and has an offensive 'fishy' odor. The odor is particularly noticeable after sexual intercourse, when alkaline semen has been deposited in the vagina. It is often a chronic condition. Irritation, dyspareunia, and dysuria are uncommon symptoms. The clinical appearance of the discharge is variable; clinical inflammation of the vagina and vulva is unusual.

There have now been numerous studies of pregnant women with bacterial vaginosis that report an increased risk of preterm birth, ranging from 2.0 to 6.9%[18]. There is also a likely link between bacterial vaginosis and upper genital tract infection in pregnancy, including chorioamnionitis. As it is estimated that 15–20% of pregnant women have bacterial vaginosis[19], significant numbers of otherwise healthy women are at risk.

The optimal time for screening and treatment has not been defined. Recent randomized treatment trials with oral erythromycin and metronidazole all showed considerable reduction in the incidence of preterm labor associated with bacterial vaginosis, but only in women with a history of past preterm delivery. Bacterial vaginosis has also been associated with pelvic inflammatory disease[20], especially in the absence of *C. trachomatis* and *N. gonorrhoeae*.

CAUSATIVE ORGANISMS

Bacterial vaginosis must be considered a complex change in the normal microbiologic flora of the vagina. There is a reduction in the prevalence and concentration of hydrogen peroxide-producing lactobacilli (Doderlein bacilli) and an increase in *G. vaginalis*, anaerobic Gram-negative rods, *M. hominis*, anaerobic Gram-negative rods of the genera *Prevotella*, *Porphyromonas*, *Bacteroides*, and *Peptostreptococcus* species[21].

The massive overgrowth of vaginal anaerobes is associated with an increased production of proteolytic carboxylase enzymes. These act to break down vaginal peptides to a variety of amines which, in the presence of a high pH, are transformed into volatile malodorous amines. It is not known, however, whether the loss of lactobacilli precedes or follows this upheaval in flora. Most of the microorganisms are traditionally found in low numbers in the healthy vagina.

DIAGNOSIS

The diagnosis of bacterial vaginosis rests on four factors:

1 A vaginal pH greater than 4.5
2 A homogeneous, thin, vaginal discharge
3 A positive amine ('whiff') test. A small amount of discharge is placed on a microscope slide and a drop of 10% potassium chloride is added to it. A fish-like

amine odor is noticed immediately, similar to that produced by the action of the relatively alkaline seminal fluid on the vaginal contents.

4 The presence of 'clue cells' in wet or Gram-stained vaginal preparations. Clue cells are epithelial cells covered in bacteria, usually curved rods. The appearance is very striking, sometimes giving a 'scratched edge' appearance to the cells.

As well as these features, a large number of microorganisms are often seen in the background in wet or Gram-stained smears of vaginal secretion. These are usually curved motile rods of *Mobiluncus* spp. Bacterial culture does not play a part in the diagnosis of bacterial vaginosis, although it may be needed to exclude other pathogens. In particular, the isolation of *G. vaginalis* on bacterial culture is not diagnostic of bacterial vaginosis.

TREATMENT

As no specific microorganism is responsible for the clinical syndrome of bacterial vaginosis, it is not surprising that no treatment is 100% effective.

Metronidazole is the most commonly prescribed antibiotic, with a success rate of over 90% for a 7-day course of 800–1200 mg daily. If this fails, oral ampicillin (or amoxycillin) is the drug of second choice (mean cure rate 66%). Topical therapy with 2% clindamycin once daily for 7 days, or with metronidazole gel 0.75% twice daily for 5 days, has been shown to be as effective as oral metronidazole[22]. After therapy with oral metronidazole, about 30% of those patients initially responding to treatment experience recurrence of symptoms within 3 months[11]. Although reasons for recurrence are unclear, it is thought that this may represent vaginal relapse with failure to eradicate the offending organisms at the same time that the normal protective lactobacillus-dominant vaginal flora fails to re-establish itself.

It is now considered that asymptomatic bacterial vaginosis should be treated before pregnancy, in women with cervical abnormalities, and before elective gynecologic surgery. Most clinicians do not treat male partners routinely, as there has been no documented reduction in recurrence rates in women with bacterial vaginosis whose partners have been treated.

REFERENCES

1 Nyirjesy, P. Vaginitis in the adolescent patient. *Pediatr. Clin. North Am.* 1999; **46**: 733–745.

2 Hawes, S. E., Hillier, S. L., Benedetti, J., *et al*. Hydrogen peroxide-producing lactobacilli and acquisition of vaginal infections. *J. Infect. Dis.* 1996; **174**: 1058.

3 Sobel, J. D. and Chaim, W. Vaginal microbiology of women with acute recurrent vulvovaginal candidiasis. *J. Clin. Microbiol.* 1996; **34**: 2497.

4 Jaquiery, A., Stylianopoulos, A., Hogg, G. and Grover, S. Vulvovaginitis: clinical features, aetiology, and microbiology of the genital tract. *Arch. Dis. Child.* 1999; **81**: 64–67.

5 Hillier S. L. and Lau R. J. Vaginal microflora in postmenopausal women who have not received estrogen replacement therapy. *Clin. Infect. Dis.* 1997; **25**: S123–126.

6 Odds, F. C. Candidiasis of the genitalia. In: Odd, R. C. (ed.) *Candida and Candidosis: A Review and Bibliography*, 2nd edn, pp. 124–135. Ballière Tindall, London, 1988.

7 Horowitz B. J., Giaquinta D. and Ito S. Evolving pathogens in vulvovaginal candidiasis: implications for patient care. *J. Clin. Pharmacol.* 1992; **32**: 248–255.

8 Nyirjesy P., Vazquez J. A., Ufberg D. D., *et al. Saccharomyces cerevisiae* vaginitis: transmission from yeast used in baking. *Obstet. Gynecol.* 1995; **86**: 326–329.

9 Eckert L. O., Hawes S. E., Stevens C. E., *et al*. Vulvovaginal candidiasis: clinical manifestations, risk factors, management algorithm. *Obstet. Gynecol.* 1998; **92**: 757–765.

10 Foxman B. Epidemiology of vulvovaginal candidiasis: risk factors. *Am. J. Publ. Health* 1990; **80**: 329–331.

11 Sobel J. D. Vulvovaginitis in healthy women. *Comp. Ther.* 1999; **25**: 335–346.

12 Sobel J. D. and Chaim W. Treatment of *candida glabrata* vaginitis: a retrospective review of boric acid therapy. *Clin. Infect. Dis.* 1997; **24**: 649–652.

13 Sobel J. D. Epidemiology and pathogenesis of recurrent vulvovaginal candidiasis. *Am. J. Obstet. Gynecol.* 1985; **152**: 924–934.

14 Fidel, P. J. Jr. and Sobel J. D. Immunopathogenesis of recurrent vulvovaginal candidiasis. *Clin. Microbiol. Rev.* 1996; **9**: 335–348.

15 Spinillo A., Carrata L. and Pizzoli G. Recurrent vulvovaginal candidiasis: results of a cohort study of sexual transmission and intestinal reservoir. *J. Reprod. Med.* 1992; **37**: 342–347.

16 Reef, S., Levine, W. C., McNeil, M. M., *et al*. Treatment options for vulvovaginal candidiasis. Background paper for development of 1993 STD treatment recommendations. *Clin. Infect. Dis.* 1995; **20**(Suppl): 580–590.

17 Hammil H. A. Trichomonas vaginalis. *Obstet. Gynecol. Clin. North Am.* 1989; **16**: 531–540.

18 Oleen-Burkey M. A. and Hillier S. L. Pregnancy complications associated with bacterial vaginosis and their estimated costs. *Infect. Dis. Obstet. Gynecol.* 1995; **3**: 149–157.

19 Eschenbach D. A. Bacterial vaginosis: emphasis on upper genital tract complications. *Obstet. Gynecol. Clin. North Am.* 1989; **16**: 593–610.

20 Hillier S. L., and Holmes K. K. Bacterial vaginosis. In: Holmes, K. K., Mardh, P. A., Sparling, P. F., *et al*. (eds) *Sexually Transmitted Diseases*, pp. 547–560. McGraw-Hill, New York, 1990.

21 Hill G. B. Microbiology of bacterial vaginosis. *Am. J. Obstet. Gynecol.* 1993; **169**: 450–454.

22 Ferris D. G., Litaker M. S., Woodward L., *et al*. Treatment of bacterial vaginosis: a comparison of oral metronidazole: metronidazole vaginal gel and clindamycin vaginal cream. *J. Fam. Pract.* 1995; **41**: 443–449.

13 Vulvar Anatomy

Peter Braude

INTRODUCTION

The vulva comprises the structures that form the female external genitalia (**13.1**), namely:

- The mons pubis
- The labia majora and minora
- The clitoris
- The vestibule
- The Bartholin (greater vestibular) glands

It lies centrally within the anterior perineal triangle. This is the region defined by the symphysis pubis anteriorly, the pubic rami laterally, and the transverse perineal muscles posteriorly. A sling of fibers derived from the levator ani muscle sweeps behind the vagina to form the sphincter vaginae, with the remaining space laterally filled by the urogenital diaphragm.

LABIA MAJORA

The labia majora correspond to the scrotum in the male, and form two thick folds of skin lateral to the vaginal orifice. Anteriorly, they fuse to form the mons pubis overlying the pubic bone; posteriorly, they blend into the perineal skin. The lateral aspects contain numerous hair follicles and apocrine sweat glands, with sebaceous glands lying predominantly within the medial walls.

LABIA MINORA

The labia minora are two vascular, rugose slips of skin, which lie just within the labia majora. The lateral portions of the inner minora contain tiny sebaceous glands, which are seen as small yellowish papules when the skin is stretched. Devoid of hair follicles and adipose tissue, the labia minora are hyperpigmented in the adult and may vary considerably in size (**13.2**).

Anteriorly, they fuse around the clitoris, forming the prepuce above it and the frenulum below. Posteriorly, they form a lip of skin known as the fourchette. At birth, under the influence of maternal estrogens,

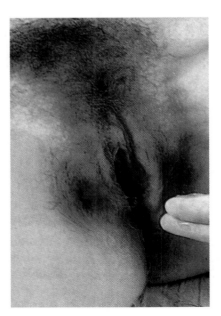

Fig 13.2 Normal vulva.

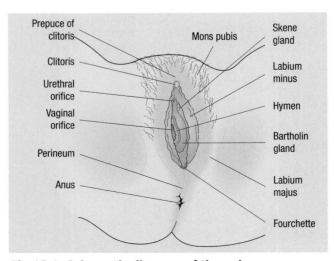

Prepuce of clitoris — Mons pubis — Skene gland
Clitoris — Labium minus
Urethral orifice — Hymen
Vaginal orifice — Bartholin gland
Perineum — Labium majus
Anus — Fourchette

Fig 13.1 Schematic diagram of the vulva.

the female genitalia are prominent and occasionally pigmented. Throughout infancy, the labia majora and mons pubis gradually lose their generous layer of adipose tissue and remain devoid of hair.

CLITORIS

This sensitive and erectile organ is the homolog of the male penis. With the exception of a urethra, it contains all the structures found in the penis, with the following less developed and thus less easily demonstrated, namely:

- The spongy, vascular corpora cavernosa (originating from the inferior pubic rami), which form most of the body
- The vestigial ischiocavernosus and bulbospongiosus muscles, which insert into the body and root, respectively

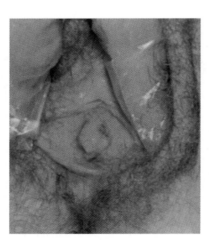

Fig 13.3 Separation of the labia minora reveals the vestibule.

Densely supplied by cutaneous branches of the pudendal nerve, the clitoris becomes engorged and highly sensitive during intercourse.

VESTIBULE

Parting of the labia reveals the oval orifice known as the vestibule (13.3), into which opens the urethra anteriorly, the ducts of Skene glands lateral to the urethra, the ducts of Bartholin glands posterolaterally, and the vagina. At the posterior fourchette, tiny finger-like projections (papillae) may often be seen. Sweeping around the vestibule on each side, rudimentary fibers of the bulbospongiosus muscles envelop a rich plexus of veins and loose areolar tissue called the bulb of the vestibule (13.4), which becomes engorged during sexual arousal and may become varicose during pregnancy.

At the posterior base of each bulb, about two-thirds of the way down the lateral wall, lie the mucus-secreting Bartholin glands. Normally impalpable, their 2 cm ducts may easily become blocked in adulthood resulting in dramatic swelling and infection (*see Chapter 22*).

PERINEAL BODY

The fibromuscular perineal body, formed from the common insertion of the superficial muscles of the perineal pouch, both supports the lower part of the vagina and divides it from the anal canal. The perineal body is often the subject of trauma at delivery, as a result of tearing or episiotomy, and afterwards the fourchette may be left deficient (13.5)

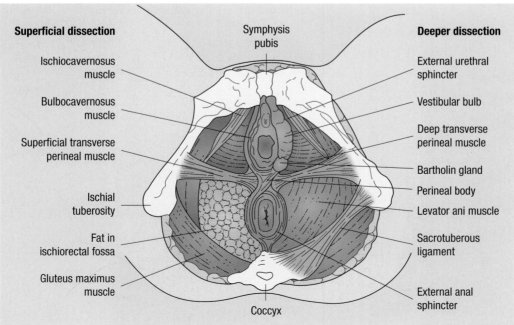

Superficial dissection

Ischiocavernosus muscle

Bulbocavernosus muscle

Superficial transverse perineal muscle

Ischial tuberosity

Fat in ischiorectal fossa

Gluteus maximus muscle

Symphysis pubis

Coccyx

Deeper dissection

External urethral sphincter

Vestibular bulb

Deep transverse perineal muscle

Bartholin gland

Perineal body

Levator ani muscle

Sacrotuberous ligament

External anal sphincter

Fig 13.4 Dissection of the perineum shows the superficial muscles, the position of the Bartholin gland, and the vestibular bulb.

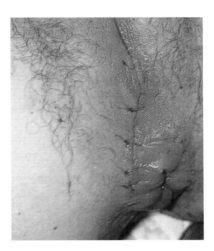

Fig 13.5 Repair of episiotomy following instrumental delivery.

EMBRYOLOGY OF THE LOWER GENITAL TRACT

Until 5 weeks' gestation, the urogenital and alimentary systems share a common reservoir, the cloaca. This is derived from the caudal region of the hindgut (**13.6**), and is separated from the surface by the cloacal membrane. Between 5 and 7 weeks' gestation, mesoderm migrates distally to become the urogenital septum, dividing the cloaca into the larger urogenital sinus and the anorectal canal. The septum eventually fuses with the cloacal membrane to produce the anal membrane and the urogenital membrane, with the genital tubercle superiorly (**13.7**). The close embryologic derivation of the vulva and anus is reflected in the common blood supply and nerve supply of these areas, and the numerous dermatologic conditions that afflict both organs in a similar manner.

The mesonephric ducts (Wolffian ducts) open into the cloaca on about day 26 of gestation. This subdivides the urogenital sinus into a cranial portion continuous with the allantois (the vesicourethral canal), which subsequently forms the bladder and part of the urethra, and a caudal portion, the urogenital sinus 'proper', which gives rise to the lower one-third of the vagina. Two solid outgrowths of the sinus – the sinovaginal bulbs – elongate as the fetus grows, eventually meeting the lower tip of the fused paramesonephric (Müllerian) ducts to form a solid epithelial column that represents the future vagina.

Canalization of the vagina occurs relatively late (at approximately 26 weeks' gestation), with the formation of lacunae that progressively coalesce. The process is occasionally incomplete, resulting in vaginal septae, or more rarely, partial or total occlusion. The hymen is thought to represent the region between the urogenital sinus and the canalized derivatives of the sinovaginal bulbs. In rare cases, the hymen may be imperforate, causing the retention of menstrual blood behind it and giving rise to a hematocolpos (**13.8**).

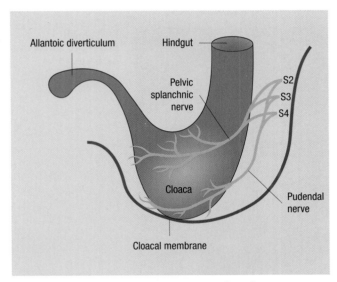

Fig 13.6 The cloaca at about 5 weeks of intrauterine life.

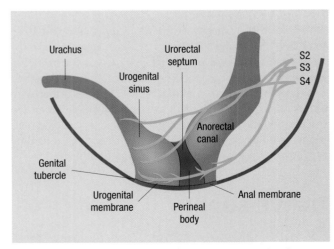

Fig 13.7 The cloaca after the seventh week of intrauterine life.

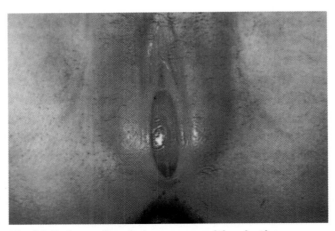

Fig 13.8 Imperforate hymen resulting in the accumulation of menstrual blood.

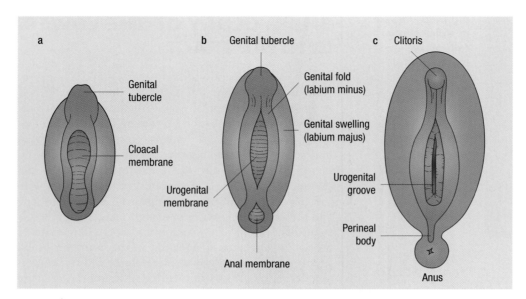

Fig 13.9 Stages in the development of external genitalia in the female: a at 5 weeks; **b** at 7 weeks; **c** at 12 weeks.

The external genitalia of the male and female are structurally indistinguishable (the indifferent stage) until about 12 weeks of gestation. By about 7 weeks, the cloacal membrane is divided into a urogenital membrane and an anal membrane (13.9), with an anterior genital tubercle, two symmetric genital folds and two genital swellings. The secondary sex characteristics appear earlier in the male than in the female fetus, probably reflecting the earlier functional activity in the testis. The Y chromosome induces the gonad to become a testis in the genetically male fetus. The differentiation of the external genitalia in the female occurs because this male-determining effect is not present. Exposure to exogenous or endogenous androgens at this critical stage will result in a variable degree of masculinization (13.10).

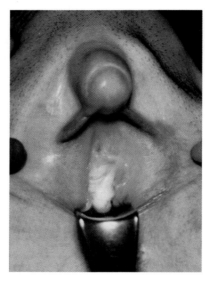

Fig 13.10 Enlarged clitoris as a result of virilization.

BLOOD SUPPLY

The arterial supply to the vulva is derived largely from the internal pudendal artery, a terminal branch of the internal iliac artery. Entering the buttock beneath the gluteus maximus muscle, it arches round the ischial spine, passes through the lesser sciatic notch, and approaches the perineum in the roof of the ischiorectal fossa, lying in company with the pudendal nerve in the pudendal (Alcock) canal (13.11). The named terminal branches, from posterior to anterior, are:

- The inferior rectal artery, passing medially from the pudendal canal to supply the anal canal and sphincter
- The perineal and transverse perineal branches, passing anteromedially over the ischiorectal fossa, and piercing the superficial perineal muscles to supply the anal and vaginal sphincters, anterior fibers of the levator ani muscle, and the skin of the perineal body and posterior labia

- The artery of the bulb, passing through the urogenital diaphragm to the bulb of the vestibule
- Two terminal branches, the dorsal and deep arteries, to the clitoris

There is also a supply from the superficial and deep external pudendal arteries, which arise from the femoral artery. The pudendal artery and its branches are accompanied by a rich network of veins, ultimately draining into the internal iliac veins. This, together with extensive anastomoses to the peripheral branches of the inferior gluteal and external pudendal arteries, ensures a plentiful blood supply and accounts for the rapid healing of the vulva following trauma, such as childbirth.

NERVE SUPPLY

The nerve supply to the vulva and perineum arises mainly from the anterior rami of the five sacral and coccygeal nerves, with a small input from the fifth

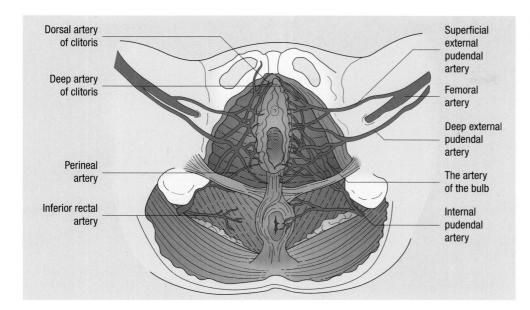

Fig 13.11 Blood supply of the vulva.

Labels on figure:
- Dorsal artery of clitoris
- Deep artery of clitoris
- Perineal artery
- Inferior rectal artery
- Superficial external pudendal artery
- Femoral artery
- Deep external pudendal artery
- The artery of the bulb
- Internal pudendal artery

lumbar nerve via the ilioinguinal nerve. The vulva itself is supplied by branches of the pudendal nerve, formed from the second, third, and fourth sacral nerve roots, and representing the largest component of the anterior sacrococcygeal plexus. Lying just medial to the pudendal artery, the nerve follows an almost identical path through the pudendal canal to reach the vulva (**13.12**). Recognized branches are:

- The inferior rectal nerve, supplying the external anal sphincter and the perianal skin
- The perineal nerve, divided into a superficial branch (supplying the skin over the perineal body) and a larger deep branch, supplying the levator ani muscle, the external sphincters, the vaginal muscles, and ultimately the erectile tissue of the bulb

- The dorsal nerve to the clitoris, running close to the pubic arch to enter the root of the clitoris

All the nerves communicate extensively and there is considerable overlap with the ilioinguinal nerve anteriorly, the posterior cutaneous nerve of the thigh centrally, and the anococcygeal nerve posteriorly.

A knowledge of the course through the pudendal canal is important in producing a pudendal block using local anesthetic agents. Access can be gained through the skin lateral to the perineal body, or through the lateral wall of the vagina, using a specially guarded pudendal needle (**13.13**).

Labels on Fig 13.12:
- Pudendal nerve leaves the pelvis through the greater sciatic notch
- Nerve behind ischial spine – anesthetized here in pudendal black
- Dorsal nerve of clitoris
- Nerve enters canal by passing through lesser sciatic notch
- Inferior rectal nerve
- Perineal nerve

Fig 13.12 Course of the pudendal nerve.

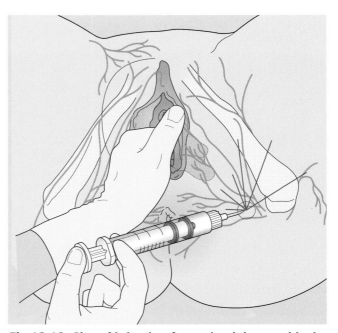

Fig 13.13 Site of injection for pudendal nerve block. Practically, the needle would be inserted through the vaginal wall and not through the skin as shown, which is done simply for clarity.

LYMPHATIC DRAINAGE

The vulva, in common with the lower trunk and back, the buttock, the perineum, and the anus (below the mucocutaneous junction), drains via superficial lymphatic channels to the superficial inguinal (groin) nodes. These lie just distal to the inguinal ligament on each side. From here, drainage occurs through the saphenous opening in the fascia lata femoris to the deep inguinal (femoral) nodes that lie in the femoral triangle (13.14).

A constant feature is the medially placed Cloquet node, guarding the entrance to the femoral canal. Lymph channels then pass beneath the inguinal ligament to reach the external iliac nodes, and subsequently the common iliac nodes, and thence the para-aortic nodes. Drainage from the labia occurs predominantly to the ipsilateral inguinal nodes, whereas midline structures, the fourchette, and particularly the clitoris may drain bilaterally.

ACKNOWLEDGEMENTS

Figures **13.2**, **13.5** and **13.8** are reproduced from E.M. Symonds and M.B.A. Macpherson *Color Atlas of Obstetrics and Gynaecology* (Figs 1.25, 7.48 and 10.1), Mosby–Wolfe, London, 1994.
Figures **13.3** and **13.10** are reproduced from V.R. Tindall *Colour Atlas of Clinical Gynaecology* (Figs 6 and 27), Wolfe, London, 1981.

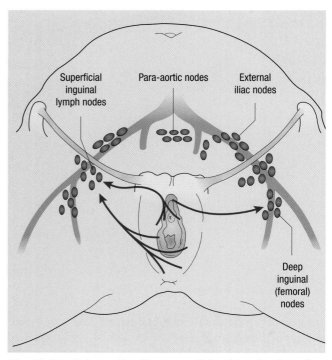

Fig 13.14 Schematic diagram of the lymphatics of the vulva. Extensive intercommunication exists between the lymphatics of each side.

14 Classification of Cutaneous Vulvar Disorders – International Society for the Study of Vulvovaginal Disease (ISSVD)

C. Marjorie Ridley

INTRODUCTION

Attempts to distinguish between cutaneous vulvar diseases began to be made towards the end of the nineteenth century. A profusion of terms arose which were devised by dermatologists and gynecologists, but without mutual understanding. In the twentieth century several efforts were made to formulate a classification; they are summarized below and described in more detail elsewhere[1]. They have been unsatisfactory, foundering on a failure to recognize that the skin of the vulva is exclusively subject to cutaneous conditions occurring on the skin elsewhere. This is a concept easy to understand for the dermatologist, but less so for the gynecologist; the pathologist must also come to realize it. In accordance with this tenet, a simpler, more rational, scheme will be formulated in the early years of the twenty-first century.

EVOLUTION OF EARLY SCHEMES

The main aims were:

- To clarify the entity of lichen sclerosus, a name chosen uncontroversially to replace lichen sclerosus et atrophicus.
- To recognize lichen simplex and lichenification; that is, thickening of the skin in response to itching and rubbing, the former being a primary event, the latter a secondary condition superimposed on an itching dermatosis.
- To declare redundant many terms used up to that time, for example leucoplakia, erythroplasia of Queyrat, kraurosis vulvae, etc.

The outcome was that described originally by Gardner and Kaufman, and formalized as that of the International Society for the Study of Vulvovaginal Disease (ISSVD)[2]. The ISSVD is a multidisciplinary body that came into being (as the International Society for the Study of Vulvar Disease) in 1970.

The original scheme (**Table 14.1**) had two drawbacks. It was essentially histopathologic and omitted consideration of many known cutaneous disorders, the diagnosis of which is of obvious clinical and academic importance. For example, lichen simplex and lichenification were concealed under 'hyperplastic dystrophy', and the term 'dystrophy' itself is not meaningful. Moreover, with its categories of 'atypia' it encroached into neoplastic disease. This trespass was emphasized by the increased recognition and frequency of vulvar intraepithelial neoplasia (VIN) in subsequent years.

Table 14.1 ISSVD Classification of Vulvar Dystrophies 1976[2].

1 Hyperplastic dystrophy
  (a) Without atypia
  (b) With atypia

2 Lichen sclerosus

3 Mixed dystrophy (lichen sclerosus with foci of epithelial hyperplasia)
  (a) Without atypia
  (b) With atypia

A detailed histologic definition and description were given for each of the conditions noted above. Atypia was classified as mild, moderate, or severe, and with or without dystrophy.
This classification is no longer recommended.

CLASSIFICATION OF VULVAR INTRAEPITHELIAL NEOPLASIA

In turn, efforts were made to create a satisfactory classification of VIN, and to try to note in it the significance of human papillomavirus (HPV). The outcome, jointly agreed by the ISSVD and the International Society of Gynecologic Pathologists (ISGYP) is set out in **Table 14.2**[3]. The grades of VIN 1, 2 and 3 correspond to what had been referred to previously as mild and moderate atypia (VIN 1 and 2) and severe atypia, carcinoma *in situ* (VIN 3). VIN was defined as follows:

'VIN is characterized by loss of epithelial cell maturation with associated nuclear hyperchromasia, pleomorphism, cellular crowding and abnormal mitosis. Dyskeratotic cells, 'corps ronds', hyperkeratosis and parakeratosis may be present.

- VIN 1. Nuclear hyperchromasia is present, with cellular disarray involving the lower one third of the epithelium; mitoses within the lower third of the epithelium are often seen and are abnormal.
- VIN 2. Nuclear hyperchromasia is present, with cellular disarray involving up to the lower two thirds of the epithelium; mitoses are often seen and are usually abnormal.
- VIN 3. Nuclear hyperchromasia is present, with cellular disarray involving more than the lower two thirds of the epithelium; mitoses within the area of cellular disarray are often seen and are usually abnormal; the term carcinoma *in situ* is usually reserved for cases that have near-full or full-thickness epithelial changes' (**14.1**).

Further comments elaborated on these definitions:

'The term *differentiated type* (i.e. VIN 3, severe dysplasia, differentiated type) is recommended for those cases that have cells with prominent eosinophilic cytoplasm, often with keratin or "pearl-like" changes within the involved epithelium. These changes are usually seen near the tips of the rete ridges in the lower third of the epithelium [**14.2**]. The epithelial cell nuclei in these areas usually have prominent nucleoli with vesicular, rather than coarsely clumped, chromatin. The more superficial epithelium may show some maturation. It is recommended that cases with such findings be classified as VIN 3.

'Although the terms *Bowen's disease*, *erythroplasia of Queyrat* and *carcinoma simplex* are included under the general heading of VIN, they are not preferred terms. The term *bowenoid papulosis*, though controversial, is not accepted as a pathologic term, although it is recognized that the term, as used by some dermatologists, refers to cases of VIN associated with multiple papule formation. Use of

Category	Description
VIN 1	Mild dysplasia
VIN 2	Moderate dysplasia
VIN 3	Severe dysplasia, carcinoma *in situ*

Table 14.2 Classification of Vulvar Intraepithelial Neoplasia 1986[3].

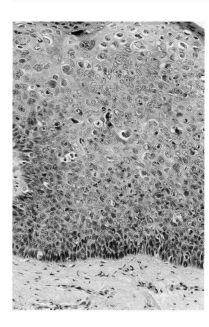

Fig 14.1 VIN 3. Full-thickness changes.

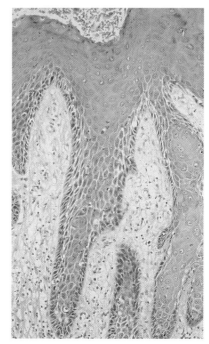

Fig 14.2 VIN 3. Differentiated type. Note that the changes are confined to the basal and parabasal area, with keratin pearls in the rete ridges.

the terms *bowenoid papulosis* or *bowenoid dysplasia* is not recommended by the Society (ISSVD) for either clinical or pathologic use. The association of condyloma acuminatum should not influence the diagnosis or grading of VIN. When koilocytic change or condyloma acuminatum occurs adjacent to or within a VIN lesion, it is recommended that a statement to that effect be made and that such terms as *condylomatous dysplasia* not be used.'

This classification will probably be modified in the next few years. It was drawn up, in part, on a false analogy with cervical intraepithelial neoplasia: the vulva has no transformation zone, nor is it a mucosa, and there is no inevitable progression from VIN 1 to VIN 3 – indeed in some cases, the three grades coexist in the same specimen. There is some evidence[4] that a solitary lesion of VIN in an older patient is of more clinical significance in relation to malignancy than are the multiple, often HPV-related areas in younger patients, and this judgement is not reflected in the purely histologic terminology described. Moreover, no attention is paid to the state of the surrounding skin – whether normal or showing evidence of lichen sclerosus or HPV infection. It is thought that the differentiated type of VIN 3 has special significance as a forerunner of squamous cell carcinoma in lichen sclerosus, yet, because its changes are confined to the lower third of the epithelium, it may be confused with VIN 1. A more logical system would describe VIN, as is the case with intraepithelial neoplasia on the rest of the body, as being of high or low grade.

EXTRAMAMMARY PAGET'S DISEASE AND MELANOMA IN SITU (NON SQUAMOUS VIN)

The classification of VIN also includes extramammary Paget's disease (**14.3**) and melanoma *in situ* (i.e. non-squamous VIN). Although they are often difficult to diagnose clinically and histologically, their inclusion in the scheme has been uncontroversial.

SQUAMOUS CELL CARCINOMA OF THE VULVA

Agreement has been reached between the ISSVD and the International Federation of Obstetricians and Gynecologists (FIGO) on staging (**Table 14.3**)[5]. This listing will aid the clinician to select therapies that are more individualized and less uncompromisingly radical than is often now the case. The superficially invasive stage Ia lesion, for example, is not associated with lymphatic involvement and may therefore be treated by excision unaccompanied by lymphadenectomy. When carcinomas are excised, it is also important to pay attention to any underlying vulvar condition.

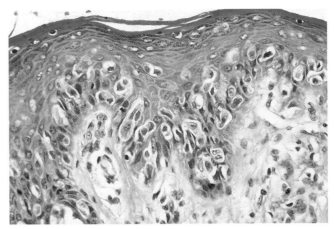

Fig 14.3 Extramammary Paget's disease.

Table 14.3 Vulva Cancer Staging[5].

Stage[a]	Clinical findings
I	Lesions 2 cm or less, confined to the vulva or perineum. No lymph node metastases
Ia	Lesions 2 cm or less, confined to the vulva or perineum with stromal invasion no greater than 1.0 mm[b]. No nodal metastases
Ib	Lesions 2 cm or less, confined to the vulva or perineum and with stromal invasion greater than 1 mm[b]. No nodal metastases
II	Tumor confined to the vulva and/or perineum or more than 2 cm in greatest dimension, with no nodal metastases
III	Tumor of any size arising on the vulva and/or perineum with (1) adjacent spread to the lower urethra and/or the vagina or anus, and/or (2) unilateral regional lymph node metastases
IVa	Tumor invading any of the following: upper urethra, bladder mucosa, rectal mucosa, pelvic bone, and/or bilateral regional nodal metastases
IVb	Any distant metastasis, including pelvic lymph nodes

[a] The more advanced stages (II–IV) are as defined previously.
[b] Depth of invasion is defined as measurement of the tumor from the epithelial stromal junction of the adjacent most superficial dermal papilla to the deepest point of invasion.

CURRENT CLASSIFICATION OF NON-NEOPLASTIC CONDITIONS

Following the separation of VIN from the non-neoplastic conditions, a new scheme for the latter, agreed by the ISSVD and the ISGYP, was drawn up (**Table 14.4**)[6]. Additional comments on it were made in the form of footnotes as follows:

> 'Mixed epithelial disorders may occur. In such cases, it is recommended that both conditions be reported. For example lichen sclerosus with associated squamous cell hyperplasia (formerly classified as mixed dystrophy) should be reported as lichen sclerosus with squamous cell hyperplasia. Squamous cell hyperplasia with associated VIN (formerly hyperplastic dystrophy with atypia) should be diagnosed as VIN ... Squamous cell hyperplasia is used for those instances in which hyperplasia is not attributable to a more specific tissue process. Specific lesions or dermatoses involving the vulva (e.g. psoriasis, lichen planus, lichen simplex chronicus, *Candida* infection, condyloma acuminatum) may include squamous cell hyperplasia, but should be diagnosed specifically and excluded from this category because of their pathognomonic characteristics.'

This scheme was never wholly acceptable to dermatologists. Squamous cell hyperplasia appears out of place in conjunction with the other headings. Epithelial cell hyperplasia is a preferable term and would best be considered as a descriptive feature of some underlying dermatological condition, in lichen sclerosus, indeed, it is often a harbinger of malignancy.

At the 1999 Congress of the ISSVD, an agreement was reached (to be published in due course) that was satisfactory to all disciplines involved. This will be a simple listing of conditions to be found at the vulva, as they are found elsewhere, using clinical and histologic criteria. The list may be numbered in accordance

---

Table 14.4 Non-neoplastic Epithelial Disorders of Skin and Mucosa 1989[6].

1 Lichen sclerosus

2 Squamous cell hyperplasia (formerly hyperplastic dystrophy)

3 Other dermatoses

This scheme is currently in use but is to be replaced.

Table 14.5 Current Classification of Vulvar Disorders.

1 Vulvar dermatoses
Visible skin changes classified according to SNOMED

2 Vulvar dysesthesia (vulvodynia)
  (a) Generalized
  (b) Localized
    (i) Vestibulodynia
    (ii) Clitorodynia
    (iii) Other

Approved at the 1999 ISSVD World Congress in Santa Fe, as a 'working' scheme.

---

with the SNOMED system (College of American Pathologists Systematized Nomenclature of Medicine). An added advantage of this plan is that there is provision for functional disorders, so vulvodynia (*see Chapter 20*) will be accommodated; at the same Congress it was agreed that this may be conveniently categorized as vulval dysesthesia (vulvodynia), and subdivided into two forms, generalized and localized, the latter comprising vestibulodynia (previously vulvar vestibulitis), clitorodynia, etc. (**Table 14.5**).

These new approaches will undoubtedly lead to a more logical assessment of vulvar disease in the new millennium.

REFERENCES

1 Ridley, C. M. and Neill, S. M. Non-infective cutaneous conditions of the vulva. In: Ridley, C. M. and Neill, S. M. (eds) *The Vulva*, pp. 121, 154–156. Blackwell Scientific, Oxford, 1999.

2 Friedrich, E. G. New nomenclature for vulval disease. *Obstet. Gynecol.* 1976; **47**: 122–124.

3 Wilkinson, E. J., Kneale, B., and Lynch, P. J. Report of the ISSVD terminology committee. *J. Reprod. Med.* 1986; **31**: 973–974.

4 Leibowitch, M., Neill, S., Pelisse, M., *et al.* The epithelial changes associated with squamous cell carcinoma of the vulva: a review of the clinical, histological and viral findings in 78 women. *Br. J. Obstet. Gynaecol.* 1990; **97**: 135–139.

5 Shepherd, J. H. Cervical and vulva cancer: changes in FIGO definitions of staging. *Br. J. Obstet. Gynaecol.* 1996; **103**: 405–406.

6 Ridley, C. M., Frankman, O., Jones, I. S. C., *et al.* New nomenclature for vulval disease; report of the committee on terminology. *Am. J. Obstet. Gynecol.* 1989; **160**: 769.

ACKNOWLEDGEMENTS

Figure 14.2 has been reproduced by kind permission of Dr C. H. Buckley, and Figures 14.1 and 14.3 by kind permission of Dr P. H. McKee.

15 Vulvar Manifestations of Skin Disorders

Marilynne McKay

INTRODUCTION

This group of disorders includes conditions that are familiar to dermatologists trained to seek diagnostic clues elsewhere on the skin. With practice, the nondermatologist can recognize and treat these diseases with greater ease. **Table 15.1** summarizes the differential diagnosis of the vulvar disorders discussed in this chapter, and also outlines treatment.

PSORIASIS

(See also Chapter 8)

Psoriasis (15.1–15.3) is usually easy to recognize, but lesions can look different on various parts of the body. Red plaques have silvery scales on dry skin, such as the elbows and knees, but appear gray-white and macerated in intertriginous areas, where fissures and cracks often cause discomfort. Acute generalized flares of psoriasis may result in intense vulvar erythema (*see also* **15.25**). 'Pinking' of the gluteal cleft is common, and nail pitting may be a diagnostic clue, even when skin involvement is minimal. *Psoriatic arthritis* occurs in less than 15% of patients. It is similar to rheumatoid arthritis, but is predominantly distal, involving the fingers and toes. Reiter disease should be considered when arthritis, acropustulosis, and ankylosing spondylitis occur with psoriasiform genital lesions. *Pustular psoriasis* is an unusual type of psoriasis that looks very much like *Staphylococcus* or *Candida* infection. Reiter disease (**15.4**) may also have a pustular component.

TREATMENT

For lesions on the extremities and trunk, topical therapy with a mid- to high-potency steroid cream or ointment is the usual mainstay of treatment. Vulvar

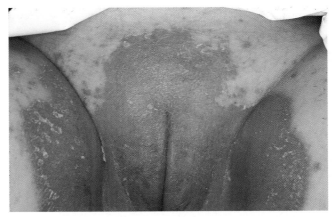

Fig 15.1 Intertriginous psoriasis. Extensive scaling and erythema of gluteal cleft and vulva. The patient should be examined carefully for other stigmata of psoriasis (plaques on the knees, elbows, scalp; nail pitting).

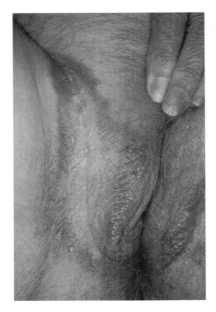

Fig 15.2 Intertriginous psoriasis. Thick scaly plaques in intertriginous folds with a sharply defined border are typical of psoriasis. These areas are easily traumatized and fissuring is common. Note: ungloved fingers in these photographs are the patient's own.

Table 15.1 Differential Diagnoses of Vulvar Dermatoses.

Diagnosis	Onset	Symptoms	Appearance	Other areas	Treatment
Psoriasis	Chronic and recurrent	Painful if fissured	Thick, red scaly plaques with distinct margins	Scalp, knees, elbows, sacrum, nails	Topical steroids (triamcinolone 0.1%), systemic therapy if severe
Seborrheic dermatitis	Chronic and recurrent	Minimal	Thin reddish plaques with greasy scale	Scalp, central face, axillae	Antidandruff shampoos, hydrocortisone 1% cream
Pityriasis versicolor	Chronic and recurrent	Minimal	Thin reddish plaques with furry scale	Trunk, shoulders; pigment variable	Topical imidazole creams twice daily until clear for 1 week
Intertrigo (chafing)	Acute	Tender	Erythema, sometimes petechiae	May follow clothing lines	Cool compress, bland emollient or hydrocortisone; avoid allergens
Intertrigo (chronic)	Ongoing and recurrent; common in obese	Moderate itching	Thin reddish patches (erythrasma); if pruritic, may lichenify	Axillae	For erythrasma, topical or systemic erythromycin; mild soaps, talc, cortisone cream
Dermatitis (irritant or allergic contact)	Acute; may be recurrent	Itching	Vesicular eruption becomes dry and scaly; lasts 2–3 weeks	Other areas of contact	Cool compress, bland emollient or hydrocortisone; avoid allergens
Steroid rebound dermatitis	Occurs after using steroids for several months	Burning	Pebbly, fine-textured erythema; accentuation of sebaceous glands	Similar lesions can occur on face if steroids have been applied there	Discontinue topical steroid – may need to taper by decreasing potency and/or frequency
Tinea (dermatophytosis)	Acute or chronic	Itching, variable	Scaly plaques with inflammatory border	Usually spreads to adjacent areas	Topical imidazole creams twice daily until clear for 1 week; systemic antifungal if extensive
Candida vulvitis	Acute; may be recurrent in susceptible patients	Itching and burning	Bright erythema, swelling, statellite pustules; vaginal discharge may be absent	Inflammatory area, sometimes axillae. Oral thrush	Topical imidazole creams for vulva and vagina for 1 week; systemic fluconazole if persistent
Cyclic vulvovaginitis	Recurrent, often cycles with menses	Postcoital irritation, swelling	Mild edema, erythema; fissures with intercourse; normal between flares	Vaginal discharge rare	Vaginal antiyeast cream twice weekly for 4–6 months or oral fluconazole weekly for 2 months, then monthly for 6 months
Lichen simplex chronicus	Chronic	Intense bouts of itching	Thick leathery plaques with enhanced skin markings, diffuse margins	May occur elsewhere if patient has a history of atopic dermatitis	Clobetasol 0.05% ointment twice daily for 1 month then daily for 1 month, then 1–3 times weekly as needed; check often for vaginal *Candida*
Lichen planus	Chronic	Sometimes itchy, soreness at introitus	Erosive mucosal surfaces; violaceous papules or white reticulate pattern and/or adhesions	Lacy white oral and and vulvar mucosa; sometimes erosions and/or adhesions	Biopsy for diagnosis; topical steroids, cream or suppositories
Lichen sclerosus	Chronic	May itch or burn; often asymptomatic	White, wrinkly, atrophic, often petechial. Perianal 'keyhole' pattern	Usually none. Rarely generalized with confetti white spots on trunk, extremities	Clobetasol 0.05% ointment twice dailyfor 1 month then daily for 1 month, then 1–3 times weekly as needed
Paget's disease	Chronic and progressive	Minimal	Red, moist-appearing plaque with scaling	Local cutaneous spread; tumor cells may involve adjacent structures	Surgical excision; topical agents (e.g. 5-fluorouracil) are not curative

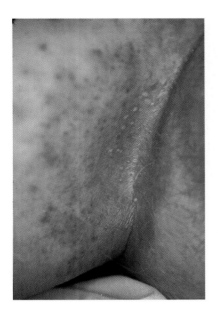

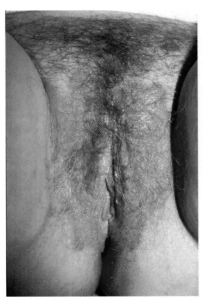

Fig 15.3 Pustular psoriasis of the vulva and inner thigh. This eruption may be indistinguishable from that of Reiter's disease, especially when there are symptoms of arthritis together with pustular lesions of the palms and soles. (These pustules were sterile and continued to erupt despite anticandidal treatment.)

Fig 15.4 Reiter's disease on the vulva. This patient had pustular lesions on the palms and soles as well as symptoms of arthritis. Radiographic examination of the spine revealed ankylosing spondylitis.

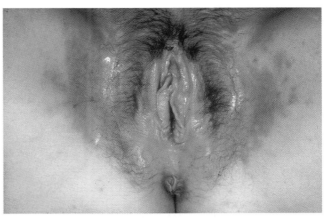

Fig 15.5 Seborrheic dermatitis, showing erythema of the vulva and intertriginous areas. This looks very much like psoriasis, but the typical scale is lacking. The patient also had lesions on the face and inframammary area, which were typical of seborrheic dermatitis. If there had also been scaling psoriatic plaques on the knees and elbows, this would have been called 'sebo-psoriasis'.

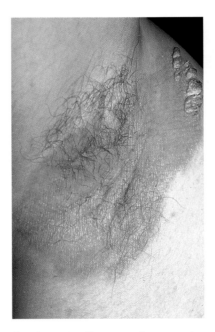

Fig 15.6 Axillary psoriasis. This would be indistinguishable from axillary seborrheic dermatitis, without the characteristic thick psoriatic scales at the edge of the lesion. The rest of the skin should be examined for typical lesions.

lesions typically respond well to mid-potent steroids (e.g. triamcinolone acetonide 0.1%) and should be tapered rapidly to hydrocortisone 1% or 2.5%. Ultraviolet light therapy, while effective for the rest of the body, is difficult to administer to vulvar lesions. With severe involvement of the entire body, systemic therapy may be required (e.g. methotrexate, oral retinoids).

SEBORRHEIC DERMATITIS

Scaling and erythema are the most common signs of seborrhea, but immunosuppressed patients may have particularly active lesions, with extensive red plaques and heavy dry scaling (15.5–15.7). It is rare for seborrheic dermatitis to occur only on the genitalia. Other areas that should be examined include the eyebrows, nasolabial folds, and the periauricular and posterior

hairline. Axillary involvement is common when genital lesions are present. A potassium hydroxide preparation of lesional scale may reveal the short hyphae and spores of tinea versicolor (*Pityrosporum ovale*, previously *Malassezia furfur*). This is probably a commensal organism that thrives in an environment rich in sebaceous oils.

TREATMENT

Topical treatment is usually effective. Mainstays of therapy are keratolytic agents ('dandruff' shampoos containing selenium sulfide, zinc pyrithione, or ketoconazole) and/or anti-inflammatory topical hydrocortisone preparations (hydrocortisone 1%, cream or lotion).

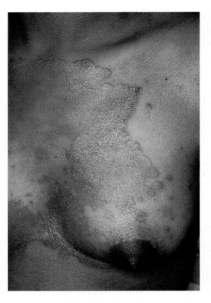

**Fig 15.7
Extensive trunkal seborrheic dermatitis.**
There is postinflammatory pigmentation in this postpartum patient, who developed this eruption during the last trimester of pregnancy. Although inframammary involvement is common, central chest lesions are uncommon in women. There was no evidence of *Pityrosporum ovale* in scale taken from the lesions.

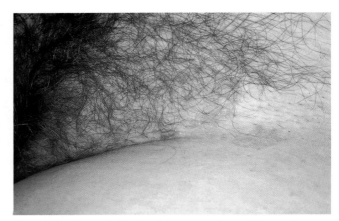

Fig 15.8 Tinea (pityriasis) versicolor of the vulva.
The fine scale and salmon patches are very similar to seborrhea, but microscopic examination of lesional scale revealed *Pityrosporum ovale*. There were no lesions on the trunk.

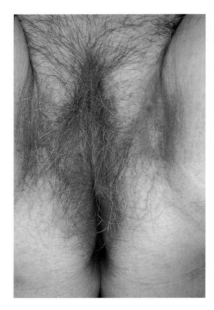

Fig 15.9 Intertrigo. The patient complained of irritation with heat and tight clothing. There was no evidence of *Candida* or tinea infection, and her condition improved with the use of cornstarch powder and loose cotton underwear.

PITYRIASIS (TINEA) VERSICOLOR

This common fungal infection (15.8) of the topmost layer of the skin (stratum corneum) recurs in susceptible individuals. There is some evidence that the responsible microorganism, *P. ovale*, may grow preferentially where sebaceous gland output is highest. Superinfection with *P. ovale* might explain why seborrheic dermatitis is so active in immunosuppressed patients, who are presumably less able to control the inflammatory response. It is unclear, however, whether the organisms are the cause of the increased seborrheic output, or are simply found in greater concentration where there is greater sebaceous gland production.

TREATMENT

Treatment with topical antifungals or keratolytic agents, such as sulfur and salicylic acid-containing soaps, is usually effective, but treatment must often be repeated monthly, especially in climates where temperature and humidity are high. Systemic antifungals may be given for severe or persistent infections.

INTERTRIGO

This term refers to the skin changes that develop in intertriginous areas (**15.9, 15.10**) because of chafing and chronic inflammation. Obese sedentary individuals

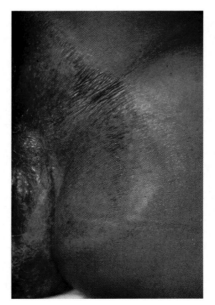

Fig 15.10 Chronic intertrigo. Postinflammatory hypopigmentation and hyper-pigmentation of chronic intertrigo. Variations in pigmentation may be seen as inflammatory cutaneous conditions flare and resolve, especially in patients with darkly pigmented skin.

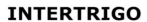

and active athletes are both likely to have problems with intertrigo; the common factor is occlusion and rubbing together of skin surfaces. Deep body folds are less able to dry out after perspiration, however, and the obese are more likely to develop a secondary intertriginous fungal or bacterial infection, usually tinea, *Candida*, or *Corynebacterium minutissimum* (erythrasma).

TREATMENT

Keeping the area clean and dry, reducing friction with talcum powder, and treating secondary infection with the appropriate medication are all effective ways to control the problem.

CONTACT DERMATITIS

There are two different types of contact dermatitis: allergic and irritant. Allergic contact dermatitis is due to a cell-mediated (type IV) allergic reaction; the rash develops some 48–72 hours after the exposure. Only someone sensitized to a substance will develop allergic contact dermatitis, and the dermatitis will occur every time the patient encounters that substance (**15.11**, **15.12**). Contact urticaria is an immediate hypersensitivity reaction that can cause intense edema of the vulva without dermatitis; it will not be considered here (*see* **Table 22.2**).

An irritant reaction, on the other hand, occurs only if the skin's barrier function is compromised; it will happen to almost everyone under the same circumstances (like the stinging of vinegar on chapped hands). When the skin is intact, the irritant reaction is reduced or eliminated. The complaint of immediate stinging when something is applied to the skin is typical of an irritant reaction; although the skin may be sensitive, this does not mean the patient is truly allergic to that substance (i.e. will react every time it is encountered).

The cutaneous eruption of allergic contact dermatitis lasts for between 2 and 3 weeks. Outbreaks lasting only a few days are more likely to be eczema. If episodes seem to be continuous, patch testing may be necessary to discover the allergen, which may be a medication that is being used to treat the problem. Medications that cause allergic contact dermatitis in susceptible individuals include topicals containing the preservative ethylenediamine, the antibacterial agent neomycin, or the local anesthetic benzocaine. A suspected medication allergy can be tested by means of a 'use test'. This involves applying a possible allergen-containing medication to the forearm under an elastic bandage for 48 hours. Development of a rash may confirm the diagnosis. Caustic materials, such as powdered detergents, should not be tested in this way.

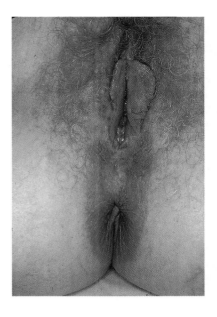

Fig 15.11 Allergic contact dermatitis of the vulva. The patient intermittently used a topical medication containing neomycin, to which she was allergic.

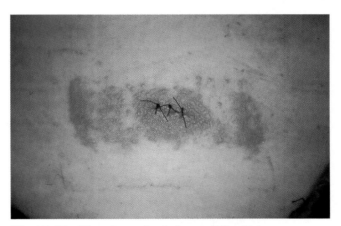

Fig 15.12 Allergic contact dermatitis. This was a reaction to an ointment containing neomycin, which had been applied under an adhesive plaster following excision of a nevus. The typical pattern where an allergen has touched the skin is a clue to diagnosis.

Treatment of irritant dermatitis is with mild topical steroids (hydrocortisone 1%, preferably in an ointment base that contains few additives), or with easily obtainable bland emollients, such as milk compresses or vegetable shortening. Cool water or plastic icepacks (wrapped in a cloth) can help provide rapid relief of itching and swelling. Treatment of severe allergic contact dermatitis may require a tapering course of systemic steroids (prednisone or prednisolone, starting with 40–60mg and decreasing over a 2-week course). Mid- to high-potency topical steroids can be used for 2 weeks to control an allergic reaction to a known substance, but the long-term use of topical steroids is discouraged for nonspecific dermatitis.

STEROID REBOUND DERMATITIS

Characterized by intense erythema and the complaint of stinging or burning, this problem is the result of 'rebound' from high-potency topical steroids (15.13, 15.14). These preparations cause local vasoconstriction. When the effect wears off, vessels relax and dilate, with resulting erythema. Patients may interpret this as a worsening of their condition, and thus apply steroids more often than is recommended.

Almost all high potency or 'superpotent' steroids will cause rebound dermatitis, but susceptible individuals (those with rosacea-like complexions) may develop steroid rebound from mid- or even low-potency preparations. Hydrocortisone 1% or 2.5% rarely causes

problems with steroid rebound, even if used daily. Superinfection with *Candida* can also be a problem when using steroids, so, if itching accompanies erythema, a vaginal culture should be considered. (*See Appendix B for a discussion of steroid potencies*).

DERMATOPHYTE (TINEA CRURIS)

Tinea infections (15.15–15.17) typically begin as inflammatory blisters or pustules which spread concentrically. The center of the lesion dries, becomes scaly, and heals, while the periphery continues to expand with small blisters or pustules. It may be difficult to find fungal hyphae at the active border because the inflammatory reaction is too great; lesional scale is best for identifying tinea.

Inadequate treatment of tinea often results in recurrence. Topical treatment typically takes about a month, which surprises many patients. It is good advice to recommend twice-daily treatment 'for at least a week after it looks like the rash has gone'. This will be more likely to eradicate hyphae that have penetrated hair follicles – a frequent source of reinfection.

CANDIDA VULVOVAGINITIS

(*See also Chapter 12*)

Candida vulvovaginitis (15.18–15.20) is very common and is usually associated with suppression of the normal cutaneous and gastrointestinal flora with antibiotic therapy. Immunosuppression is another factor, and diabetics are very likely to have problems with recurrent candidiasis (*see also* **19.3**). The typical eruption is

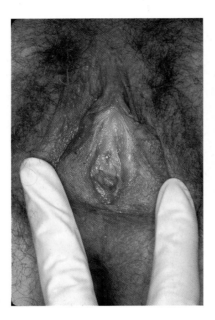

Fig 15.13 Steroid rebound dermatitis with burning of the inner labia minora after a high-potency topical steroid (fluocinonide 0.05% cream) had been applied for 2 months to skin that was not lichenified and only mildly symptomatic.

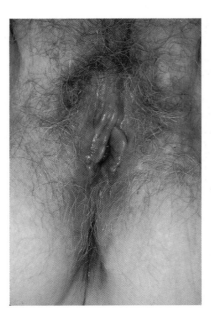

Fig 15.14 Steroid rebound dermatitis with burning of the labia majora after a high-potency topical steroid (triamcinolone 0.5% cream) had been applied for 3 months for treatment of erosive vaginitis.

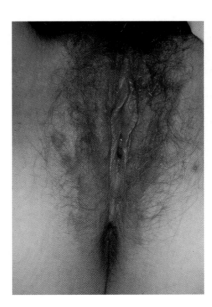

Fig 15.15 Annular margin of tinea on the vulva. Lesions of tinea are often subtle in women with normal immune systems. A high index of suspicion should be maintained and appropriate diagnostic tests should be done before treating lesions with topical steroids.

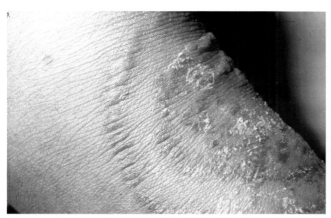

Fig 15.16 Annular tinea lesion. Vesicles and pustules at the advancing edge of a typical scaly plaque represent an inflammatory reaction, which subsequently subsides, leaving dry scales behind. Microscopic examination of the blister roof or dry scales may reveal fungal hyphae.

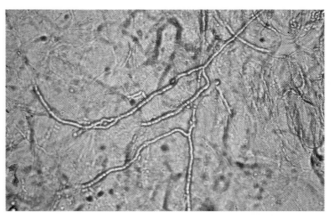

Fig 15.17 Dermatophyte (tinea cruris), showing a microscopic view of branched hyphae among cleared keratinocytes as they appear in a positive potassium hydroxide (KOH) preparation of lesional scale.

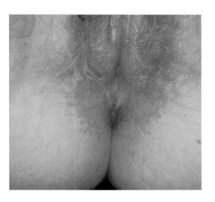

Fig 15.18 Acute *Candida* vulvovaginitis. Intense erythema and edema around the introitus, perineum, and perianal areas. The discrete erythematous macules at the active borders are resolving pustules.

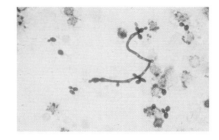

Fig 15.19 *Candida*. Periodic acid–Schiff (PAS) stain of budding yeast and pseudohyphae seen in *Candida albicans* vulvovaginitis.

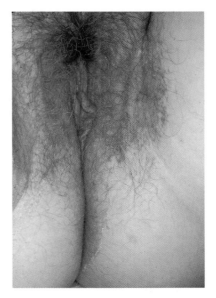

Fig 15.20 Recurrent *Candida* vulvovaginitis. Relatively mild erythema and peeling of the gluteal cleft and satellite pustules in the inguinal folds.

a bright erythema with edema around the vagina and vulva. Pustules on an erythematous base are often dotted at the periphery of the primary plaque or erosive area. Gram staining of a pustule will generally reveal budding yeast forms, confirming the diagnosis.

CYCLIC VULVOVAGINITIS

This is recurrent or recalcitrant vulvovaginitis, with or without typical, microscopically confirmed, monilial discharge (15.21–15.23). The patient usually confirms that she has occasional pain-free days and/or that symptoms are worse at a particular time during the menstrual cycle. Dyspareunia is typically described as 'irritation afterwards'. Inflammatory symptoms suggest a local tissue hypersensitivity to *Candida*, with an exaggerated response to the presence of a very low concentration of the organism. Although there is often swelling and itching, these patients rarely have a typical 'cottage-cheese' discharge and the diagnosis may not have been considered. The temptation to apply a potent steroid to red, itchy, or burning skin should be firmly resisted. Patients with a history of monilial vaginitis and cyclic symptoms should be given a trial of *Candida* suppression therapy.

TREATMENT

The patient should be treated with low-dose, long-term anticandidal agents – either a vaginal cream or oral medication. A vaginal cream should be inserted every night for 10 days, followed by 1/2 applicator on Monday, Wednesday, and Friday, for 2–4 months. Maintenance therapy can be very helpful in some patients; vaginal cream should be used nightly for only the 3–5 days before menses each month.

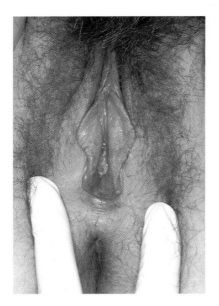

Fig 15.21 Cyclic vulvovaginitis. There is minimal involvement of the labia majora, but the minora are red and swollen. There is vaginal erythema, without a 'cottage cheese' discharge. The patient complained of burning and itching after intercourse and monthly just prior to menses.

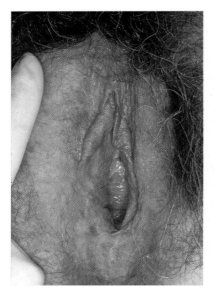

Fig 15.22 Cyclic vulvovaginitis. This postmenopausal patient was on estrogen replacement therapy. She complained of recurrent episodes of burning which were relieved by anticandidal vaginal creams. There is minimal vaginal discharge, but *Candida* was cultured from the erythematous area near the clitoris.

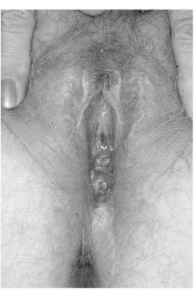

Fig 15.23 Cyclic vulvovaginitis. Low-grade erythema of the vulva with no evidence of vaginal discharge. The patient complained of postcoital irritation, with swelling and itching around the time of menses. She had asthma and often took oral corticosteroids. A potassium hydroxide (KOH) smear and vaginal culture revealed *Candida albicans*.

Oral medications (e.g. ketoconazole or fluconazole) may be given daily for a short time (1–4 weeks for keto-conazole), then tapered to an intermittent dosage (e.g. every other day) for 2–4 months. When using keto-conazole, liver function tests should be performed monthly. Fluconazole is metabolized by the kidneys, not the liver, and so is less toxic. Once- or twice-weekly doses of fluconazole appear to be effective in suppress-ing *Candida* (see also Chapter 12).

LICHEN SIMPLEX CHRONICUS

Lichen simplex chronicus (LSC) (15.24, 15.25) is the most common of the vulvar dermatoses that contain the word 'lichen' in their name. This word is merely descriptive, and was originally used to evoke the botan-ical image of a rough-surfaced lichen heaped on a smooth-surfaced rock, emphasizing the difference in textures.

Each of the three skin diseases (LSC, lichen sclerosus (LS), and lichen planus (LP) is histologically distinct. A dermatopathologist should have no difficulty in distin-guishing between them, so it is reasonable to do a biopsy if the diagnosis is unclear. With experience, however, one can usually be distinguished from another clinically. A pathology report noting 'hyperkeratosis and parakeratosis' usually refers to LSC. This non-specific description is of the cutaneous change seen when the patient has persistently rubbed or scratched the skin, producing the secondary change called licheni-fication. Clinically, the skin has a leathery appearance with accentuation of the normal skin markings.

LICHEN PLANUS

LP (15.26, 15.27) occurs in two forms. The classic description of the 'five Ps: Purple Polygonal Papules and Plaques that are Pruritic' is characteristic of lesions on the inner wrists and anterior shins. The second, or erosive, form of LP occurs on the oral and vulvar mucosa, and patients with this form of LP may have lesions only in this area (see Chapter 18).

LICHEN SCLEROSUS

LS (15.28, 15.29) is one of the major vulvar dermatoses. The epidermis is atrophic, white, and wrinkly, whereas the dermis is thickened and sclerotic. Typically, the disorder involves only the vulva and/or anus (keyhole pattern), but the trunk can also be involved with morphea-like white plaques. If a patient has had vulvar LS for many years, it is less likely that she will develop generalized LS (see Chapter 17).

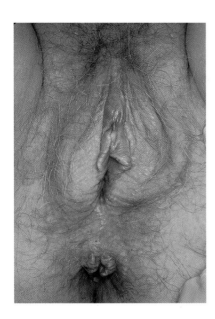

Fig 15.24 Lichen simplex chronicus (LSC). Leathery changes of intertriginous skin as a result of chronic rubbing and scratching. Note the accentuation of normal skin lines, one of the hallmarks of LSC.

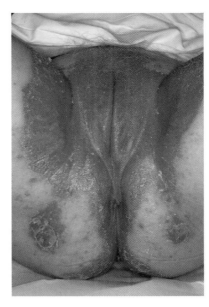

Fig 15.25 Psoriasis. Thick plaques with typical intense erythema and peripheral scale. Unlike the plaques of LSC, psoriasis plaques are sharply demarcated and patients rarely complain of itching.

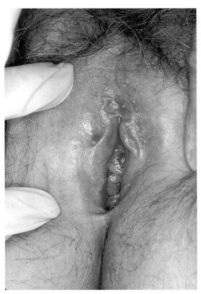

Fig 15.26 Vulvar lichen planus. Mucosal erosions of the vulvar vestibule and vagina are typical. Apparent loss of the posterior labia minora is due to adhesions developing after cutaneous erosion. This patient also had oral lesions of LP.

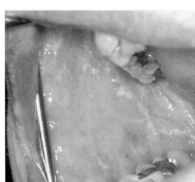

Fig 15.27 Oral lichen planus. Thin whitish linear streaks (Wickham striae) are seen on the buccal mucosa. This is not usually symptomatic unless it is erosive.

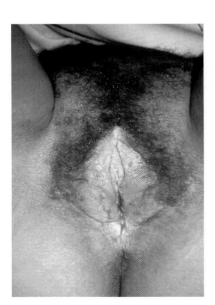

Fig 15.28 Lichen sclerosus. In this patient there is well-circumscribed, white, atrophic change around the vulva and perianal skin. It can be distinguished from vitiligo because the latter is simply loss of pigment from normal skin, whereas LS also shows scarring and loss of vulvar architecture.

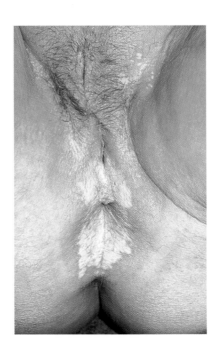

Fig 15.29 Lichen sclerosus. This patient complained of itching. Lichen simplex chronicus is superimposed on LS; biopsies confirmed LS and hyperkeratosis. There was no evidence of malignancy.

PAGET'S DISEASE

A biopsy should be taken of any solitary plaques (15.30, 15.31) of oozy, crusted skin on the nipple or perianal area which grow slowly, do not itch, and do not resolve with topical steroids. While the diagnosis is usually suspected with chronic unilateral nipple eczema, perineal lesions are often neglected for months or years. Several punch biopsies should be taken from representative areas, preferably the thickest part of a lesion rather than the base of an ulcer or erosion.

About 15% of patients have an associated carcinoma of an adjacent structure, such as the cervix, rectum, or urinary tract. The prognosis is worse in this group. In the remaining 85% of patients, tumor cells arise within the epidermis of the adjacent skin, probably from apocrine duct cells or pluripotential germinative cells.

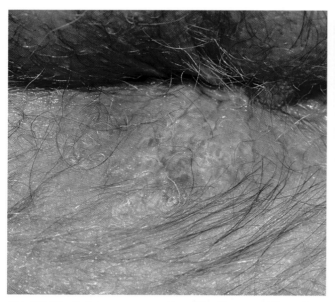

Fig 15.30 Extramammary Paget's disease. There is an asymmetric plaque of red, papillomatous skin with a white, oozy surface. There were no symptoms and the lesion did not respond to topical steroids.

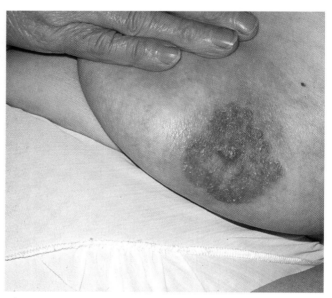

Fig 15.31 Paget's disease of the breast. An eczematous appearance is seen here, involving the entire areola and spreading on to the skin of the breast. This disorder should be suspected in any unilateral eruption affecting the areolar skin.

FURTHER READING

Gardner, S.S. and McKay, M. Seborrhea, psoriasis and the papulosquamous dermatoses. *Prim. Care* 1989; **16**: 739–763.

McKay, M. Vulvodynia and pruritus vulvae. *Semin. Dermatol.* 1989; **8**: 40–47.

McKay, M. Vulvar dermatoses: common problems in dermatological and gynaecological practice. *Br. J. Clin. Pract.* 1990; **44**: 5–10.

McKay, M. Vulvar dermatoses. *Clin. Obstet. Gynecol.* 1991; **34**: 614–629.

McKay, M. Vulvitis and vulvovaginitis: cutaneous considerations. *Am. J. Obstet. Gynecol.* 1991; **165**: 1176–1182.

Pincus, S.H. Vulvar dermatoses and pruritus vulvae. *Dermatol. Clin.* 1992; **10**: 297–308.

Pincus, S.H. and McKay, M. Disorders of the female genitalia. In: Fitzpatrick, T.B., Eisen, A.Z., Wolfe, K. *et al.* (eds) *Dermatology in General Medicine*, 4th edn, pp. 1463–1482. McGraw-Hill, New York, 1993.

Ridley, C.M. General dermatological conditons and dermatoses of the vulva. In: Ridley, C.M. (ed.) pp. 138–211. *The Vulva*, Churchill Livingstone, Edinburgh, 1988.

Sobel, J. Recurrent vulvovaginal candidiasis: a prospective study of the efficacy of maintenance ketoconazole therapy. *N. Engl. J. Med.* 1986; **315**: 1455–1458.

Witkin, S.S., Jeremias, J. and Ledger, W.J. A localized vaginal allergic response in women with recurrent vaginitis. *J. Allergy Clin. Immunol.* 1988; **81**: 412–416.

ACKNOWLEDGEMENTS

Figure **15.1** is reproduced from G.M. Levene and S.K. Goolamali *Diagnostic Picture Tests in Dermatology* (Fig 127), Wolfe, London, 1986. Figures **15.6**, **15.29**, **15.30** and **15.31** are reproduced from C.M. Lawrence and N.H. Cox *Color Atlas and Text of Physical Signs in Dermatology* (Figs 8.15, 8.29, 8.20 and 8.18), Wolfe, London, 2001.

16

Pediatric Vulvar Disorders

Lynette J. Margesson

INTRODUCTION

Vulvar conditions in children cover a wide spectrum from congenital malformations at birth to infections, dermatoses, and tumors. Nondermatologic disorders are more familiar to specialized gynecologists and pediatricians, and a full discussion of these conditions is beyond the scope of this text.

CONGENITAL VULVAR ABNORMALITIES

Female genital tract developmental abnormalities are rare. They may involve only the external genitalia or the whole reproductive tract (**Tables 16.1 and 16.2**).

Table 16.1 Ambiguous External Genitalia.

Clinical Presentation	Diagnosis	Etiology
Clitoromegaly or variable phallus formation with ventral opening; variable labial formation with opening or scrotal sac formation	Female pseudohermaphroditism	
	Congenital adrenal hyperplasia	Enzyme deficiencies (recessive) 21-Hydroxylase deficiency 11-Hydroxylase deficiency (rare)
	Exogenous hormones	Maternal androgen-producing tumor Exogenous androgen exposure
	Male pseudohermaphroditism	Lack of gonadotropin Enzyme defect in testosterone synthesis Target tissue androgen receptor defect

Table 16.2 Abnormalities of External Genitalia.

Disorder	Clinical Presentation	Treatment
Labial hypertrophy	Long labia minora	Surgery
Hymenal abnormalities	Variable hymenal openings or complete closure	Surgery
Hemangiomas	Red to purple vascular macules, nodules or plaques with or without erosions or ulcers	Reassurance; laser destruction if extensive or ulcerated
Congenital nevi	Small to large pigmented macules or plaques	Biopsy if atypical; close observation as indicated

AMBIGUOUS EXTERNAL GENITALIA

At birth the external genital organs in these conditions are not clearly male or female, thus the sexual ambiguity. Eighty per cent of ambiguous genitalia are due to female pseudohermaphroditism with androgenization of the female fetus. Such infants present with an enlarged phallus alone or associated with some degree of labioscrotal fusion because of a recessive, congenital, enzymatic defect of adrenal steroid biosynthesis. The most common cause is a 21-hydroxylase deficiency resulting in overproduction of cortisol and androgen that virilizes the fetal female external genitalia. Rarely this can be caused by an 11-hydroxylase deficiency. Exogenous hormones from a maternal androgen-producing tumor or maternal ingestion of androgen can also produce virilization of a female fetus.

Male pseudohermaphroditism is far less common and represents only 15% of cases of ambiguous genitalia. In these infants there is a partial or complete block in the masculinization process during development due to a lack of gonadotropins, an enzyme defect in testosterone biosynthesis, or a defect in the androgen-dependent target tissue response (e.g. androgen receptor defect or 5α-reductase deficiency). Clinically these children present with varying degrees of phallus formation, scrotal sac formation, and with varying genital openings (**16.1, 16.2**)[1–3].

CONGENITAL LABIAL HYPERTROPHY

This relatively common developmental abnormality is typically noted at puberty. Rarely it may develop as a result of lymphostasis or chronic physical pulling of the labia. Patients complain of difficulties with hygiene or local irritation with physical activity and sexual intercourse. The problem may be unilateral or bilateral labial hypertrophy (**16.3**). Treatment is with surgical reduction.

LABIAL ADHESIONS

Superficial fusion of the labia minora occurs in 1–2% of prepubertal girls. The cause is unknown, but local irritation, poor hygiene, and lack of estrogen may all play a role. The result is inflammation and adherence of skin surfaces on either side of the labia, giving the vulva a flat appearance. Localized posterior fusion is often

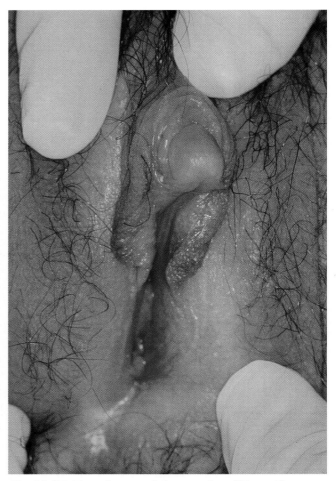

Fig 16.1B Female pseudohermaphroditism. Eleven-year-old girl with increasing facial hirsutism, thick genital hair, normal vagina, and clitoromegaly as a result of a 21-hydroxylase deficiency.

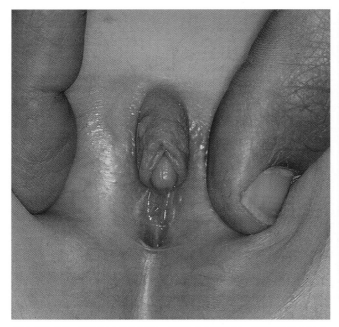

Fig 16.1A Clitoromegaly with posterior labial fusion in congenital adrenal hyperplasia. An example of female pseudohermaphroditism.

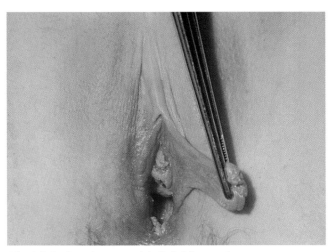

Fig 16.3 An elongated left labium minus.

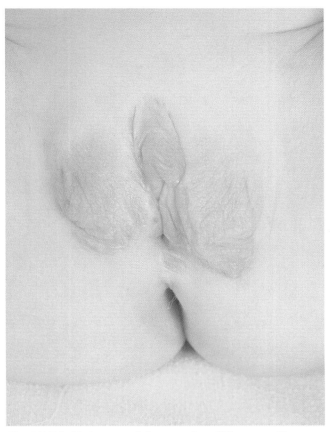

Fig 16.2A Male pseudohermaphroditism resulting from partial androgen insensitivity. Ambiguous genitalia in a XY child raised as a girl.

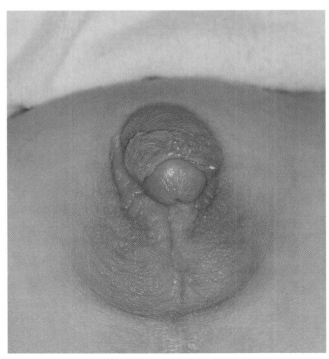

Fig 16.2B Ambiguous genitalia in an XY child with partial androgen insensitivity.

minor and asymptomatic. Although this condition resolves spontaneously with pubertal estrogenization, extensive fusion leaving only a pinhole opening can result in urine retention, urinary infection, genital irritation and burning. The first line of therapy is topical conjugated estrogen (Premarin) cream, used two or three times a day with gentle traction for 2–3 weeks if needed. If extensive, surgery may be required[4,5].

HYMENAL ABNORMALITIES

The thin membrane of connective tissue over the entrance of the vagina normally has a round or crescentric opening. There can be several microperforations, giving a cribriform or fenestrated hymen or no opening at all (imperforate hymen). With only partial opening of the hymen at the time of menarche, secretions can be trapped, resulting in infection. An imperforate hymen presents as primary amenorrhea and there will be lower abdominal discomfort with progressive cyclical lower abdominal pain (**16.4, 16.5**). Treatment is surgical[6,7].

HEMANGIOMAS

These benign tumors of the vascular endothelium form pink to reddish papules or plaques anywhere on the body. They usually start within a few days of birth with a flat red patch that gradually enlarges. The proliferative phase of rapid growth lasts about 8–9 months, then the lesion stabilizes for a time. Involution starts at about 2 years of age, and most of these lesions flatten into a whitish scar by the age of 9 years. Symptoms depend on size: large tumors can create considerable discomfort with ulcers, erosions, and bleeding (**16.6, 16.7**). Treatment depends on the degree of involvement, and asymptomatic lesions may be left to resolve on their

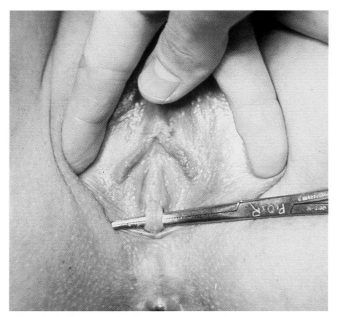

Fig 16.4 Septate hymen.

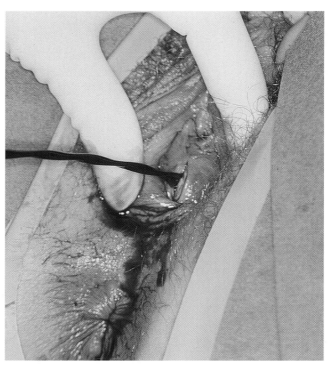

Fig 16.5B The patient's imperforate hymen is incised and the old blood is released.

MELANOCYTIC NEVI

Congenital melanocytic nevi ('moles') are not common on the vulvar area. These melanocytic hamartomas may present at birth, when they can show varying degrees of pigmentation. Flat tan-colored macules or papules with varying degrees of pigmentation often grow and darken as the patient ages. Giant nevi present at birth (**16.8**) are more likely to undergo malignant transformation (*see Chapter 21*). Most nevi have little risk of malignant change, although rare cases of vulvar malignant melanoma have been reported in prepubertal girls. Treatment is observation with biopsy of suspicious lesions.

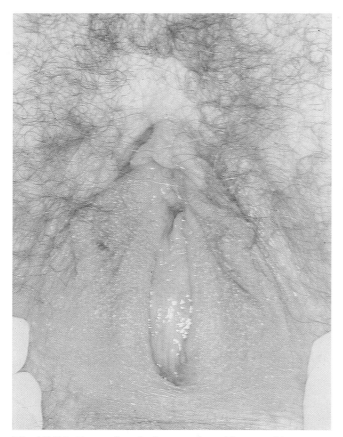

Fig 16.5A Imperforate hymen in a 13-year-old adolescent who presented with an acute abdomen.

DERMATOSES

Many childhood vulvar problems (**Table 16.3**) are associated with estrogen depletion. Estrogen is an important factor in vulvar skin reactions to irritants, infection, etc. Estrogen is present and effective in the first 1–2 years of life and then again at 2–3 years before menarche. In the interval, the vulva is relatively estrogen deficient. In this state, the labia minora and the vulvar epithelia are thin with a visible capillary network. This tissue is susceptible to irritants but resistant to candida. The estrogenized vulva is resilient and pink with plump labia minora and well-moisturized vulvar introital epithelium. This results in resistance to chemical and physical irritants but increased susceptibility to candida.

own. Hemangiomas that bleed or ulcerate may respond well to early pulsed dye laser treatment. For severe cases, co-management with a pediatric dermatologist is recommended[8–10].

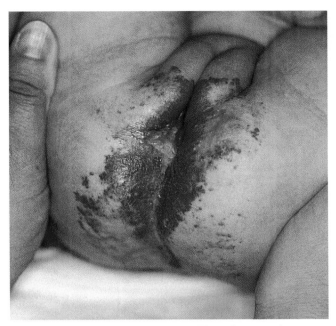

Fig 16.6A Rapidly growing capillary hemangioma on the perineum in a 1-month-old baby.

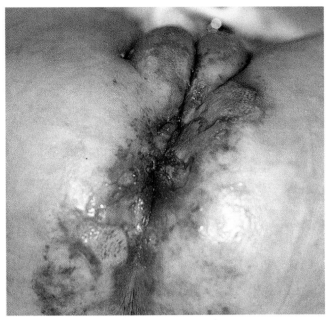

Fig 16.6B Capillary hemangioma. Eroded ulcerated perineum 10 days after the second pulsed dye laser treatment. The first pulsed dye laser treatment was at 1 month of age, the second at 2 months of age. After laser treatment, the ulcers resolved in 3 weeks. The interval between **Figs. 16.6 A** and **B** was six weeks.

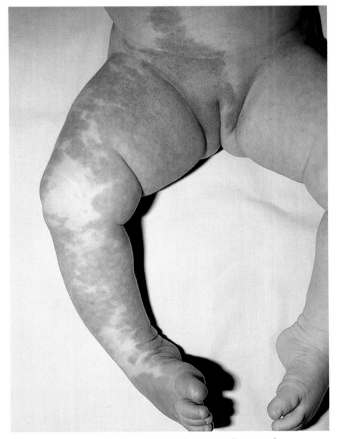

Fig 16.7 Extensive capillary hemangioma of abdomen, vulva, and right leg in a 2-month-old with Klippel–Trenaunay–Weber syndrome.

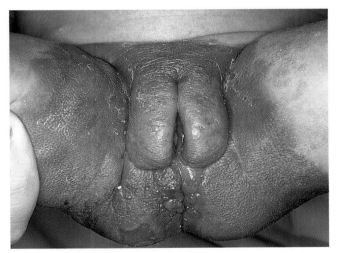

Fig 16.8 Giant pigmented nevus of the vulva, thighs, and buttocks in a baby with an eroded diaper rash.

CONTACT DERMATITIS

Contact dermatitis is an inflammation resulting from an external agent that acts either as an irritant or an allergen, producing an erythematous rash that may be either acute (blistering, itching, oozing), subacute (chapping and cracking), or chronic (thickening of the skin with varying degrees of scaling). Primary irritant contact dermatitis is due to prolonged or repeated exposure to an irritating product such as soap, detergent, or urine. There is no immune reactivity. The problem is the caustic or physically irritating effect of the substance.

123

Table 16.3 Pediatric Vulvar Dermatoses.

Condition	Clinical Presentation	Etiology	Other Areas/Factors	Diagnosis	Treatment
Dermatoses					
Diaper dermatitis	Red, shiny to chapped skin on friction areas, spares skin folds	Moisture from urine and feces; candida may be present	Tendency to eczema or psoriasis	Clinical pattern; culture for secondary infection	Stop irritants; improve hygiene, 1% hydrocortisone ointment with imidazole cream
Irritant dermatitis	Inflamed red chapped skin on friction areas	Detergents, soaps, baby wipes, etc.	Other skin areas where irritant used	Clinical pattern; family with psoriasis or atopy	Stop irritants, hydrocortisone ointment
Allergic contact dermatitis	Red itchy rash at sites of allergen contact	Allergen: neomycin, benzocaine, perfume	Other skin areas where allergen used	Careful history, patch test	Stop allergen, triamcinolone 0.1% ointment
Seborrheic dermatitis	Greasy, red-orange skin rash in folds	*Malassezia furfur*	Scalp, face, behind ears, other body folds; note secondary infection	Clinical pattern	Hydrocortisone 1% plus imidazole cream
Psoriasis	Patchy to diffuse red rash, including folds	Familial defect in skin, worsened with friction and moisture	Scalp, ears, elbows, knees, other body folds, gluteal cleft; nail pits	Clinical pattern plus family history	Hydrocortisone 2.5% ointment; brief treatments with more potent topical steroids; treat secondary infection
Atopic dermatitis	Patchy, red, chapped rash on labial and gluteal surfaces	Familial with history eczema, hay fever, asthma	Itchy red rashes on face, extensor areas in babies; antecubital fossae, behind knees in older children	Clinical pattern; note family history of atopy	Stop irritants; corticosteroid ointment of low to mid potency
Lichen sclerosus	White papules and plaques in 'figure of, eight' pattern, vulvar and perianal; purpura	Autoimmune	Other area of skin in 20%	Clinical pattern; biopsy	Potent to superpotent steroid for 6–12 weeks then maintenance 2–3 times per week; close follow-up; condition chronic
Vitiligo	White groin skin	Autoimmune	In folds of skin, face, hands, elbows, knees	Clinical pattern; biopsy	Mild topical steroid; observation

Table 16.3 (continued)

Condition	Clinical Presentation	Etiology	Other Areas/Factors	Diagnosis	Treatment
Infections					
Bacterial					
Impetigo	Superficial erosions and peeling red areas	*Staphylococcus aureus*, sometimes streptococcus	May be localized, primary, secondary, or generalized	Culture positive for organism	Dicloxacillin, cephalosporin, erythromycin
Streptococcal infection	Acute, burning, red, eroded perianal or vulvar rash	*Streptococcus pyogenes*		Culture for streptococci	Penicillin
Viral					
Herpes simplex	Acute onset of burning with groups of vesicles and pustules; erosions; recurrent	Herpes simplex virus (HSV)	Primary or secondary	Culture for HSV	Valaciclovir, famciclovir
Molluscum	Itchy, skin-colored, umbilicated papules isolated and in groups	Molluscum contagiosum	Other lesions scattered on body	Clinical; smear	Local destruction or removal (e.g. cryotherapy)
Genital warts	Warty papules or cauliflower-like clusters	Human papilloma virus (HPV)	May have warts on hands, etc.	Clinical	Observation only or local destruction
Fungal					
Candida	Itchy, burning rash, erythematous, swollen patches with satellite pustules	*Candida albicans*	Often associated with diaper dermatitis	KOH; culture	Topical imidazole cream
Tinea	Circular, red rash around edges of genitalia	*Trichophyton rubrum* or *T. mentagrophytes*	Scaling fourth–fifth toewebs in parent or sibling with tinea	KOH; culture	Topical imidazole or terbinafine cream
Infestations					
Scabies	Scattered, very itchy papules and nodules; look for tracks	*Sarcoptes scabiei*	Tracks in finger web; other family member itchy	Scrapings of tracks for KOH	Permethrin 5% cream; 6% precipitated sulfur in petrolatum for infants
Pinworms	Nocturnal scratching with perianal and vulvar itching	*Enterobius vermicularis*	Other siblings itchy	Examine cellophane tape applied to perianal area for eggs	Oral mebendazole, pyrantel pamoate

Table 16.3 (continued)

Condition	Clinical Presentation	Etiology	Other Areas/Factors	Diagnosis	Treatment
Foreign Body Vaginitis	Red, itchy, sore vulva with discharge	Foreign body; peanut, tissue	None	Locate foreign body	Remove foreign body, treat secondary infection
Sexual Abuse	Red, sore vulva with or without discharge; lacerations or distortion of introitus or anus	Typically male with access to child, not necessarily father	May have bruises in acute cases, chronic cases may develop psychologic problems	Requires investigative team if suspected by physician	Remove offender from household or remove child from situation; counseling
Bullous Diseases					
Linear IgA disease	Large, tense bullae in circular plaques around the groin	Autoimmune	Perioral; may be generalized	Biopsy for histology and immunofluorescence	Avlosulfone
Erythema multiforme	Blisters and erosions	Hypersensitivity to infection (e.g., HSV) or drugs (e.g., sulfa)	Mucous membranes, mouth, eye; may be generalized	Clinical pattern; biopsy	Minor disease – no treatment; major blistering – early use of cyclosporine
Miscellaneous					
Acrodermatitis enteropathica	Sharply marginated, vesicular, pustular, or eroded rash in the groin	Zinc deficiency	Perioral, nose, eyes, flexural areas; hair loss, irritability; diarrhea	Serum zinc levels	Oral zinc
Langerhans cell histiocytosis	Greasy, yellowish, scaly papules in the diaper area and buttock; sometimes ulcers, purpura	Excess proliferation of histiocytes	In infants, brown, crusted areas, scalp, ears, perioral; fever, anemia, etc.; erosive papules with vulvar ulcers; associated diabetes insipidus		Chemotherapy
Labial adhesions	Variable fusion of labia minora	Local inflammation	None	Clinical	Topical estrogen

Allergic contact dermatitis is caused by a specific allergy (type IV delayed hypersensitivity reaction) to even a small amount of a chemical substance such as a perfume, benzocaine, neomycin, or poison ivy.

DIAPER DERMATITIS

This term means any dermatitis in the diaper area, usually due to repeated contact irritation from urine, feces, and friction. This is an irritant contact dermatitis. The skin is pink to red, with shiny or chapped areas of friction. Typically the mons pubis, the labia majora, and the buttocks are irritated; the skin folds are usually spared (16.9). Children with atopic dermatitis or a tendency to psoriasis are more susceptible. With time, the skin may become red, chapped, and raw, and open ulcers may develop. There can be secondary infection with bacteria, and candida may produce scattered satellite pustules or desquamating papules. Treatment is to stop the irritants and change the diapers more frequently and, when possible, to leave the infant without a diaper. Routine cleansing should be with bare or vinyl-gloved hands in plain water with a soapless cleanser (Cetaphil, unscented Dove bar or super-fatted soap) followed by a thorough rinse, then 1% hydrocortisone ointment. An imidazole cream (clotrimazole) is added for secondary yeast. For diaper changes away from home, cleansing with plain water or light mineral oil on a soft tissue or cotton ball is permitted[11-14].

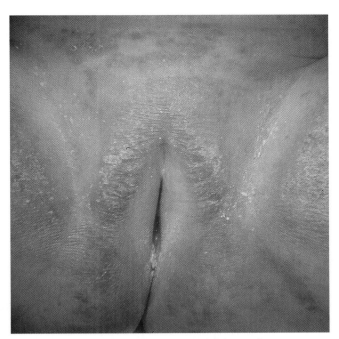

Fig 16.9 Extensive diaper dermatitis on the mons, convex surfaces of the labia majora and thighs with erythema, scaling and crusting, in a 6-month-old baby girl. Note sparing of the folds, secondary candida, and satellite pustules in the mons area.

IRRITANT DERMATITIS

Repeated exposure to caustic or physically irritating products, usually a soap, cleanser, or wipe, may result in erythema, itching, and burning of the labia and perineum. Children who have this problem often have a background history of atopic dermatitis or eczema, making their skin more sensitive and more easily irritated. Most vulvar contact dermatitis in children is due to irritants. The irritants must be stopped and topical hydrocortisone ointment prescribed.

ALLERGIC CONTACT DERMATITIS

This is not a common problem in children but, when an allergen is found, the most common causes are neomycin, benzocaine, perfumes, or preservatives such as parabens. There may be an acute blistering eruption or a more chronic picture with erythema and scaling. Other sites may be involved if the allergen has been applied elsewhere. Patch testing may confirm the diagnosis. The condition improves over 2–3 weeks when the allergen is stopped. For severe reactions, a topical corticosteroid ointment such as triamcinolone 0.1% might be needed. If there is blistering, systemic prednisone could be used starting at 1 mg/kg daily for 4–5 days, then decreasing over 10 days[15,16].

SEBORRHEIC DERMATITIS

This condition produces erythema and greasy, yellowish scaling around the vulva and the labiocrural fold. In the first 3 months of life, it is often associated with a greasy dandruff-type rash in the scalp, around the ears, down the central part of the face and in the axillae. The cause is *Malassezia furfur*, a lipophilic yeast that thrives in areas rich in sebaceous glands that have been activated before birth by maternal or placental hormones. Treatment is with topical imidazole, such as clotrimazole cream with 1% hydrocortisone added[17,18].

PSORIASIS

Psoriasis is a common, hereditary, red, scaly rash of the skin. In infants, it may present as a very chronic diaper dermatitis with bright red, sharply outlined plaques around the mons pubis and labia majora through the perineum and often up into the gluteal cleft with varying degrees of fissuring. In young infants it often presents as a diaper dermatitis that is resistant to therapy. The white scales typical of psoriasis are not present in body folds, but may occur on elbows, knees, or scalp. A history of psoriasis in other family members helps to make a diagnosis[19].

Treatment involves avoiding trauma such as irritating soaps and lotions, and keeping the area cool and dry. Cleanse with a bland product such as Cetaphil Cleanser or unscented Dove bar or super-fatted soap. A low-potency steroid ointment (hydrocortisone 2.5%, desonide 0.05%) may be used twice a day initially, tapering to 1% hydrocortisone ointment with response. In more severe cases, mid- or even high-potency topical corticosteroids may be necessary for 1–2 weeks followed by long-term management with intermittent use of low-dose hydrocortisone. For concurrent secondary infection antiyeast topical clotrimazole and antibacterial mupirocin ointment may be needed.

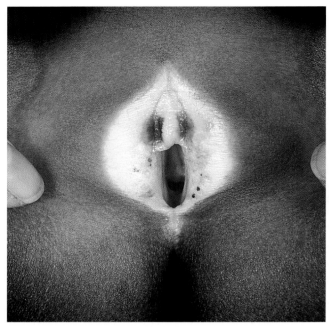

Fig 16.10 Hypopigmentation in lichen sclerosus.

ATOPIC DERMATITIS

This eruption consists of a dry itchy rash that occurs in patients who usually have a personal or family history of one or more atopic conditions: asthma, allergic rhinitis ('hay fever'), or eczema. Infants with atopic dermatitis present with chapped red skin over the cheeks and extensor surfaces of the extremities. Older children show involvement of the antecubital fossae and behind the knees. Although the typical rash is not common on the vulva, children with a background history of atopic dermatitis have much more easily irritated skin and may present with an irritant dermatitis or a diaper dermatitis. Treatment combines avoidance of harsh, irritating soaps and cleansers, and the application of mild corticosteroid ointment, as for diaper dermatitis[20,21]. (For general management principles, *see also Chapter 10*.)

LICHEN SCLEROSUS

This is a common cutaneous disease of the genitalia resulting in marked hypopigmentation, skin thinning, and scarring. Some 10–15% of cases develop in childhood, as early as 1–2 years of age. Often, the condition is asymptomatic, but some children chronically rub and scratch, developing raw areas with pain and dysuria. Typical lesions are small white papules that coalesce into plaques of parchment-like skin. Lesions of the vulva, perineum, and perianal area may be patchy or form a white 'figure of eight' pattern. With time, there is atrophy with loss of labia, scarring, and loss of the clitoris. Scratching causes purpura, erosions, and excoriations which can be confused with sexual abuse (**16.10, 16.11**). Treatment is with topical steroids[22-24]. (For further discussion, *see Chapter 17*.)

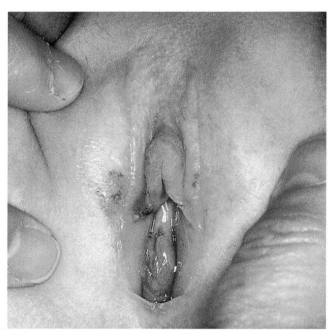

Fig 16.11 Lichen sclerosus. Scarring and mild purpura (mistaken for sexual abuse).

VITILIGO

This is an acquired loss of pigmentation on an autoimmune basis that often starts in childhood, although it may occur at any age. Irregularly shaped patches of hypopigmentation present around orifices (eyes, nose, mouth, vagina) and over the extensor areas of the body, most usually sites of trauma such as the backs of the hands, knees, and body folds. There is no surface skin change, just color loss. For involvement of the vulvar area, no treatment may be recommended[25,26].

INFECTIONS
BACTERIAL

IMPETIGO

Staphylococcus aureus infection may occur anywhere on the body. It may involve the vulva and perineum in a young child, producing fragile blisters that rapidly evolve into red, round, desquamating erosions. Associated streptococcal infection may produce honey-colored crusts that may be dry or wet and oozy. Treatment with oral antibiotics is recommended: dicloxacillin, a cephalosporin, or erythromycin. For localized lesions, topical mupirocin ointment can be used[27,28].

STREPTOCOCCAL INFECTION

Streptococcus (*Group A β-hemolytic streptococcus*) can cause a vulvitis and/or a perianal dermatitis. Classically, there is a burning, red rash in the perianal area that may be associated with perianal fissures and painful defecation. Similar lesions may be seen in the vulvar area. Treatment is with oral penicillin or erythromycin and topical mupirocin ointment. This can be mistaken for chronic yeast, eczema, psoriasis, pinworms, or abuse[29,30].

VIRAL

(See also Chapter 11)

HERPES SIMPLEX (HSV)

Although herpes simplex infections are usually found in sexually active adolescents or adults, they can sometimes present in infancy or childhood, acquired from an infected caregiver or from sexual abuse. In primary disease there are groups of small vesicles or pustules with surrounding erythema and swelling (**16.12**). These rapidly break, leaving tender erosions that may last for up to 2 weeks. Recurrence is common, and these lesions are much less extensive, with a shorter duration, mild swelling, a few vesicles, pustules, and erosions. If herpes is suspected, immunofluorescent testing or culture for HSV typing should be done. If a genital lesion is due to HSV type I, there is less chance of recurrence; HSV type II has a recurrence rate of up to 95%. Treatment is with oral valaciclovir or famciclovir. In children with eczema, herpes simplex can spread all over the body, yielding 'eczema herpeticum'[31].

MOLLUSCUM CONTAGIOSUM

This poxvirus infection of the skin presents with discrete, firm, 1–3 mm flesh-colored, umbilicated papules anywhere on the body (**16.13**). It spreads in children and

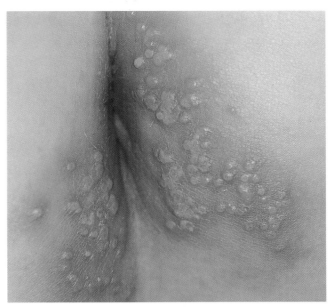

Fig 16.12 Primary herpes simplex on the perineum and buttocks with groups of vesicles.

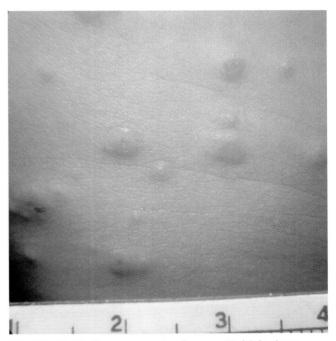

Fig 16.13 Molluscum contagiosum. Multiple dome-shaped pink papules.

young adults by autoinoculation or through fomites. A few initial papules are easily spread by scratching. Diagnosis is usually clinical but a direct smear of the whitish material from one of these lesions can confirm the diagnosis. Mollusca resolve spontaneously in 6–12 months in young children, so no treatment may be needed. Treatment involves destruction with liquid nitrogen, curettage, or keratolytics[32].

GENITAL WARTS

Genital warts are caused by human papilloma virus (HPV). As the incidence of condylomata has increased in adults, there has been an increased prevalence of this condition in children, and oral or laryngeal lesions may be transmitted to infants through the birth canal. Transmission of the virus is usually from infected caregivers or rarely autoinoculation from warts on the hand. HPV is the most common sexually transmitted disease in the United States. Because 30–40% of cases in children have been associated with abuse, this must always be ruled out (*see below*). Pinhead-sized papules that grow into filiform papules or plaques are usually found symmetrically on opposing skin surfaces. The lesions can be small or large, skin-colored to reddish, and may grow into confluent, cauliflower-like clusters. Diagnosis is based on the clinical picture.

No treatment for HPV guarantees a cure. In young children, treatment may be simple observation. Treatment is undertaken if there are symptoms of itching, burning, spread, disfiguring lesions, or bleeding. Treatment with caustic agents, as in adults, is not usually appropriate. If treatment is needed, electrodessication or laser surgery under general anesthesia is recommended. Imiquimod, a new topical agent, is currently being studied in children[33–35].

EPSTEIN–BARR VIRUS

Epstein–Barr virus may occasionally cause vulvar ulcers in teenagers and young adults. The illness has an inconsistent prodrome of fever, fatigue, sore throat, oral ulcers, and swollen cervical glands. Deep, painful, punched-out ulcerations appear on the labia minora. Lesions are solitary or multiple, with erythema surrounding an irregular grayish ulcer base with a serous or purulent exudate (**16.14**). The differential diagnosis includes herpes simplex, aphthosis, human immunodeficiency virus, and Behçet's disease. Diagnosis is made by serology for Epstein–Barr virus. This shows an increase in immunoglobulin (Ig) M levels that may not be detectable until 1–2 weeks after the onset of infection. The monospot test may be negative[36,37].

Treatment is symptomatic. The lesions resolve in 2 weeks.

FUNGAL

CANDIDA

The majority of vulvovaginal yeast infections are due to *Candida albicans*, often occurring after a course of oral antibiotics. Candida vulvitis is red swollen, and itchy with satellite pustules (**16.15**) or dried collarette scales; fissures are common. Secondary candidal infection can occur in diaper dermatitis or other chronically moist rashes, and should be a consideration in vulvar

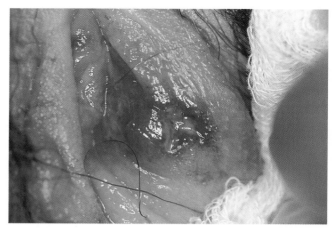

Fig 16.14 Epstein–Barr virus infection. A painful punched-out, red-rimmed vulvar ulcer in a 15-year-old girl.

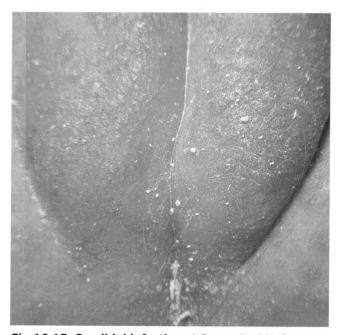

Fig 16.15 Candidal infection. A 3-month-old infant with red swollen labia majora studded with red papules and pustules of candida, with satellite pustules.

dermatitis not responding to topical steroid therapy. Diagnosis is made by culture or potassium hydroxide examination showing the budding yeast. Topical imidazole cream, miconazole or clotrimazole, is the routine treatment. If vaginitis is also present, oral fluconazole is indicated.

TINEA

This superficial dermatophyte infection is not common in infancy or childhood. Commonly called 'ringworm', tinea may occur on other areas of the body as well. It presents as a circular, red rash that clears in the center to leave a ring-like pattern. Diagnosis is made with a potassium hydroxide examination showing the typical fungal hyphae. Treatment is with a topical imidazole or terbinafine cream[38].

INFESTATIONS
SCABIES

This highly contagious skin infestation is caused by the mite, *Sarcoptes scabiei*. It is spread among children and young adults by skin-to-skin contact and also by fomites. Patients describe intense itching that is worse at night. It typically involves body creases, fingerwebs, wrists, axillary and groin folds. Tiny linear tracks may be visible in fingerwebs or groin areas, but excoriated and sometimes crusted papules are typical. In infants, there may be nodules on the mons pubis, thighs, buttocks, axillae, and even the head and scalp. For diagnosis, a scraping for examination under oil or potassium hydroxide must be taken from papules or tracks. Treatment for children aged 2 months or more is with topical 5% permethrin cream. For younger infants, 6% precipitated sulfur in a petrolatum base can be applied twice a day for 2 days. All members of a household and those in contact with the child must be treated to avoid reinfestation by this very contagious mite[39,40].

PINWORMS

Infestation by *Enterobius vermicularis* results in nocturnal itching as the worms migrate out onto the perianal skin to lay eggs. Clinically there may be little rash, but scratching may result in chronic skin changes from the perianal area to the vulva. Diagnosis is made with cellophane tape applied to the perianal skin in the morning to collect the eggs, which are identified in a potassium hydroxide preparation. The whole family needs treatment with oral mebendazole or pyrantel pamoate with one retreatment 1–2 weeks later.

VAGINITIS DUE TO A FOREIGN BODY

Foreign bodies inserted into the vagina may cause chronic vaginal discharge with an irritant dermatitis. The whole vaginal area may be swollen with varying degrees of burning, itching, and soreness. Treatment for infection does not help. Finding the foreign body may be difficult: the most common cause is toilet tissue (16.16), but peanuts or any small item may be found. In young adults, forgotten tampons can cause copious malodorous discharge with secondary infection. Treatment is removal of the foreign body[41].

SEXUAL ABUSE

Sexual abuse refers to the involvement of a dependent, developing, immature child or adolescent in sexual activities by an older person for their own sexual stimulation or for gratification of others as in pornography and prostitution. Sexual abuse involves the misuse of power and the betrayal of the child's trust by an older person. Activities involve oral–genital, genital–genital, and anogenital contact including exhibitionism, sexual kissing, fondling, masturbation, and digital or object penetration of the vagina and anus.

Being aware that sexual abuse is a common problem should alert the physician to consider this when examining children who present with an infection (condyloma acuminata, herpes simplex, gonorrhea, or other sexually transmitted diseases) or with trauma that includes scratches, bruising or hematoma, lacerations or fissures (16.17), scars, and gaping of the anus or introitus[42].

Major long-term problems occur with sexually abused children and their families. Obtaining an appropriate history requires interview techniques used by specially trained personnel. Children who have been abused are often withdrawn or may even act out. Sometimes they are very anxious to please.

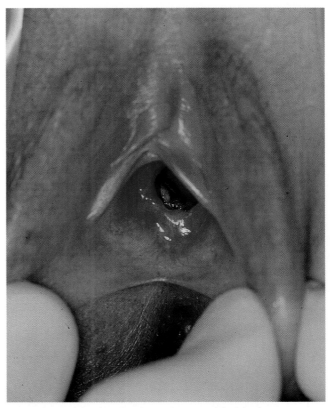

Fig 16.16 Foreign body. A 6-year-old girl who presented with scratching, pain, bleeding, and vaginal discharge showed an intact red hymenal ring with tissue paper just inside the opening.

131

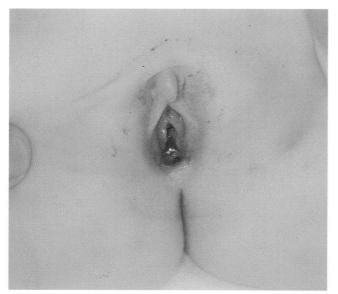

Fig 16.17 Perineal laceration through the hymen and posterior fossa with hematoma formation and surrounding bruising in a raped child.

Examination of these children involves specific local protocols. Total physical examination is necessary plus cultures for all sexually transmitted infections where indicated. The hymen is usually annular or crescentic in normal children. A variety of notches and bumps is quite normal. After trauma there can be a variety of different changes. Healed transections of the hymen between 4 and 8 o'clock (**16.18**), and sometimes partial hymenal loss, may be seen. Unfortunately, the majority of sexual abuse cases may not show evidence of forcible trauma, as abrasions, lacerations, and bruising often heal quickly. If there is any question, children should be referred to the proper authorities. Treatment is best managed by a specialized team.

BULLOUS DISEASES

LINEAR IgA DISEASE

Linear IgA disease of children is also referred to as chronic bullous disease of childhood. This condition presents as tense bullae and erosions forming an annular

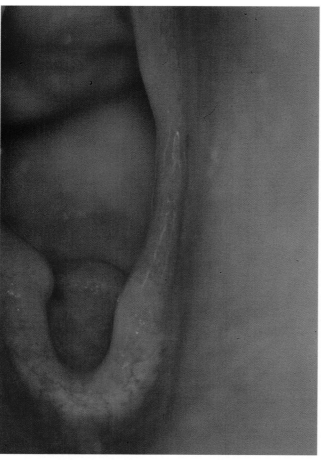

Fig 16.18A Sexual abuse. A 5-year-old girl with a typical keyhole deformity of the hymenal ring at the 6 o'clock position resulting from penetration, laceration, and scarring.

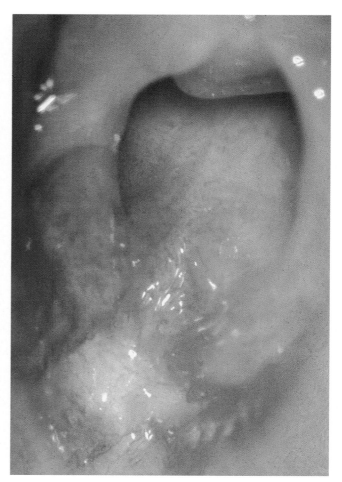

Fig 16.18B Sexual abuse. Same child as in **16.18A** (supine position) 2 years later with a healed scar at 6 o'clock.

pattern around the vulva and perianal areas. Often these are grouped in dense clusters with varying degrees of erosions and scarring. The condition can become generalized[43,44]. (*See Chapter 18.*)

ERYTHEMA MULTIFORME

Erythema multiforme is a cutaneous hypersensitivity phenomenon due to infections (herpes simplex, streptococcus, and mycoplasma in children) and sometimes drugs (sulfonamides, penicillin or phenytoin). In the mild form, there are few or no symptoms, and crops of iris or target-like lesions (**16.19**) erupt anywhere on the body, classically on hands, feet, elbows, knees, and perineum. These disappear gradually over 2–4 weeks and no treatment may be needed. A more severe form (Stevens–Johnson syndrome) presents with extensive blistering that can start in the mouth, around the eyes, and in the perianal area. There is painful erythema and erosion with blistering (**16.20**), which can become generalized with fever and malaise.

Treatment is to identify and manage the underlying condition. Local care is nonspecific. If the condition is diagnosed within 72 hours, systemic corticosteroids may be instituted, but this treatment is controversial. A rare, serious, variant is toxic epidermal necrolysis (TEN). This is usually due to drugs and starts in the body folds of the groin and around the neck, with a full-thickness desquamation. This can be life threatening; aggressive early therapy with cyclosporine (5 mg/kg/day) is warranted[45–47].

MISCELLANEOUS

ACRODERMATITIS ENTEROPATHICA

This is a rare disorder. It may be caused by a zinc-deficient diet or an autosomal recessive failure of zinc absorption. The clinical triad consists of (1) acral dermatitis (scaling, redness, and irritation) with (2) diarrhea and (3) alopecia. These infants present with diarrhea and persistent 'diaper rash' that will not heal (**16.21**). A variable degree of anorexia, alopecia, and irritability is associated. A low serum zinc level makes the diagnosis. Management is with oral zinc gluconate[48,49].

LANGERHANS CELL HISTIOCYTOSIS

This neoplastic proliferation of the epidermal Langerhans cells can result in a spectrum of disease in

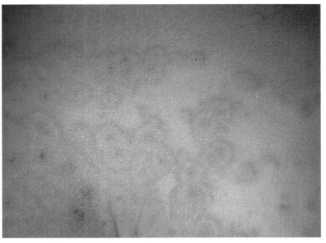

Fig 16.19 Erythema multiforme. Iris or target lesions on the buttock.

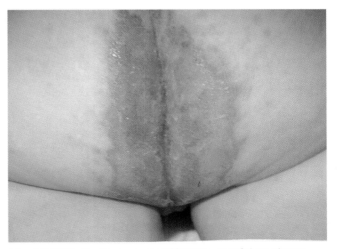

Fig 16.20A Erythema multiforme. Painful erythema and erosion of the perianal skin extending to the vulva.

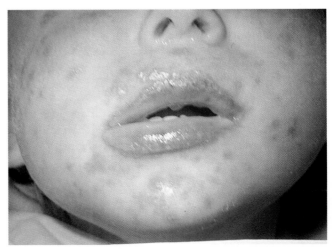

Fig 16.20B Erythema multiforme. Same child as in **16.20A**, showing blistering and erosion of the lips and face.

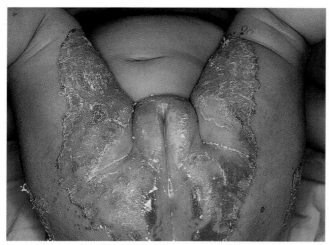

Fig 16.21 Acrodermatitis enteropathica. Well demarcated scaling plaque of the whole diaper area with erosion and perianal bleeding.

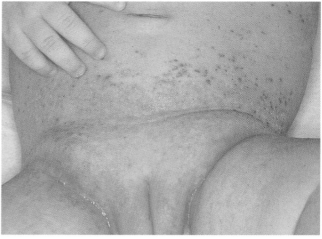

Fig 16.22 Langerhans cell histiocytosis. A baby with extensive erythematous papules on the lower abdomen, vulva, and inner thighs with petechiae and erosion in the inguinal crease.

young children or young adults. In infants, it is often confused with a seborrheic dermatitis or chronic diaper dermatitis. Brown crusty papules can involve the diaper area (16.22) and buttock, as well as the scalp, behind the ears and even around the mouth. In older children there may be extensive hemorrhagic

papules on the labia minora and majora, sometimes forming confluent sheets and/or well-defined ulcers. Diagnosis is by histopathological examination. Management depends on the case and may include prednisone and/or chemotherapy. Co-management with a pediatric oncologist is suggested[50,51].

REFERENCES

1 Hewitt, J., Pelisse, M., and Paniel, B. J. Congenital malformations of the vulva. In: Hewitt, J., Pelisse, M., and Paniel, B. J. (eds) *Diseases of the Vulva*, pp. 64–71. McGraw-Hill, London, 1991.

2 Ridley, C. M. and Neill, S. M. Embryology and congenital abnormalities of the vulva. In: Ridley, C. M., and Neill, S. M. (eds) *The Vulva*, pp. 1–36. Blackwell Scientific, Oxford, 1999.

3 Margesson, L. J. Congenital malformations of the vulva. In: Fisher, B. K., and Margesson, L. J. (eds) *Genital Skin Disorders: Diagnosis and Treatment*, pp. 108–114. Mosby, St Louis, 1998.

4 Capraro, V. J. and Greenberg, H. Adhesions of the labia minora. A study of 50 patients. *Obstet. Gynecol.* 1972; **39**: 65–69.

5 Jenkinson, S. D. and MacKinnon, A. E. Spontaneous separation of fused labia minora in prepubertal girls. *B.M.J.* 1984; **289**: 160–161.

6 Pokorny, S. F., Pediatric vulvovaginitis. In: Kaufman, R. H., and Faro, S. (eds) *Benign Diseases of the Vulva and Vagina*, Vol. 4, pp. 47–49. Mosby, St Louis, 1994.

7 Anania, C. and Malinak, L. R. Developmental anomalies of the vulva and vagina. In: Kaufman, R. H., and Faro, S. (eds) *Benign Diseases of the Vulva and Vagina*, Vol. 3, pp. 26–29. Mosby, St, Louis, 1994.

8 Powell, J. Update on hemangiomas and vascular malformations. *Curr. Opin. Pediatr.* 1999; **11**: 457–463.

9 Richards, K. A. and Garden, J. M. The pulsed dye laser for cutaneous vascular and non-vascular lesions. *Semin. Cutan. Med. Surg.* 2000; **19** (4): 276–286.

10 Drolet, B. A., Esterly, M. B., and Frieden, I. J. Hemangiomas in children. *N. Engl. J. Med.* 1999; **341**: 173–181.

11 Hayakawa, R. and Matsunaga, K. Common conditions and factors associated with diaper dermatitis. *Pediatrician* 1987; **14**(Suppl 1): 18–20.

12 Boiko, S. Treatment of diaper dermatitis. *Dermatol. Clin.* 1999; **17**: 235–240.

13 Sires, U. I. and Mallory, S. B. Diaper dermatitis. How to treat and prevent. *Postgrad. Med.* 1995; **98**: 79–84, 86.

14 Singalavanija, S. and Frieden, I. J. Diaper dermatitis. *Pediatr. Rev.* 1995; **16**: 142–147.

15 Marren, P., Wojnarowska, F., and Powell, S. Allergic contact dermatitis and vulvar dermatoses. *Br. J. Dermatol.* 1992; **126**: 52–56.

16 Lynch, P. J. and Edwards, L., Pediatric problems: red plaques with eczematous features. In: Lynch, P. J., and Edwards, L. (eds) *Genital Dermatology*, pp. 27–55. Churchill Livingstone, New York, 1994.

17 Skinner, R. B., Jr., Noah, P. W., Zanolli, M. D., *et al*. The pathogenic role of microbes in seborrheic dermatitis. *Arch. Dermatol.* 1986; **122**: 16–17.

18 Heng, M. C., Henderson, C. L., Barker, D. C., *et al*. Correlation of *Pityrosporum ovale* density with clinical severity of seborrheic dermatitis as assessed by a simplified technique. *J. Am. Acad. Dermatol.* 1990; **23**: 82–86.

19 Farber, E. M. and Nall, L., Childhood psoriasis. *Cutis* 1999; **64**: 309–314.

20 Boerio, M., Brooker, J., Freese, L., *et al*. Pediatric dermatology: that itchy scaly rash. *Nurs. Clin. North Am.* 2000; **35**: 147–157.

21 Wuthrich, B., Clinical aspects, epidemiology, and prognosis of atopic dermatitis. *Ann. Allergy Asthma Immunol.* 1999; **83**: 464–470.

22 Fischer, G. and Rogers, M. Treatment of childhood vulvar lichen sclerosus with potent topical corticosteroid. *Pediatr. Dermatol.* 1997; **14**: 235–238.

23 Ridley, C. M. Genital lichen sclerosus (lichen sclerosus et atrophicus) in childhood and adolescence. *J. R. Soc. Med.* 1993; **86**: 69–75.

24 Meffert, J. J., Davis, B. M., and Grimwood, R. E. Lichen sclerosus. *J. Am. Acad. Dermatol.* 1995; **32**: 393–416.

25 Halder, R. M., Childhood vitiligo. *Clin. Dermatol.* 1997; **15**: 899–906.

26 Janniger, C. K. Childhood vitiligo. *Cutis* 1993; **51**: 25–28.

27 Darmstadt, G. L. and Lane, A. T. Impetigo: an overview. *Pediatr. Dermatol.* 1994; **11**: 293–303.

28 Hogan, P. Pediatric dermatology. Impetigo. *Aust. Fam. Physician* 1998; **27**: 735–736.

29 Krol, A. L., Perianal streptococcal dermatitis. *Pediatr. Dermatol.* 1990; **7**: 97–100.

30 Kokx, N. P., Comstock, J. A., and Facklam, R. R. Streptococcal perianal disease in children. *Pediatrics* 1987; **80**: 659–663.

31 Annunziato, P. W. and Gershon, A. Herpes simplex virus infections. *Pediatr. Rev.* 1996; **17**: 415–423.

32 Smith, K. J., Yeager, J., and Skelton, H. Molluscum contagiosum: its clinical, histopathologic, and immunohistochemical spectrum. *Int. J. Dermatol.* 1999; **38**: 664–672.

33 Moscicki, A. B. Human papilloma virus infection in adolescence. *Pediatr. Clin. North. Am.* 1999; **46**: 783–807.

34 Obalek, S., Jablonska, S., and Orth, G. Anogenital warts in children. *Clin. Dermatol.* 1997; **15**: 369–376.

35 Armstrong, D. K. and Handley, J. M. Anogenital warts in prepubertal children: pathogenesis, HPV typing and management. *Int. J STD AIDS* 1997; **8**: 78–81.

36 Sisson, B. A. and Glick, L. Genital ulceration as a presenting manifestation of infectious mononucleosis. *J. Pediatr. Adolesc. Gynecol.* 1998; **11**: 185–187.

37 Taylor, S., Drake, S. M., Dedicoat, M. J., *et al.* Genital ulcers associated with acute Epstein–Barr virus infection. *Sex. Transm. Infect.* 1998; **74**: 296–297.

38 Rudy, S. J. Superficial fungal infections in children and adolescents. *Nurse Pract. Forum.* 1999; **10**: 56–66.

39 Chosidow, O. Scabies and Pediculosis. *Lancet* 2000; **355**: 819–826.

40 Peterson, C. M. and Eichenfield, L. F. Scabies. *Pediatr. Ann.* 1996; **25**: 97–100.

41 Pokorny, S. F. Long-term intravaginal presence of foreign bodies in children. A preliminary study. *J. Reprod. Med.* 1994; **39**: 931–935.

42 Kaufman, R. H. and Faro, S. Traumatic lesions of the vulva and vagina. In: Kaufman, R. H. and Faro, S. (eds) *Benign Diseases of the Vulva and Vagina*, 4th edn, pp. 391–396. Mosby, St Louis 1994.

43 Rabinowitz, L. G. and Esterly, N. B. Inflammatory bullous diseases in children. *Dermatol. Clin.* 1993; **11** 565–581.

44 Kulthanan, K., Akaraphanth, R., Piamphongsant, T., *et al.* Linear IgA bullous dermatosis of childhood: a long-term study. *J. Med. Assoc. Thai.* 1999; **82**: 707–712.

45 Martin Mateos, M. A., Roldan Ros, A. and Munoz-Lopez, F. Erythema multiforme: a review of twenty cases. *Allergol. Immunopathol. (Madr.)* 1998; **26**: 283–287.

46 Weston, W. L. What is erythema multiforme? *Pediatr. Ann.* 1996; **25**: 106–109.

47 Arevalo, J. M., Lorente, J. A., Gonzalez-Herrada, C. *et al.* Treatment of toxic epidermalnecrolysis with cyclosporin A. *J. Trauma* 2000; **48** (3): 473–478.

48 Kumar, S., Sehgal, V. N. and Sharma, R. C. Acrodermatitis enteropathica. *J. Dermatol.* 1997; **24**: 135–136.

49 Piela, Z., Szuber, M., Mach, B., *et al.* Zinc deficiency in exclusively breast-fed infants. *Cutis* 1998; **61**: 197–200.

50 Huang, F. and Arceci, R. The histiocytoses of infancy. *Semin. Perinatol.* 1999; **23**: 319–331.

51 Howarth, D. M., Gilchrist, G. S., Mullan B. P., *et al.* Langerhans cell histiocytosis: diagnosis, natural history, management, and outcome. *Cancer* 1999; **85**: 2278–2290.

ACKNOWLEDGEMENTS

Figures **16.1B**, **16.2B**, **16.4**, **16.5A**, **16.5B**, **16.16**, **16.17**, **16.18A**, **16.18B** are reproduced by kind permission of Dr G. D. Oliver, Hospital for Sick Children, University of Toronto, Toronto, Canada. Figure **16.3** is reproduced by kind permission of Dr P. Bryson, Kingston General Hospital, Queen's University, Kingston, Canada. Figure **16.10** is reproduced by kind permission of Dr B. Krafchik, Hospital for Sick Children, University of Toronto, Toronto, Canada. Figures **16.1–16.8**, **16.10–16.12**, **16.16–16.22** are from *Genital Skin Disorders: Diagnosis and Treatment*. Fisher, B. K. and Margesson, L. J. (eds) Mosby, St Louis, 1998.

17 Vulvar Lichen Sclerosus

Sallie M. Neill

HISTORICAL BACKGROUND

Lichen sclerosus (LS) is a chronic inflammatory skin condition, which was first recognized as a possible variant of lichen planus by Hallopeau and Darier in 1887[1]. It can occur at any site, but has a predilection for the genital area, particularly in women. Coincidentally, in 1885, Breisky[2] reported the same condition in the vulva, but called it kraurosis vulvae. This led to the misunderstanding that vulvar lichen sclerosus and kraurosis vulvae were two separate conditions. The nomenclature was further complicated for many years by the additional terms, leucoplakic vulvitis and vulvar dystrophy. The International Society for the Study of Vulvovaginal Disease (ISSVD), together with the International Society of Gynecological Pathologists (ISGYP), has recommended changes in the terminology of vulvar disorders (*see Chapter 14*). As a result, the terms vulvar dystrophy, leucoplakic vulvitis, and kraurosis vulvae have been abandoned, and lichen sclerosus et atrophicus has been abbreviated to lichen sclerosus.

INCIDENCE

The incidence of LS is unknown, but the prevalence has been suggested as between 1 in 300 and 1 in 1000 of the population[3]. There are two ages at which the disease is most likely to present: prepuberty and perimenopause or postmenopause. However, asymptomatic disease is sometimes found coincidentally in women of childbearing age at routine examination and cervical screening.

ETIOLOGY

The etiology is uncertain. In some instances, LS may be familial, affecting siblings and their parents in successive generations. There have been conflicting reports of an association with some types of human leucocyte antigen (HLA)[4,5]. A possible association with autoimmune disease was first recognized when raised titers of antibodies to thyroid cytoplasm and gastric parietal cells were found in patients with lichen sclerosus[6]. Further reports, supporting an autoimmune basis, have described patients with LS and at least one other autoimmune disease, including vitiligo, lichen planus, morphea, bullous pemphigoid, and thyroid disease[7]. Other immunologic evidence includes fibrin and immunoglobulin deposited along the basement membrane of involved skin[8] and increased numbers of epidermal Langerhans cells[9].

SYMPTOMS

The major symptom of LS is intense pruritus, so severe that it interferes with sleep. In some cases, however, the patient may be unaware of the disease for years. Pain is an unusual feature, but does occur with deep excoriations and erosions, particularly if there is secondary bacterial infection and cellulitis. Dyspareunia may be a presenting symptom in patients with atrophy posteriorly around the fourchette and consequent tearing at the posterior labial commissure (17.1). In children with perianal involvement, painful fissuring of the skin occurs with defecation and the child may then present with constipation.

CLINICAL SIGNS

The initial cutaneous signs are usually pallor, thickening, and excoriations (17.2), with edema and shrinkage of the labia minora (17.3). The skin gradually begins to lose all pigmentation and acquires a thinned texture with characteristic 'cigarette paper' wrinkling (17.4). There may be purpura and extensive ecchymoses (17.5), which occasionally have been mistaken for signs of child abuse. Blistering may be seen, but it is an

137

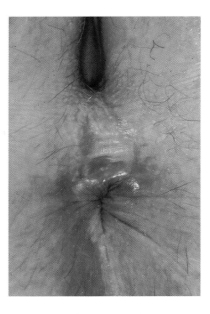

Fig 17.1 Lichen sclerosus, affecting the posterior labial commissure, with involvement of the perianal skin and fissuring.

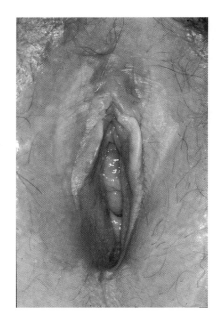

Fig 17.4 Lichen sclerosus. The epithelium in the interlabial sulci shows the characteristic pallor with involvement of the labia minora and clitoral hood.

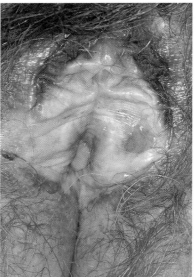

Fig 17.2 Lichen sclerosus. Excoriations on a background of lichen sclerosus.

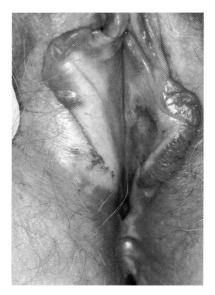

Fig 17.5 Lichen sclerosus. There is some asymmetry with more pallor on the left but there is purpura on both sides.

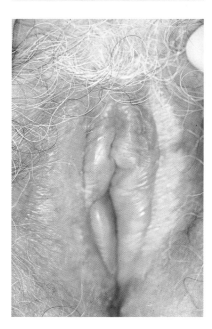

Fig 17.3 Lichen sclerosus. There is marked edema of the labia minora and clitoral hood. The skin of the interlabial sulci is white, shiny, and atrophic.

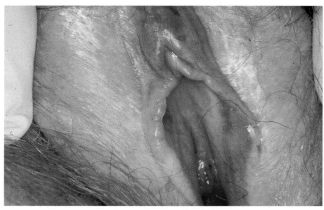

Fig 17.6 Lichen sclerosus. The clitoral hood is swollen and small blisters can be seen on the edge of the left labium minus.

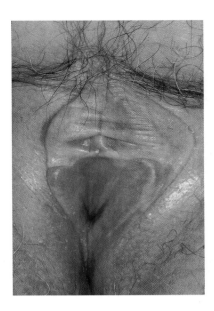

Fig 17.7 Lichen sclerosus. There is fusion anteriorly, with burying of the clitoris. The labia minora are merging into the surrounding epithelium and there is some narrowing of the introitus.

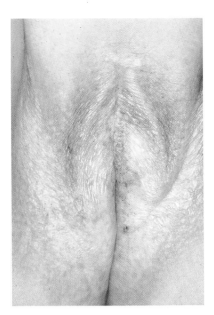

Fig 17.10 Lichen sclerosus. extending laterally into the genitocrural folds.

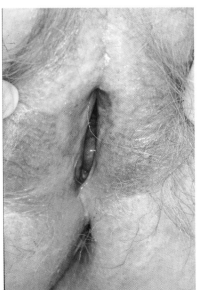

Fig 17.8 Lichen sclerosus. The vulva has become featureless with loss of the labia minora, clitoris, and clitoral hood.

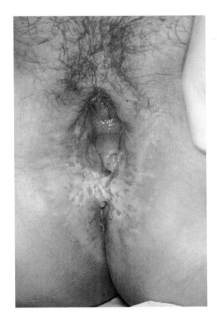

Fig 17.11 Lichen sclerosus. The skin across the posterior labial commissure is hyperkeratotic with multiple small erosions.

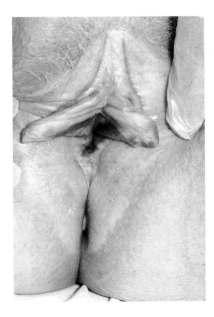

Fig 17.9 Lichen sclerosus. involving the vulva and extending perianally.

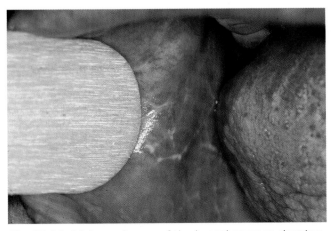

Fig 17.12 Lichen planus of the buccal mucosa showing white striae in a reticulate pattern.

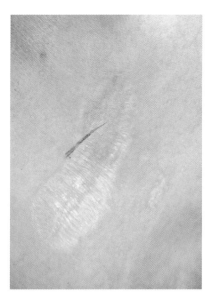

Fig 17.13 Lichen sclerosus. affecting the lateral chest wall.

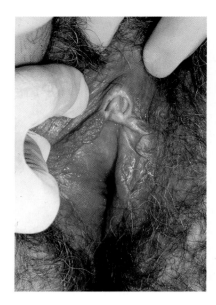

Fig 17.14 Localized lichen sclerosus. The area involved may be very limited, as in this patient who has disease localized to the clitoris only.

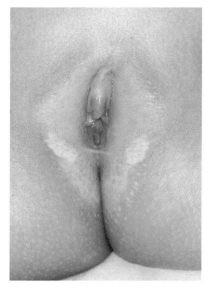

Fig 17.15 Childhood lichen sclerosus. There is generalized pallor of the vulvar skin with two symmetrically arranged plaques of LS either side posteriorly. The clitoral area is also involved.

unusual feature (17.6). Eventually, there is architectural distortion with burying of the clitoris under the clitoral hood, loss of the labia minora, and in some cases narrowing of the introitus (17.7). There may be a total loss of all the characteristic anatomic features (17.8). Lesions of LS often extend around the perianal area (17.9) or into the genitocrural folds (17.10). The skin in some cases has a warty appearance due to marked hyperkeratosis (17.11). LS does not seem to occur on the noncornified stratified squamous epithelium (i.e. mucosal surfaces), and thus the vagina is spared. There are anecdotal reports of oral involvement, but many of these are probably of lichen planus (LP) (17.12). Extragenital involvement occurs in less than one-third of patients (17.13). There is also an increased incidence of morphea and LP occurring at extragenital sites in patients with vulvar LS. Postinflammatory hyperpigmentation is uncommon.

NATURAL HISTORY

There is great variation in the both the area of skin involved and the architectural distortion associated with this condition. Some women have only minimal changes (17.14), while in other cases all structure is lost with almost total closure of the introital opening. It was originally believed that childhood LS (17.15) went into remission spontaneously with the onset of puberty, but this is no longer believed to be the case. Many patients continue to have the disease, although they may become less symptomatic[10]. It is also interesting that many patients improve with pregnancy, but relapse in the puerperium.

About 6% or less of patients with LS develop squamous cell carcinoma. However, LS has been found in about 60% of vulvectomy specimens with squamous cell carcinoma[3,11]. Thus, there would seem to be an important association between LS and squamous cell carcinoma, even though malignancy is a rare complication.

HISTOLOGY

The typical histologic appearance is of a thinned, effaced epidermis, with or without overlying hyperkeratosis. In the reticular dermis, immediately beneath the epidermis, there is a band of homogenized collagen. An associated lymphocytic infiltrate may be seen just beneath this abnormal dermis (17.16). Occasionally, this lymphocytic infiltrate is high in the dermis, occurring along the dermoepidermal junction with areas of basal cell liquefaction very similar to the changes seen in LP[12]. In some cases, the epidermis is acanthotic showing squamous cell hyperplasia (17.17). It has been suggested that this type of LS is more frequently associated with squamous cell carcinoma[13].

MANAGEMENT

MEDICAL TREATMENT

The treatment of choice is a potent topical cortico-steroid, such as clobetasol propionate 0.05%[14,15]. This is applied to the affected skin once daily, usually at night, until there is an improvement, after which the frequency may be reduced. Patient information and instruction leaflets are invaluable (*see Appendix D*). It is important to monitor the amount of topical steroid used. A 30-g tube should last for 3 months, but considerably less is required once the disease is under control.

Despite the high incidence of LS at the time of the menopause and the apparent improvement in pregnancy, both systemic and topical exogenous estrogens are ineffective in the treatment of LS. Similarly, topical testosterone acts mainly as an emollient and is no longer a recognized treatment[16]. There are anecdotal reports of systemic and topical synthetic retinoids being used to treat vulvar LS, but these should probably be reserved for cases that fail to respond to topical corticosteroids. A soap substitute, such as aqueous cream, is a useful adjunct to treatment. (*See also Appendix D*).

Psychosexual problems are common in all women with a chronic vulval disorder and these must also be addressed and managed appropriately.

SURGERY

A vulvectomy should never be performed for treatment of this disorder, except when it has been complicated by the development of squamous cell carcinoma (**17.18**). Otherwise, surgical intervention should be considered only when there has been such extensive labial fusion that it is necessary to reconstruct an introitus (**17.19**). A vulvoperineoplasty is then recommended which uses part of the posterior vaginal wall in the reconstruction[17].

DIFFERENTIAL DIAGNOSIS

Leucoplakia literally means 'white plaque' and is not a diagnosis in itself. It should therefore be used only as a descriptive term. LS is only one of a number of conditions that result in the formation of white plaques associated with pallor, scarring, and atrophy. These changes can also represent the endstage appearance for many dermatoses (*see Chapter 15 and Appendix A*).

Human papillomavirus infection, with or without vulvar intraepithelial neoplasia (**17.20**), may be another cause of white plaques, but atrophy and scarring would be unusual features. A skin biopsy is always important to establish a definite diagnosis, and direct and indirect immunofluorescence studies should be done if there are diagnostic difficulties.

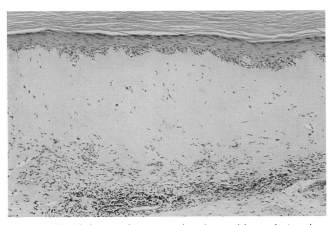

Fig 17.16 Lichen sclerosus showing epidermal atrophy with overlying hyperkeratosis, and upper dermal hyalinization with cellular infiltrate underneath (hematoxylin and eosin stain; ×40).

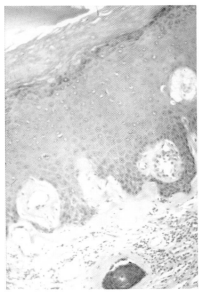

Fig 17.17 Lichen sclerosus with squamous cell hyperplasia.

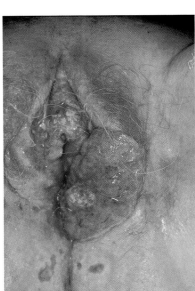

Fig 17.18 Squamous cell carcinoma. A large fungating squamous cell carcinoma arising on a background of lichen sclerosus which had not previously been diagnosed or treated.

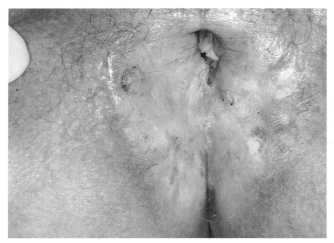

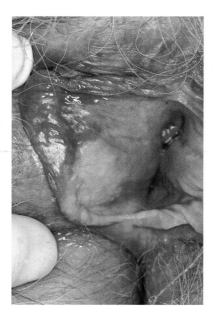

Fig 17.20 Vulvar intraepithelial neoplasia (VIN). Biopsy of these white plaques showed full-thickness atypia, consistent with the diagnosis of VIN 3.

Fig 17.19 Severe introital narrowing which interfered with micturition. In younger patients, this degree of narrowing would affect sexual function.

REFERENCES

1 Hallopeau, H. Lichen plan sclereux. *Ann. Dermatol. Syph* 1889; **10**: 447–449.

2 Breisky, D. Uber kraurosis vulvae. *Z. Heilkd.* 1885; **6**: 69–80.

3 Wallace, H.J. Lichen sclerosus et atrophicus. *Trans. St. John's Dermatol. Soc.* 1971; **57**: 9–30.

4 Purcell, K.G., Spencer, L.V. Simpson, P.M. *et al.* HLA antigens in lichen sclerosus et atrophicus. *Arch. Dermatol.* 1990; **126**: 1043–1045.

5 Marren, P., Yell, J., Charnock, F.M., Bunce, M., Welsh, K. and Wojnarowska, F. The association between lichen sclerosus and antigens of the HLA system. *Br. J. Dermatol.* 1995; **132**: 197–203.

6 Goolamali, S.K., Barnes, E.W., Irvine, W.J. *et al.* Organ specific antibodies in patients with lichen sclerosus. *BMJ* 1974; **iv**: 78–79.

7 Harrington, C.I. and Dunsmore, I.R. An investigation into the incidence of autoimmune disorders in patients with lichen sclerosus et atrophicus. *Br. J. Dermatol.* 1981; **104**: 563–566.

8 Dickie, R.J., Horne, C.H.W. and Sutherland, H.W. Direct evidence of localized immunologic damage in lichen sclerosus et atrophicus. *J. Clin. Pathol.* 1982; **35**: 1395–1399.

9 Carli, P., Cattaneo, A., Pimpenelli N. *et al.* Immunohistochemical evidence of skin immune system involvement in vulvar lichen sclerosus et atrophicus. *Dermatologica* 1991; **182**: 18–22.

10 Ridley, C.M. Genital lichen sclerosus (lichen sclerosus et atrophicus) in childhood and adolescence. *J. R. Soc. Med.* 1993; **86**: 69–75.

11 Leibowitch, M., Neill, S., Pelisse, M. *et al.* The epithelial changes associated with squamous cell carcinoma of the vulva: a review of the clinical, histologic and viral findings in 78 women. *Br. J. Obstet. Gynaecol.* 1990; **97**: 1135–1139.

12 Hewitt, J. Histologic criteria for lichen sclerosus of the vulva. *J. Reprod. Med.* 1986; **31**: 781–787.

13 Rodke, G., Friedrich, E.G. and Wilkinson, E.J. Malignant potential of mixed vulvar dystrophy (lichen sclerosus associated with squamous cell hyperplasia). *J. Reprod. Med.* 1988; **33**: 545–550.

14 Dalziel, K., Millard, P.R. and Wojnarowska, F. The treatment of vulvar lichen sclerosus with a very potent topical corticosteroid (clobetasol propionate 0.05%) cream. *Br. J. Dermatol.* 1991; **124**: 461–464.

15 Garzon M.C. and Paller, A.S. Ultrapotent topical corticosteroid treatment of childhood lichen sclerosus. *Arch Dermatol.* 1999; **135**: 525–528.

16 Sideri, M., Origoni, M., Spinaci, L. and Ferrari, A. Topical testosterone in the treatment of vulvar lichen sclerosus. *Int. J. Gynecol. Obstet.* 1994; **46**: 53–56.

17 Paniel, B.J., Truc, J.B., de Margerie, V. *et al.* La vulvo-perineoplastie. *J. Gynecol. Obstet. Biol. Reprod.* 1984; **1**: 91–99.

FURTHER READING

Meffert, J.J., Davis, B.M. and Grimwood, R.E. Lichen sclerosus. *J. Am. Acad. Dermatol.* 1995; **32**: 393–416.

Powell, J.J. and Wojnarowska, F. Lichen sclerosus. *Lancet* 1999; **353**: 1777–1783.

Ridley, C.M. and Neill, S.M. (eds) *The Vulva* pp. 154–164, Blackwell Science, Oxford, 1999.

Erosive Vulvovaginitis

Jenny Powell,
Pauline Marren,
Fenella Wojnarowska

INTRODUCTION

Erosion is the loss of epidermis and can occur with a variety of inflammatory, bullous, infective, and neoplastic processes. Ulcers are deeper than erosions, although there is overlap in the differential diagnoses (*see Appendix A*). The diagnosis is often difficult, as lesions may be generalized, limited to the mucosa, or localized to one region. Examination of the vulvovaginal area must be combined with a thorough examination of the skin, all mucosal sites, hair, and nails, so that the diagnosis is based on a complete clinical picture.

Erosions may form after loss of a fragile blister roof (pemphigus), or from intertriginous rubbing and breakage of tense, otherwise resilient, blisters (bullous pemphigoid). Excoriations are erosions caused by the patient's scratching, and are a secondary feature of pruritic vulvar dermatoses. In the past 20 years much progress has been made in the differential diagnosis of 'erosive vaginitis', but some cases still cannot be classified clinically or histologically. These idiopathic forms may represent vulvovaginal diseases that have not yet been characterized.

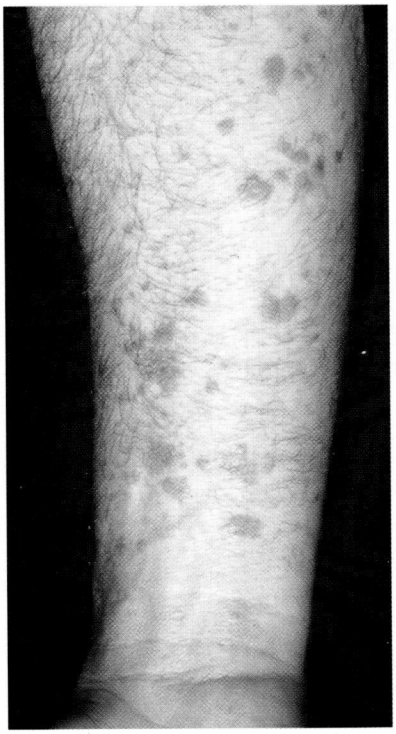

Fig 18.1 Lichen planus with typical violaceous papules on skin surfaces.

EROSIVE LICHEN PLANUS

Mucocutaneous lichen planus (LP) is a relatively common condition characterized by itchy, violaceous, flat-topped papules on cutaneous sites (18.1), and less clearly defined reticulated, white, and violaceous papules or plaques on oral and vulvar skin (18.2, 18.3). Cutaneous and oral involvement is common, either separately or in combination, but the frequency of benign vulvar involvement is unknown[1].

Erosive LP (vulvovaginal–gingival syndrome) was first described as a distinct entity in 1982[2], and is a well-defined, although uncommon, subgroup. The characteristic feature is severe and extensive erosion and ulceration at affected sites with a prolonged clinical course, which represents a difficult therapeutic challenge. It is generally believed that patients with erosive LP will develop erosive lesions at vulvar, vaginal, and gingival sites, at some stage in the course of the disease, although all three sites may not be affected concurrently. The site of the presenting symptom determines the referring physician: gynecologist, dermatologist, or oral specialist. About 20–30% of these patients also have evidence of cutaneous or scalp involvement. Lichen planus is uncommon in childhood[3], and the erosive form has been described only in adults.

Vulvar symptoms are often severe and unremitting. Patients complain of pain, burning, dyspareunia, and postcoital bleeding. Frank erosion may vary in degree and extent, but can encircle the entire introitus (18.4, 18.5). Eroded areas may be surrounded by a reticulated

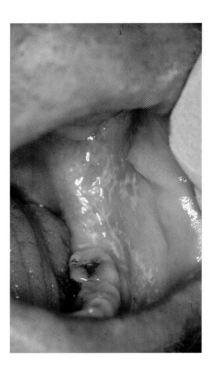

Fig 18.2 Lichen planus of the mouth with reticulated white plaques.

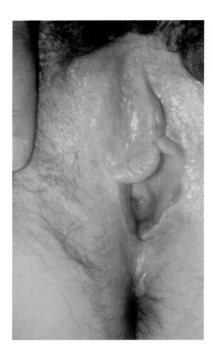

Fig 18.3 Lichen planus of the vulva with violaceous border.

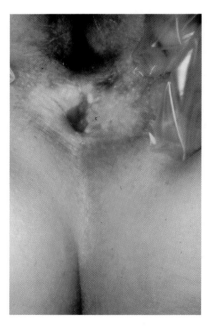

Fig 18.4 Erosive lichen planus of the vulva.

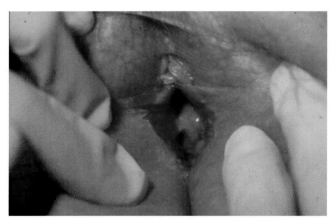

Fig 18.5 Erosive lichen planus of the vulva.

white border. Vulvar adhesions and labial atrophy with fusion and clitoral burial, together with loss of tissue mass, are common. The keratinized skin in the perineal and perianal area tends to show the classic violaceous papules and plaques of LP, which may be helpful in diagnosis (18.6).

One-half to two-thirds of patients with erosive LP have vaginal involvement during the course of the disease[4,5]. Episodes of vaginitis do not necessarily correlate in time with the appearance of vulvitis, and symptoms vary in severity, with periods of regression. The insertion of a vaginal speculum may be exceedingly painful, and

sometimes impossible, because of vaginal adhesions. There may be either a generalized vaginitis that is friable, desquamative, and hemorrhagic, or less extensive erosions with an overlying white lacy network. The cervix can be friable and desquamative, and may be obscured from view by stenosis of the upper vagina.

Although tender, friable gingivitis is an uncommon presenting complaint, it will develop at some time during the course of the disease in two-thirds to three-quarters of patients. Gingival erosion and desquamation may be localized or generalized, and erosions are sometimes surrounded by a white rim (18.7).

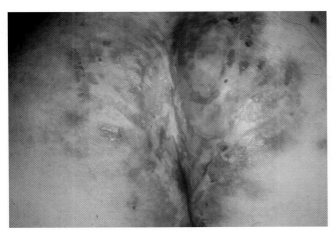

Fig 18.6 Erosive lichen planus of the buttocks and perianal skin.

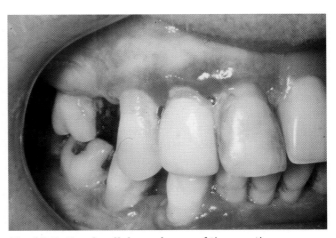

Fig 18.7 Erosive lichen planus of the mouth.

DIAGNOSIS

Biopsies should be taken from the border of an eroded area for histopathology and direct immunofluorescence (IF). An experienced dermatopathologist can be extremely helpful in the interpretation of mucosal sections. The typical histologic features of LP are a subepidermal band-like inflammatory infiltrate and some basal cell degenerative changes, with or without cytoid bodies (18.8). Direct IF with colloid bodies may support the diagnosis, while the typical clinical morphology and distribution of LP lesions can support the diagnosis when histology is equivocal.

DIFFERENTIAL DIAGNOSIS

Autoimmune blistering diseases may also present with an erosive gingivitis, vulvitis, cervicitis, or vaginitis. Of these, cicatricial pemphigoid is clinically most like

erosive LP (*see below*). A general physical examination is essential to exclude evidence of either disease at other sites. Direct and indirect IF studies are helpful in differentiating these disorders. Vulvitis circumscripta plasmacellularis (plasma cell vulvitis, Zoon erythroplasia) may present with well demarcated erosions on the labia minora, but oral and vaginal involvement are not characteristic[6] and histologic findings tend to be more specific. Erosive vaginitis with adhesions has been described in many patients with graft-versus-host disease (GVHD), a condition also associated with lichenoid cutaneous eruptions. Biopsy is recommended to differentiate between the variety of possible diagnostic considerations[7] (*see Appendix A*). Even with histologic examination, diagnosis of widespread erosive vulval disease may be difficult (18.9), and in some cases it is only after some time – perhaps years – that a diagnosis of lichen planus is confirmed.

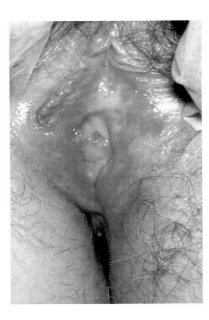

Fig 18.9 Widespread vulval erosions. Histological findings were not diagnostic and the diagnosis remained uncertain.

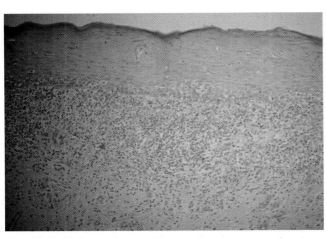

Fig 18.8 Lichen planus. Biopsy of oral mucosa showing features of lichen planus.

MANAGEMENT

Erosive LP is chronic and recalcitrant. These patients probably also have an increased risk of developing squamous cell carcinoma. This supposition is based on the well-documented risk of squamous cell carcinoma in erosive oral and penile LP[8,9]. It would be logical to assume that patients with vulvovaginal lesions share a similar risk. Certainly, patients should be monitored carefully throughout the course of their disease. There is no ideal treatment for this disorder, but several possible therapies have proved helpful in some cases. (*See also Appendix D.*)

TOPICAL TREATMENT

Aqueous cream emollients are soothing, and the discomfort of towel drying can be avoided by using a hand-held hairdryer at low temperature. Some patients find that potent topical steroids (e.g. clobetasol propionate 0.05%) are very helpful. Rectal preparations such as hydrocortisone acetate 10% in the form of a 'foam', and prednisolone suppositories, are useful for vaginal lesions. In one series, only about 25% of patients showed satisfactory improvement with topical preparations[3]. Although topical cyclosporin 'swish and spit' therapy has been helpful in treating erosive oral LP[10–12], topical treatment has been disappointing in vulvovaginal lesions[13] and is not widely used. Treatment is very costly and could theoretically increase the risk of malignancy. Topically applied tretinoin and isotretinoin are beneficial only for nonerosive oral lesions[14]. Their usefulness is limited by local irritation in the vulvovaginal area.

SYSTEMIC TREATMENT

Oral steroid therapy (at least 0.5 mg/kg/day) is helpful in about 50% of patients treated[3], but erosions recur on tapering. Intralesional steroid injections may be helpful in some cases. There are several reports of the use of systemic retinoids (acitretin, etretinate, isotretinoin) in mucosal LP[15–18], but these drugs are potent teratogens with prolonged half-lives, which seriously limits their use in women of childbearing age. Clearly, the efficacy of systemic retinoids for treating erosive LP at all sites requires further evaluation and the support of adequate clinical trials. In addition to teratogenicity, retinoids often cause skin fragility, hair loss, muscle cramps, headaches, increased levels of serum triglycerides, and, rarely, acute severe hepatitis.

Oral griseofulvin has been described as a useful therapy for severe LP[19–21], but not for erosive vulvar disease. There have also been anecdotal reports of the beneficial use of dapsone in severe erosive oral and acral forms of the disease[22,23], and hydroxychloroquine sulfate has been helpful in treating erosive oral LP[24]. There is no ideal treatment for erosive vulvar LP. Many systemic treatments are limited by their side effects and/or are unsuitable as maintenance therapy.

SURGERY

Juxtaposed erosive surfaces tend to form adhesions or synechiae. This is the most likely reason for recurrence in patients who have undergone surgical division of adhesions. Laser ablation is not effective[4], and the results of split-skin grafting have not yet been reported. In severe cases, in which urethral or menstrual function is compromised, blunt dissection of mucosal adhesions can be performed. Potent topical steroids should be applied after operation with vaginal dilators to minimize inflammation during healing. When only the anterior vagina is involved, function can often be restored by surgery, and maintained afterwards with topical steroids.

BULLOUS DISEASES

The autoimmune blistering diseases affect skin and mucous membrane sites, including the vulvovaginal area (**Table 18.1**). Autoantibodies directed against normal components of the epithelium and basement membrane zone (BMZ) mediate these diseases. The target antigens are those involved in the adhesion of epithelial cells to one another, or to the underlying stroma (**Table 18.2**). Their ultrastructural localization is shown in **18.10**.

At cutaneous sites, this antigen – antibody interaction provokes a characteristic blister, although erosion is more common at mucosal sites, where it may be clinically indistinguishable from erosion due to other causes. However, diagnosis is not usually a problem, as autoimmune blistering diseases usually affect both skin and mucosal sites. If, as occasionally occurs, only the mucosae are affected, then diagnosis may be difficult; appropriate laboratory investigations are essential for diagnostic accuracy in cases where a blistering disease is a possibility.

PEMPHIGUS VULGARIS

Pemphigus vulgaris is the most common type of pemphigus, affecting about 80% of patients with pemphigus. The peak incidence of occurrence is between the fourth and sixth decades. Cutaneous blisters are flaccid and fragile, rupturing to produce raw, denuded areas (**18.11**). Extensive involvement may be life threatening. Mucous membrane involvement affects 85–90% of patients (**18.12**). Other mucosal sites include the nose,

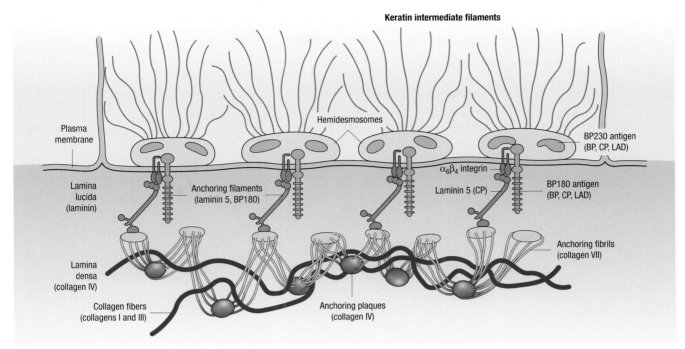

Fig 18.10 Localization of target antigens in autoimmune bullous diseases. BP, bullous pemphigoid; CP, cicatricial pemphigoid; LAD, linear IgA disease.

Table 18.1 Clinical Features of the Autoimmune Bullous Diseases.

Disease	Patients	Distribution	Mucosal lesions	Vulvovaginal lesions		Scarring	Treatment	Prognosis
Pemphigus vulgaris	Adults	Generalized	Always, major	+++ (80%)	Flaccid blisters, erosions		Steroids immuno-suppressants	Most remit
Bullous pemphigoid	Elderly (rare in children)	Trunk, limbs, flexures	Common, minor	+ (9%)	Urticated plaques, tense blisters (milia)		Steroids, dapsone, immuno-suppressants	3–4 years
Cicatricial pemphigoid	Middle to old age	Infrequent	Major, severe	+++(53%) scarring	Erosions, blisters, gingivitis, milia	+++	Steroids, dapsone, immuno-suppressants	Chronic
Linear IgA disease (CBDC and adults)	Children and elderly	Perineum, face, trunk, limbs	Majority (few severe)	++ (60%) children > adults	Urticated plaques, annular lesions, tense blisters	+ (mucosae, rare)	Dapsone, sulfonamides	3–4 years (few persist)
Epidermolysis bullosa acquisita	Adults (few children)	Generalized, variable	Some (few severe)	++ (60%)	Urticated plaques, tense blisters, milia	++	Steroids, dapsone, immuno-suppressants	Persists

CBDC, chronic bullous disease of childhood; Ig, immunoglobulin.

Table 18.2 Immunopathology of the Autoimmune Bullous Diseases.

| Disease | Immuno-fluorescence | Autoantibodies | | | |
		Isotype	Binding to split skin	Target antigens	Antigen weight (kDa)
Pemphigus vulgaris	Intraepidermal	IgG		PV antigen	130
Bullous pemphigoid	Linear BMZ	IgG, few IgA	Epidermal	BPAg-1 BPAg-2	220 180
Cicatricial pemphigoid	Linear BMZ	IgG, IgA	Epidermal Dermal	BPAg-1 BPAg-2 Epiligrin/nicein Others	220 180 600
Linear IgA disease (CBDC and adults)	Linear BMZ	IgA	Epidermal (majority) Dermal (minority)	(Few BPAg-1 and BPAg-2)	285,97 (Few 180, 220)
Epidermolysis bullosa acquisita	Linear BMZ	IgG	Dermal	Collagen VII (anchoring fibril)	290

BMZ, basement membrane zone; BPAg, bullous pemphigoid antigen; CBDC, chronic bullous disease of childhood; Ig, immunoglobulin.

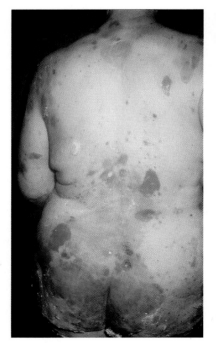

Fig 18.11 Extensive pemphigus vulgaris affecting cutaneous sites.

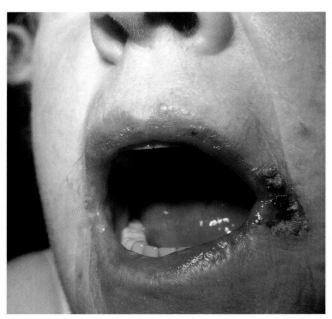

Fig 18.12 Pemphigus vulgaris affecting mucosal surfaces.

conjunctiva, larynx, pharynx, esophagus, urethra, and cervix. Vulvovaginal involvement is common[25]; lesions are erosive, painful, and may be extensive (18.13).

Histologic examination of a fresh intact cutaneous blister will show the characteristic intraepidermal blister containing rounded acantholytic cells. Immunofluorescence studies are vital in suspected cases and should be repeated if necessary. Punch biopsies are ideal for this purpose and may be performed under local anesthesia. Direct IF from perilesional skin or mucosa,

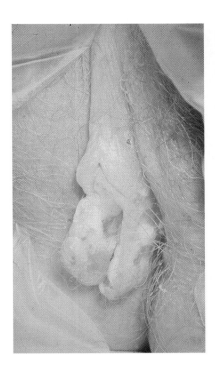

Fig 18.13 Pemphigus vulgaris with prominent vulvar erosions.

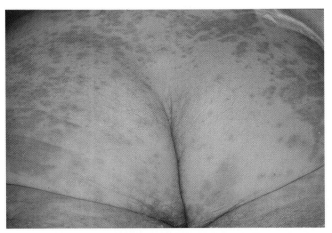

Fig 18.15 Bullous pemphigoid. Urticated plaque in the pre-blistering phase of bullous pemphigoid.

Mucosal sites are involved in over 50% of cases[25]. Labial erosions cause pain, itch, and dysuria (**18.16**). Localized vulvar pemphigoid has been described in children[26,27]. Mucosal sites affected include the vagina, oral and nasal mucosa, the pharynx, conjunctiva, esophagus, and anus. Lesions heal without scarring, so findings on examination may be normal when the disease is in control or in remission.

Histologic examination of a fresh intact cutaneous blister shows a subepidermal split at the dermoepidermal junction, with a mixed dermal inflammatory infiltrate consisting of numerous eosinophils. Direct and indirect IF studies can aid diagnosis, as shown in **Table 18.2** and in **18.17**. Antibodies to bullous pemphigoid generally bind to the roof of a split-skin preparation (**18.18**), differentiating the condition from epidermolysis bullosa acquisita in which antibodies bind to the base.

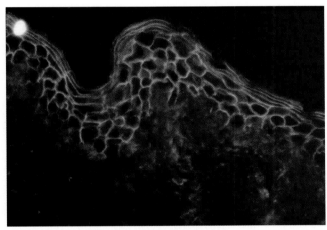

Fig 18.14 Pemphigus vulgaris. Indirect immunofluorescence with IgG deposition on the surface of epidermal cells.

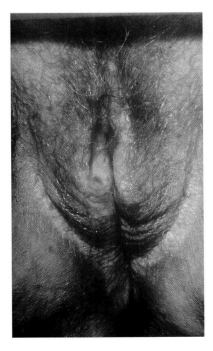

Fig 18.16 Bullous pemphigoid of the vulva with erosions.

as well as from an uninvolved site, and indirect IF of serum should be performed. IgG deposition and binding of the patient's serum to the epidermal cell surface occurs in over 90% of patients with pemphigus vulgaris (**18.14**).

BULLOUS PEMPHIGOID

Bullous pemphigoid is the commonest of all blistering diseases. Generally, it affects the elderly, although cases have been reported in childhood. Skin involvement may be localized or extensive; blisters are usually tense and may arise on normal or urticated skin (**18.15**). Two years is the average time until remission occurs.

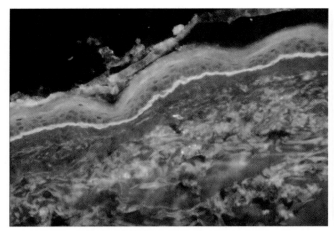

Fig 18.17 Bullous pemphigoid. Linear dermoepidermal band on indirect immunofluorescence of vaginal mucosa.

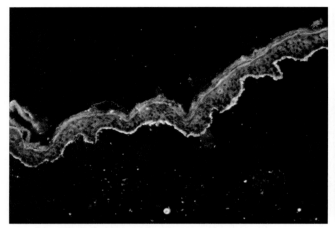

Fig 18.18 Bullous pemphigoid. Indirect immunofluorescence on bullous pemphigoid serum showing binding to the roof on salt-split skin.

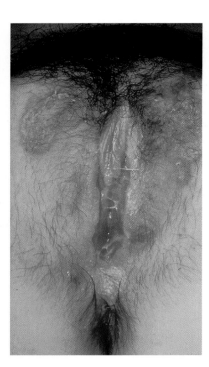

Fig 18.19 Cicatricial pemphigoid with severe vulvar erosion in a teenager.

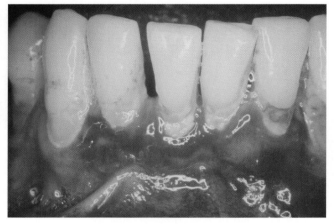

Fig 18.20 Cicatricial pemphigoid of the mouth with erosions.

CICATRICIAL PEMPHIGOID

Cicatricial pemphigoid, a scarring bullous disease, predominantly affects mucosal surfaces. Cutaneous lesions occur in only 10–25% of cases, and vulvar scarring is often indistinguishable from that of erosive LP. Although cicatricial pemphigoid usually affects the middle aged and elderly, it may present in childhood (**18.19**). Oral lesions include blisters, erosions, and/or gingivitis (**18.20**); other affected sites are the conjunctiva (**18.21**), nasal mucosa, larynx, pharynx, and esophagus. Scarring and morbidity may be significant in the eye (blindness), the larynx (stridor), and the esophagus (dysphagia).

Erosions may develop on the labia, urethra, vagina, rectum, or perianal skin (**18.19**). Patients complain of soreness, pain, itch, and urethral symptoms. Scarring with labial fusion is common, with or without clitoral burial, and vaginal introital stenosis may make intercourse difficult or impossible. Urethral stenosis may

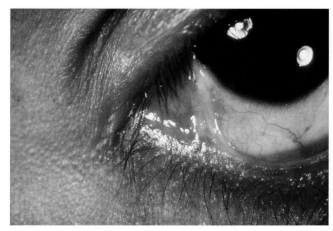

Fig 18.21 Cicatricial pemphigoid of the eyes with conjunctival scarring.

also require dilatation. The disease is typically difficult to treat and, unfortunately, there is no tendency towards spontaneous resolution.

Blistering localized to the vulva has been described in children with both cicatricial and bullous pemphigoid, and, as in adults, the cicatricial form is difficult to treat[28].

Cicatricial pemphigoid is essentially a clinical diagnosis; biopsy of a fresh intact cutaneous blister will show a subepidermal split and there may be scarring in the dermis. Direct IF is often negative, although some authors have found that biopsies from buccal and conjunctival mucosae give the best positive yield. Multiple biopsies should ideally be taken to increase the likelihood of accurate diagnosis. The use of split-skin as a substrate undoubtedly gives the highest positive yield with binding of IgG or IgA autoantibodies to the roof in most cases of cicatricial pemphigoid, although some do bind to the floor[29]. Immunoblotting is sometimes a more sensitive method for diagnosis. Despite differences in the clinical expression of the two diseases, the target antigens in cicatricial pemphigoid are shared with those in bullous pemphigoid.

EPIDERMOLYSIS BULLOSA ACQUISITA

Epidermolysis bullosa acquisita (EBA) is an uncommon blistering disease. It is characterized by skin fragility and erosion with a tendency to heal with scarring[30], and thus may be indistinguishable from bullous and cicatricial pemphigoid (18.22). Mucous membrane involvement affecting the mouth, eyes, esophagus, and larynx is common, and vulvar scarring may lead to introital stenosis and functional disability.

The histology of EBA is similar to that of pemphigoid. Direct IF shows IgG deposited in a linear band at the dermoepidermal junction, and indirect IF is positive in many patients. The use of salt split-skin improves the diagnostic yield, and the dermal binding of IgG distinguishes EBA from bullous pemphigoid[31].

LINEAR IgA DISEASE

This uncommon blistering disease has been described in both adults and children (formerly called chronic bullous disease of childhood)[32]. The most characteristic lesion of linear IgA disease is the annular polycyclic or gyrate lesion with a peripheral ring of blistering. Children present with blisters, some of which are hemorrhagic, most commonly on or near the genital or perioral area[25]. With time, blisters become more generalized, and mucosal involvement with scarring may be a feature (18.23). Some children have been mistakenly diagnosed as being victims of sexual abuse. Adults may present with widespread blistering on cutaneous and mucosal sites, including the mouth, eyes, nasopharynx, larynx, esophagus, and trachea.

Histologic examination of a fresh intact blister shows that the blister is subepidermal (18.24). Direct IF demonstrates a linear band of IgA at the BMZ in all cases. Indirect IF is positive for IgA autoantibodies in most children and some adults.

MANAGEMENT

Potent topical corticosteroid preparations and treatment of secondary infection are the mainstays of local therapy for autoimmune bullous diseases. Systemic therapy may

Fig 18.22 Epidermolysis bullosa acquisita of the hands, with fragility and erosions.

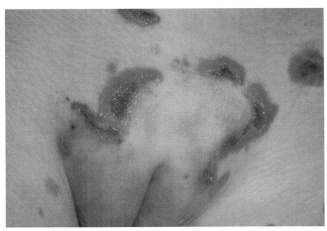

Fig 18.23 Linear IgA disease. Typical lesions of linear IgA disease (chronic bullous disease of childhood) are shown.

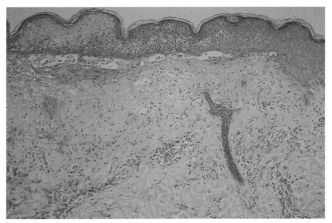

Fig 18.24 Linear IgA disease. Histologic appearance of linear IgA disease with subepidermal blistering.

be necessary in generalized or extensive disease, and is outlined in **Table 18.1**. The current armamentarium includes systemic corticosteroids, dapsone, sulfonamides, minocycline (sometimes with nicotinamide), and azathioprine. Each case must be carefully and individually assessed in the light of the patient's general health and her ability to tolerate the different treatment regimens. Multiple drug combinations are sometimes required for severe cases, and all patients need to be closely monitored for hematologic and hepatic side effects. Surgical intervention may be necessary when there is functional impairment of the vulva, esophagus, or larynx.

GENETICALLY DETERMINED BULLOUS DISEASES

EPIDERMOLYSIS BULLOSA DYSTROPHICA

Epidermolysis bullosa dystrophica is a rare blistering disease, which can be inherited as an autosomal-dominant or autosomal-recessive trait. The genetic cause is a mutation of collagen VII, which is the major component of the anchoring fibrils (*see* **18.10**). This results in faulty adhesion of the epidermis to the dermis, producing repeated blistering with dystrophic scarring and deformity. Most patients present in infancy. The involvement of mucous membranes is a constant feature of the severe form of recessive epidermolysis bullosa dystrophica. Scarring leads to a variety of complications including:

- Microstomia
- Limited mobility of the tongue
- Gingival retraction and dental decay
- Esophageal stenosis
- Corneal scarring
- Anal stenosis

Blistering, erosion, and scarring of the vulva, introitus, vagina, and perineal and perianal skin have also been

reported as leading to vaginal stenosis[33]. The diagnosis is established by electron microscopy, which is used to determine the level of separation in the BMZ, and by immunohistochemical techniques, which are used to demonstrate the absence of collagen VII in the recessive disease. Treatment is mainly supportive.

HAILEY–HAILEY DISEASE (BENIGN FAMILIAL PEMPHIGUS)

Patients with autosomal-dominant benign familial pemphigus have recurrent vesicular lesions or crusted erosions in intertriginous areas, including the axillary, inframammary, and perineal areas, and the groin[34]. The morphology varies from expanding plaques with scaly borders simulating fungal infections, to crusted erosions and vesicopustules. Hypertrophic perineal involvement may be mistaken for chronic candida infection or malignancy. Cases have been reported confined to the vulva[35]. Intact blisters are uncommon (**18.25**). Diagnosis is established histologically in cases when the typical suprabasal acantholysis can be identified. Topical steroids and the treatment of secondary infection may provide considerable amelioration, but flares and remissions are typical.

CONCLUSION

Erosive conditions of the vulva are a misery to patients and taxing to physicians. Diagnosis is often difficult, prognosis is usually uncertain, and treatment is often disappointing. The mainstay of diagnosis remains the clinical history and examination.

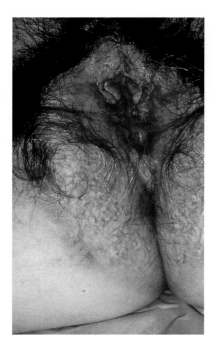

Fig 18.25 Hailey–Hailey disease of the vulva.

REFERENCES

1 Boyd, A. S. and Nelder, K. H. Lichen planus. *J. Am. Acad. Dermatol.* 1991; **25**: 593–619.

2 Pelisse, M., Leibowitch, M., Sedel, D., *et al.* Un nouveau syndrome vulvo-vagino-gingival. Lichen plan erosif plurimuqueux. *Ann. Dermatol. Venereol. (Paris)* 1982; **109**: 797–798.

3 Kanwar, A. J., Handa, S., Ghosh, S., *et al.* Lichen planus in childhood: a report in 17 patients. *Pediatr. Dermatol.* 1991; **8**: 288–291.

4 Pelisse, M. The vulvo-vaginal–gingival syndrome. A new form of erosive lichen planus. *Int. J. Dermatol.* 1989; **28**: 381–384.

5 Ridley, C. M. Chronic erosive vulval disease. *Clin. Exp. Dermatol.* 1990; **15**: 245–252.

6 Davis, J., Shapiro, L., and Baral, J. Vulvitis circumscripta plasmacellularis. *J. Am. Acad. Dermatol.* 1983; **8**: 413–416.

7 Edwards, L. Desquamative vulvitis. *Dermatol. Clin.* (vulvar diseases) 1992; **10**: 325–337.

8 Harland, C. C., Fallowfield, M. E., Marsden, R. A., *et al.* Squamous carcinoma complicating lichen planus of the lip. *Br. J. Dermatol.* 1991; **125**(Suppl 38): 96–97.

9 Marder, M. Z. and Deesen, K. C. Transformation of oral lichen planus to squamous cell carcinoma: a literature review and report of a case. *J. Am. Dent. Assoc.* 1982; **105**: 55–60.

10 Eisen, D., Griffiths, C. E. M., Ellis, C. N., *et al.* Cyclosporin wash for oral lichen planus. *Lancet* 1990; **335**: 535–536 (letter).

11 Balato, N., De Rosa, S., Bordone, F., *et al.* Dermatological application of cyclosporin. *Arch. Dermatol.* 1989; **125**: 430–431.

12 Frances, C., Boisnic, S., Etienne, S., *et al.* Effect of the local application of cyclosporin A on chronic erosive lichen planus of the oral cavity. *Dermatologica* 1988; **177**: 194–195.

13 Pelisse, M. Presented to the 11th International Congress of the International Society for the Study of Vulvar Disease. Oxford, UK, September 1991.

14 Giustina, T. A., Stewart, J. C. B., Ellis, C. N., *et al.* Topical application of isotretinoin gel improves oral lichen planus. *Arch. Dermatol.* 1986; **122**: 534–536.

15 Laurberg, G., Geiger, J. M., Hjorth, N., *et al.* Treatment of lichen planus with acitretin. *J. Am. Acad. Dermatol.* 1991; **24**: 434–437.

16 Hersle, K., Mobacken, H., Sloberg, K., *et al.* Severe oral lichen planus: treatment with an aromatic retinoid (etretinate). *Br. J. Dermatol.* 1982; **106**: 77–80.

17 Woo, T. Y. Systemic isotretinoin treatment of oral and cutaneous lichen planus. *Cutis* 1985; **35**(4): 385–393.

18 Staus, M. E. and Bergfeld, W. F. Treatment of oral lichen planus with low-dose isotretinoin. *J. Am. Acad. Dermatol.* 1984; **11**(3): 527–528.

19 Massa, M. C. and Rogers, R. S. Griseofulvin therapy of lichen planus. *Acta Derm. Venereol. (Stockh.)* 1981; **61**: 547–550.

20 Sehgal, V. N., Abraham, G. J. S., and Malik, G. B. Griseofulvin therapy in lichen planus. *Br. J. Dermatol.* 1972; **87**: 383.

21 Meyrick Thomas, R. H., Munro, D. D., and Robinson, T. W. E. Erosive lichen planus treated with griseofulvin. *Br. J. Dermatol.* 1983; **109**(Suppl 24): 97–98.

22 Falk, D. K., Latour, D. L., and King, L. E. Dapsone in the treatment of erosive lichen planus. *J. Am. Acad. Dermatol.* 1985; **12**: 567–570.

23 Beck, H. I. and Brandrup, F. Treatment of erosive lichen planus with dapsone. *Acta Derm. Venereol. (Stockh.)* 1986; **66**: 366–367.

24 Eisen, D. Hydroxychloroquine sulfate (Plaquenil) improves oral lichen planus. *J. Am. Acad. Dermatol.* 1993; **28**: 609–612.

25 Marren, P., Wojnarowska, F., Venning, V., *et al.* Vulvar involvement in autoimmune bullous diseases. *J. Reprod. Med.* 1993; **38**(2): 101–107.

26 Oranje, A. P. and Van Joost, T. Pemphigoid in children. *Pediatr. Dermatol.* 1989; **6**(4): 267–274.

27 DeCastro, P., Jorizzo, J. L., and Rajaraman, S. Localized vulvar pemphigoid in a child. *Pediatr. Dermatol.* 1985; **2**: 302–307.

28 Farrell, A. M., Kirtschig, G., Dalziel, K., *et al.* Childhood vulval pemphigoid: a clinical and immunopathological study of 5 patients. *Br. J. Dermatol.* 1999; **140**: 308–312.

29 Allen, J., Schomberg, K., Venning, V. A., *et al.* A comparison of the localization of the antibodies and antigens in cicatricial pemphigoid. *Br. J. Dermatol.* 1992; **127**: 430.

30 Roenigk, H. H., Jr., Ryan, J. G., and Bergfeld, W. F. Epidermolysis bullosa acquisita: report of three cases and review of all published cases. *Arch. Dermatol.* 1971; **103**: 1–10.

31 Yaoita, H., Briggaman, R. A., Lawley, T. J., *et al.* Epidermolysis bullosa acquisita: ultrastructural and immunological studies. J. *Invest. Dermatol.* 1981; **76**: 288–292.

32 Wojnarowska, F., Marsden, R. A., Bhogal, B., *et al.* Chronic bullous disease of childhood, childhood cicatricial pemphigoid and linear IgA disease of adults: a comparative study demonstrating clinical and immunopathological overlap. *J. Am. Acad. Dermatol.* 1988; **19**: 792–805.

33 Shakelford, G., Bauer, E., Graviss, E. R., *et al.* Upper airway and external genital involvement in epidermolysis bullosa dystrophica. *Radiology* 1982; **143**: 429–432.

34 Burge, S. M. Hailey–Hailey disease; the clinical features, response to treatment, and prognosis. *Br. J. Dermatol.* 1992; **126**: 275–282.

35 Thiers, H., Moulin, G., Rochet, Y., *et al.* Maladie de Hailey–Hailey: a localisation vulvaire predominante. Etude génétique et ultra-structurale. *Bulletin de la Société Française Dermatologie et Syphiligraphie* 1968; **75**: 352–355.

19 Vulvar Manifestations of Systemic Disease

Christine Harrington

INTRODUCTION

Vulvar symptoms usually result from a primary dermatosis, or from a generalized skin disease that involves the vulva. Occasionally, vulvar lesions are manifestations or complications of systemic disease, and, rarely, the vulva may be the site of presentation of a systemic disorder. If systemic disease is suspected, a detailed history should be taken, and the skin and mucous membranes should be examined thoroughly. Vulvar biopsy and appropriate investigations are needed to confirm the diagnosis and to guide appropriate management.

CHRONIC PRURITUS VULVAE (LICHEN SIMPLEX CHRONICUS)

Persistent scratching of the vulva causes lichenification, usually of the labia majora. The skin may be leathery and thickened (19.1), or may become eroded in severe cases (19.2). While the underlying cause is being investigated, a moderately potent topical steroid and a systemic antipruritic agent may be used to alleviate the itch[1].

IRON-DEFICIENCY ANEMIA

Iron-deficiency anemia causes chronic pruritus; occasionally, the itch is localized to the vulva. Causes of iron-deficiency anemia should be considered in the history and examination of a patient with unexplained pruritus vulvae[2]. Possible causes include a poor diet or blood loss from menorrhagia, hemorrhoids, or gastrointestinal problems. Iron replacement and correction of the underlying cause will rapidly relieve the vulvar itch.

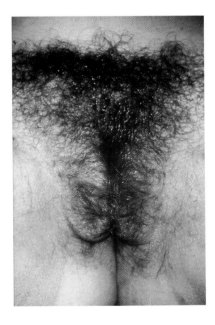

Fig 19.1 Lichen simplex, in a patient with chronic pruritus vulvae and iron-deficiency anemia.

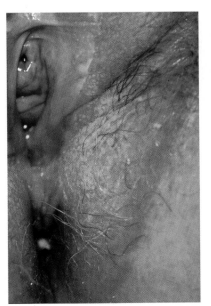

Fig 19.2 Eroded, excoriated lichen simplex, in a patient with chronic pruritus vulvae and iron-deficiency anemia.

DIABETES MELLITUS

Late-onset diabetes, especially in an obese patient, may be complicated by an inflammatory intertrigo. This may be limited to the genitocrural region and is usually associated with candidal infection (**19.3**). The lesions usually resolve once the diabetic state has been corrected.

BEHÇET'S SYNDROME

This condition, first described in 1937 by a Turkish dermatologist, is generally thought to be a viral infection causing genital ulceration. The ulcers are associated with arthritis, ulcerative colitis, thrombophlebitis, skin eruptions, and neurologic problems, and it has been suggested that the condition is an altered immune response to infection in genetically predisposed individuals[3].

Mucocutaneous lesions may be the presenting lesions in Behçet's syndrome, or arise during the course of this multisystem disease. Genital ulceration is an important diagnostic criterion for Behçet's disease (**Table 19.1**) and second only to oral ulceration in frequency of clinical features[4]. The vulvar lesions are persistent, painful ulcers, which pass deep into the vulvar skin (**19.4**). The labia minora are the most common site for these ulcers. Oral and ocular lesions may also be present. Diagnosis may be difficult in the absence of arthritic, neurologic, or thrombotic disease. The histology of the vulvar ulcers is often nonspecific, but may show thrombosed arterioles. Culture and syphilitic tests are negative and a biopsy shows chronic nonspecific inflammation.

Dapsone, systemic steroids, or cyclosporin may be indicated if systemic disease is active. Colchicine or thalidomide may benefit the genital ulcers, as may topical preparations combining triamcinolone and tetracycline. Topical steroids provide some relief from

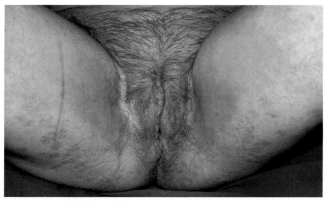

Fig 19.3 Intertrigo, complicated by candidiasis in a diabetic.

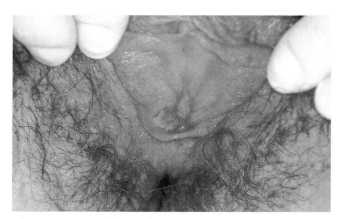

Fig 19.4 Behçet's syndrome. Sloughy, painful vulvar ulcer in Behçet's syndrome.

the painful vulvar ulcers and may speed up resolution. The lesions usually resolve spontaneously, but result in considerable scarring. Superpotent topical steroids (clobetasol) may be helpful if applied at the earliest sign of a developing ulcer.

Table 19.1 International Study Group criteria for Behçet's Disease[a].

Recurrent oral ulceration	Minor aphthous, major aphthous, or herpetiform ulceration observed by physician or patient, which recurred at least three times in one 12-month period
Plus two of the following:	
Recurrent genital ulceration	Aphthous ulceration or scarring observed by physician or patient
Eye lesions	Anterior uveitis, posterior uveitis, or cells in vitreous on slit-lamp examination or retinal vasculitis observed by ophthalmologist
Skin lesions	Erythema nodosum observed by physician or patient, pseudofolliculitis or papulopustular lesions or acneiform nodules observed by physician in postadolescent patients not receiving corticosteroid treatment
Positive pathergy test result	Read by physician at 24–48 hours

[a] *Findings applicable only in the absence of other clinical explanations.*
From Balabanova et al.[4]

CROHN'S DISEASE

Anogenital manifestations of Crohn's disease are found in up to 30% of affected patients. They may precede intestinal problems by up to several years, and can therefore be a diagnostic problem. Edema is often the first vulvar abnormality (19.5), while abscesses, ulcers, sinuses, and fistulae (19.6) are the other vulvar complications of Crohn's disease. The lesion may present as a 'knife-cut' ulcer with a thickened edge. It may communicate with the rectum and anus, rendering the patient incontinent due to fistula formation. As Crohn's disease so often mimics other conditions, it is often not diagnosed until biopsies are taken. Noncaseating epithelioid granulomas are found on biopsy, and the differential diagnosis includes other granulomatous disorders, such as sarcoidosis.

Vulvar Crohn's disease usually responds to the medical or surgical management of the intestinal symptoms. When lesions arise unrelated to gut activity, topical or intralesional steroids or topical metronidazole may be beneficial. Occasionally, it is necessary to use wide local excision, including anal resection, to improve the chances of cure. Even so, the risk of recurrence is still high. Anogenital skin lesions are much more rare in ulcerative colitis, but a pustular vegetative eruption in the groins is occasionally present[5].

SARCOIDOSIS

Granulomatous nodules of sarcoid (19.7) rarely appear on the vulva as an isolated disorder or as part of systemic sarcoidosis. Histologic confirmation should be followed by general screening to exclude other organ involvement.

PYODERMA GANGRENOSUM

'Punched-out' indolent ulcers with a purple edge should arouse suspicion of this disorder. Vulvar lesions are usually multiple and small, and arise on a vasculitic, indurated plaque. However, single lesions may be present (19.8). As histological examination shows a nonspecific inflammation, a biopsy is unlikely to be helpful.

The ulcers are 'vasculitic' and may be associated with rheumatoid arthritis, inflammatory bowel disease, and myeloma or other lymphoproliferative disorders[6]. Systemic treatment of the underlying disease usually results in resolution of the pyoderma gangrenosum, and the patient should therefore be investigated for diseases known to be associated. Lesions usually respond well to the treatment of underlying rheumatoid arthritis or ulcerative colitis. However, lesions associated with lymphoproliferative disorders are slower to respond to treatment of the underlying condition, and usually require high doses of systemic steroids. Isolated lesions may respond to intralesional steroid injection.

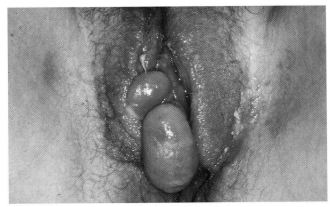

Fig 19.5 Crohn's disease. Vulvar edema in Crohn's disease.

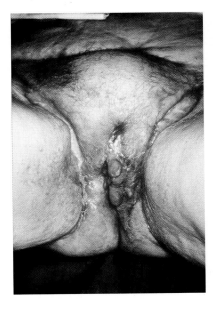

Fig 19.6 Crohn's disease. Fissures, fistulae, abscesses, and edema in severe vulvar Crohn's disease.

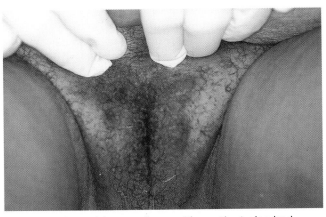

Fig 19.7 Sarcoid granuloma. The patient also had cerebral sarcoidosis.

157

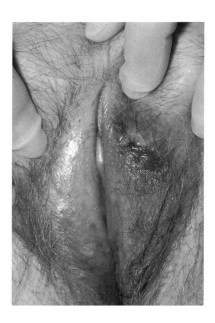

Fig 19.8 Pyoderma gangrenosum, in a patient with IgA myeloma.

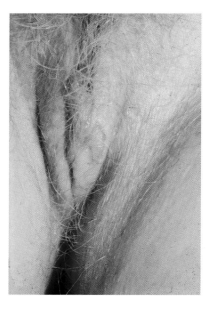

Fig 19.9 Fixed drug reaction. Pruritic, blistered patch, occurring on the vulva after each ingestion of tetracycline in a patient with acne rosacea.

FIXED DRUG ERUPTION

A patient may react to a drug by always developing a localized skin lesion at the same site after ingestion of the drug. Rarely, this reaction may occur on vulvar skin. Tetracycline and phenolphthalein (found in some laxatives) are both likely to cause fixed drug eruptions (**19.9**). The diagnosis can be made only from a detailed history[7]. The lesion will subside when the drug is withdrawn.

ERYTHEMA MULTIFORME

Erythema multiforme may result from a drug reaction or may be a complication of herpes simplex, myco-plasma, or pregnancy (*see Chapter 8*). Rarely, it is localized to the vulva. In the case shown (**19.10**), the patient developed recurrent blisters and erosions on the vulva about 10 days after repeated herpes simplex virus (HSV) infections on the face. A detailed history, examination, and biopsy are required to establish the diagnosis. Treatment is for the precipitating cause.

The speed of resolution of drug-induced erythema multiforme depends on the drug causing the problem, but may be raised by the application of potent topical steroids. Rarely, systemic steroids may be indicated if there is severe mucous membrane involvement, or if the condition progresses to toxic epidermal necrolysis[8]. Erythema multiforme following viral infection resolves spontaneously within 1 week to 10 days. Recurrent attacks of erythema multiforme after HSV infection may be halted by the immediate use of systemic acyclovir during the HSV prodrome, or by continuous administration of suppressive doses.

ACANTHOSIS NIGRICANS

The vulva and genitocrural region may be involved in any dermatosis that affects flexural sites. In particular, pigmentary disorders tend to affect the vulva. Hyperpigmentation of normal vulvar skin may be part of the flexural pigmentation of Addison's disease or neurofibromatosis. Hyperpigmentation and warty, velvety thickening of the skin should arouse suspicion of acanthosis nigricans (**19.11**). Biopsy is necessary to confirm the diagnosis. Once confirmed, an intensive history, examination, and investigation are indicated, as this disorder is a recognized cutaneous marker of underlying malignancy, especially adenocarcinoma of the stomach[9].

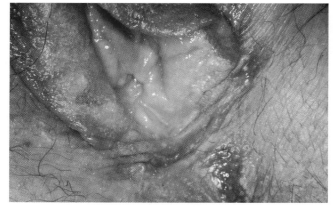

Fig 19.10 Erythema multiforme. This recurrent disorder started 10 days after repeated facial herpes simplex.

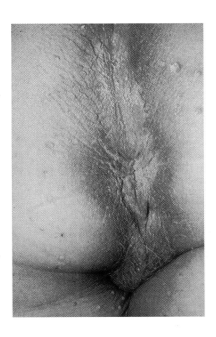

Fig 19.11 Anogenital acanthosis nigricans. This was the presenting feature in a patient with ovarian carcinoma.

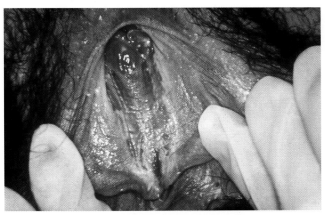

Fig 19.12 White sponge nevus syndrome. The patient presented with a white vaginal discharge. She also had oral lesions.

WHITE SPONGE NEVUS SYNDROME

Several inherited mucocutaneous disorders affect the vulva. White sponge nevus is an autosomal-dominant condition with white hyperkeratotic lesions of the oral mucosa and genitalia[10]. Occasionally, the patient may present with symptomless vulvar white patches (**19.12**).

Histologically, hyperkeratosis, acanthosis, and vacuolation of the prickle cells confirm the diagnosis. The lesions may clear upon application of a topical antibiotic such as tetracycline mouthwash.

REFERENCES

1 Pincus, S.H. and McKay, M. Disorders of the female genitalia. In: Fitzpatrick, T.B., Eisen, A.Z., Wolff, K., Freedberg, I.M. and Austen, K.F. (eds) *Dermatology in General Medicine*, 4th edn, pp. 1465–1466. McGraw-Hill, New York, 1993.

2 Adams, S.J. Iron deficiency and other hematological causes of generalized pruritus. In: Bernhard, J.D. (ed.) *Itch: Mechanisms and Management of Pruritus*, pp. 243–250. McGraw-Hill, New York, 1994.

3 Jorizzo, J.L., Behçet's's disease. In: Fitzpatrick, T.B., Eisen, A.Z., Wolff, K., Freedberg, I.M. and Austen, K.F. (eds.) *Dermatology in General Medicine*, 4th edn, pp. 2290–2294. McGraw-Hill, New York, 1993.

4 Balabanova, M., Calamia, K.T., Perniciaro, C. and O'Duffy, J.D. A study of the cutaneous manifestations of Behçet's's disease in patients from the United States. *J. Am. Acad. Dermatol.* 1999; 41: 540–545.

5 Marks, J.M. The skin and disorders of the alimentary tract. In: Fitzpatrick, T.B., Eisen, A.Z. Wolff, K., Freedberg, I.M. and Austen, K.F. (eds) *Dermatology in General Medicine*, 4th edn, pp. 2049–2050. McGraw-Hill, New York, 1993.

6 Wolff, K. and Stingl, G. Pyoderma gangrenosum. In: Fitzpatrick, T.B., Eisen, A.Z., Wolff, K., Freedberg, I.M. and Austen, K.F. (eds) *Dermatology in general medicine*, 4th edn, pp. 1171–1182. McGraw-Hill, New York, 1993.

7 Blacker, K.L., Stern, R.S. and Wintroub, B.U. Cutaneous reactions to drugs. In: Fitzpatrick, T.B., Eisen, A.Z., Wolff, K., Freedberg, I.M. and Austen, K.F. (eds) *Dermatology in General Medicine*, 4th edn. p. 1788. McGraw-Hill New York, 1993.

8 Fritsch, P.O. and Elias, P.M. Erythema multiforme and toxic epidermal necrolysis. In: Fitzpatrick, T.B., Eisen, A.Z., Wolff, K., Freedberg, I.M. and Austen, K.F. (eds) *Dermatology in General Medicine*, 4th edn, pp. 585–600. McGraw-Hill, New York, 1993.

9 McLean, D.I. and Haynes, H.A. Cutaneous manifestations of internal malignant disease. In: Fitzpatrick, T.B., Eisen, A.Z., Wolff, K., Freedberg, I.M. and Austen, K.F. (eds) *Dermatology in General Medicine*, 4th edn, pp. 2234–2235. McGraw-Hill, New York, 1993.

10 Gallagher, G.T. Biology and pathology of the oral mucosa. In: Fitzpatrick, T.B., Eisen, A.Z., Wolff, K., Freedberg, I.M. and Austen, K.F. (eds) *Dermatology in General Medicine*, 4th edn, p. 1366. McGraw-Hill, New York, 1993.

FURTHER READING

Ridley, C.M. and Neill, S.M. (eds) *The Vulva*, 2nd edn, pp. 121–186. Blackwell Science, Oxford, 1999.

20

Vulvar Dysesthesia

Ursula Wesselmann

INTRODUCTION

This chapter highlights the clinical presentation of vulvar dysesthesia and discusses treatment options. Chronic nonmalignant pain syndromes (longer than 6 months' duration) of urogenital origin are well described but poorly understood[1]. In the female patient these focal pain syndromes include vulvar dysesthesia, urethral syndrome, coccygodynia, and generalized perineal pain, and the key 'counterparts' in the male are orchialgia, prostatodynia, and chronic penile pain, as well as coccygodynia and generalized perineal pain. While the focus of this chapter is on vulvar dysesthesia, it is important to recognize that vulvar dysesthesia is one of the subgroups of the chronic nonmalignant urogenital pain syndromes, as this concept will guide the healthcare provider in making the diagnosis of a chronic pain syndrome.

Discomfort and pain in the vulvar area are usually very embarrassing for a patient, who may be afraid to discuss her symptoms with family members, friends, and healthcare providers. Except in cases in which a specific secondary cause can be identified, the etiology of vulvar dysesthesia often remains unknown. Currently available treatment options are only empirical and further research is desperately needed to understand the pathophysiological mechanisms of this disorder, in order to develop improved treatment strategies. Although cures are uncommon, it is important to recognize that some pain relief can be provided to almost all patients using currently available treatment strategies.

NEUROBIOLOGY OF THE PERINEUM

The perineum is a highly specialized area of the body, responsible for carrying out a host of basic biological functions including micturition, copulation, and reproduction. These diverse functions rely on precise nervous system control, coordinated with endocrine and other local control mechanisms. The complexity of this network has largely been considered to account for the slow progress in our understanding of the neurobiology of the perineal area compared with other areas of the body.

The innervation of the urogenital tract involves both components of the autonomic nervous system – the sympathetic and parasympathetic divisions – as well as the somatic nervous systems[2]. Dual projections from the thoracolumbar and sacral segments of the spinal cord carry out this innervation, converging mostly into peripheral neuronal plexuses from which nerve fibers ramify throughout the pelvic floor (20.1). Autonomic preganglionic efferents arise for the most part in the intermediolateral cell column, referred to as the sacral parasympathetic nucleus at sacral levels, whereas cell bodies of corresponding afferents are contained within dorsal root ganglia. The majority of the sympathetic input to the pelvic and urinary organs and the genital tract is through the superior hypogastric plexus.

Parasympathetic sacral outflow (S2–S4) consists of preganglionic nerves that are referred to as the pelvic splanchnic nerves. Parasympathetic afferent cell bodies are located in S2–S4 dorsal root ganglia and also course with the pelvic splanchnic nerve. The inferior hypogastric plexus is the major neuronal coordinating center that supplies the pelvic floor. The inferior hypogastric plexus receives sympathetic input (superior hypogastric plexus and its caudal extension, the hypogastric plexus, the sympathetic chain ganglia) and parasympathetic input (pelvic splanchnic nerve).[2] Both efferent and afferent fibers are carried in these sympathetic and parasympathetic projections[3]. Somatic efferent and afferent innervation to the pelvis originates from sacral spinal cord levels (S2–S4). Overlapping of somatic afferents with pelvic splanchnic nerve afferents on the spinal cord level have been proposed to account for the coordination of somatic and autonomic motor activity.

161

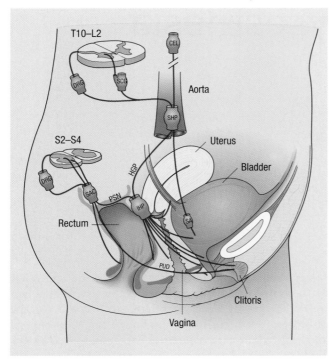

Fig 20.1 Innervation of the female perineal region.
Although this diagram attempts to show the innervation in humans, much of the anatomical information is derived from animal data. CEL, celiac plexus; DRG, dorsal root ganglion; HGP, hypogastric plexus; IHP, inferior hypogastric plexus; PSN, pelvic splanchnic nerve; PUD, pudendal nerve; SA, short adrenergic projections; SAC, sacral plexus; SCG, sympathetic chain ganglion; SHP, superior hypogastric plexus. From Wesselmann et al.[1], with permission.

Sacral nerve roots form the sacral plexus. The pudendal nerve arises from the sacral plexus as the primary efferent and afferent somatic distribution. The pudendal nerve also receives terminations of postganglionic axons arising from the caudal sympathetic chain ganglia. The inferior rectal nerve supplies the external anal sphincter and the perianal skin. The perineal nerve divides into a superficial branch supplying the skin over the perineal body and a larger deeper branch, supplying the levator ani muscle, the external sphincters, and the vaginal muscles. The dorsal nerve of the clitoris supplies the clitoris. Sensations from the perineum are conveyed mainly via the sacral somatic afferents and the sacral afferent parasympathetic system, with a far lesser afferent supply from afferents traveling with the thoracolumbar sympathetics[3]. Cholinergic nerve release likely governs the somatic mechanisms of the perineal musculature. Neuropeptide release appears to account for perineal sensations.

Despite major advances in immunohistochemical techniques over the past 10 years, there have been very few studies on the innervation of the vagina in humans. The first survey of the innervation pattern in the human vagina using a marker claimed to detect all nerves was published in 1995[4]. Free intraepithelial nerve endings were detected only in the introitus vaginae region. These very superficial free nerve endings are generally considered to be nociceptive or thermoceptive.

DEFINITIONS OF VULVAR DYSESTHESIA

Interestingly, hyperesthesia of the vulva was a well described entity in American[5] and European[6] gynecologic textbooks more than 100 years ago. Thomas[5] wrote in his textbook, *Practical Treatise on the Diseases of Women* (p. 145)

> The disease which I proceed to describe under this name, although to all appearances one of trivial character, really constitutes, on account of its excessive obstinacy and the great influence which it obtains over the mind of the patient, a malady of a great deal of importance ... This disorder, although fortunately not very frequent, is by no means very rare. So commonly it is met with at least, that it becomes a matter of surprise that it has not been more generally and fully described ... It is not a true neuralgia, but an abnormal sensitiveness; 'a plus state of excitability' in the diseased nerves.

Surprisingly, despite early detailed reports, chronic vulvar dysesthesia disappeared to a large extent from the medical literature until the early 1980s. In 1982 the International Society for the Study of Vulvar Disease (ISSVD) formed a task force to survey vulvar pain syndromes. This task force coined the term 'vulvodynia' as chronic vulvar discomfort[7], characterized by the patient's complaint of burning (and sometimes stinging, irritation, or rawness) in the vulvar area. At that time, the term vulvodynia included several disorders, all of which were thought to be factors in chronic vulvar pain: vulvar dermatoses, cyclic vulvovaginitis, vulvar vestibulitis, vulvar papillomatosis, and dysesthetic vulvodynia[8]. At the 1999 World Congress of the ISSVD a new classification system for vulvar dysesthesia (formerly vulvodynia) was proposed, namely a division into two broad categories: (1) generalized vulvar dysesthesia; (2) localized vulvar dysesthesia, including vestibulodynia (vulvar vestibulitis), clitorodynia, and others. As knowledge about the etiology and treatment of vulvar dysesthesia is advancing, definitions will probably be modified, based on emerging knowledge of the underlying pathophysiological mechanisms.

EPIDEMIOLOGY

The incidence or prevalence of vulvar dysesthesia is not known, but, as was already pointed out by Thomas[5], this pain syndrome is probably more common than generally thought. A recent survey of sexual dysfunction, analyzing data from the National Health and Social Life Survey, reported that 16% of women between the ages of 18 and 59 years living in households throughout the United States experience pain during sex[9]. When these data were analyzed by age group, the highest number of women reporting pain during sex was in the 18–29 years age group. The location and etiology of pain was not analyzed in this study. It is estimated that at least 200 000 women in the United States suffer from significant vulvar discomfort which greatly reduces their quality of life[10].

The age distribution ranges from the twenties to late sixties[11]. Goetsch[12] reported that 15% of all patients seen in her general gynecologic private practice fulfilled the definition of vulvar vestibulitis, a major subgroup of vulvar dysesthesia. Some 50% of these patients had always experienced entry dyspareunia and pain with inserting tampons, most since their teenage years. They had often wondered whether they were unique or had a hidden emotional aversion to sex. Women complaining about vulvar dysesthesia are primarily of Caucasian origin[12–14]; however, other sociocultural or socioeconomic factors could explain this observation.

ETIOLOGY

Although more than 100 years have passed since the original description of vulvar hyperesthesia, the causes and pathophysiological mechanisms of vulvar dysesthesia remain undiscovered. Despite the fact that many etiologic hypotheses have been proposed, our current understanding of vulvar dysesthesia is limited because most of the proposed causal explanations are derived from clinical case reports. Some 25–33% of women with vulvodynia know of a female relative with dyspareunia or tampon intolerance, raising the question of a genetic predisposition[12,14]. The coexistence of vulvodynia and interstitial cystitis has been reported, and it has been proposed that these syndromes represent a generalized disorder of urogenital sinus-derived epithelium[15]. Vulvar dysesthesia often has an acute onset, but sometimes no associated event can be recalled by the patient. In many cases the onset can be linked to episodes of a vaginal infection, local treatments of the vulvar or vaginal area (application of steroid or antimicrobial cream, cryosurgery, or laser surgery), or to changes in the pattern of sexual activity. However, many of these parameters are quite frequent in women anyway, and controlled prospective studies are necessary to assess whether the development of chronic vulvar discomfort is linked to a history of vaginal infection, irritation, or trauma. It could be hypothesized that, in some women, the vaginal tissue is more sensitive to these events than in others.

Histopathological studies of punch biopsies of the vulvar vestibule in patients with vestibulitis in comparison to control cases showed histopathological abnormalities in patients with vulvar vestibulitis as a result of a chronic inflammatory reaction of the mucosa of the vestibule, for which the cause remained unclear. Early reports suggested that human papillomavirus (HPV) plays a major role in the pathogenesis of vulvar vestibulitis, but this could not be confirmed by studies using molecular techniques[16]. Raised vulvar tissue levels of interleukin-1β and tumor necrosis factor α have been reported in vulvar vestibulitis, but, surprisingly, levels were lowest in the area of most severe hyperalgesia, the vulvar vestibule[17]. Interestingly, two recent studies reported vestibular neural hyperplasia in patients with vulvar dysesthesia[18,19], a finding that might provide a morphologic explanation for the pain; however, functional studies are needed to test this hypothesis.

CLINICAL PRESENTATION

On physical examination patients with vulvar dysesthesia usually present with *no visible abnormalities*. This is in contrast to patients with vulvar pain due to vulvar dermatoses where skin changes can be observed on examination of the vulvar area. Chronic infections of the vulvar area should be treated before a diagnosis of vulvar dysesthesia is considered. Further, iatrogenic, causes have to be excluded when evaluating a patient with vulvar dysesthesia. Local agents applied to the vulvar region can cause irritant reactions, which resolve after discontinuation of the irritant agent. Thus, vulvar dysesthesia is a diagnosis of exclusion. Depending on the location of the pain, a diagnosis of generalized or localized vulvar dysesthesia is made. In patients with localized vulvar dysesthesia, pain can easily be elicited or exacerbated by a simple cotton-tip applicator test: touching the dysesthetic area (typically the vulvar vestibule in patients with vulvar vestibulitis or the clitoris in patients with clitorodynia) with a moist cotton swab results in sharp, burning pain.

GENERALIZED VULVAR DYSESTHESIA

This subtype of vulvar dysesthesia seems to be more common in perimenopausal or postmenopausal women. There is diffuse, constant hyperalgesia in the vulvar area, often extending throughout the whole perineum. Patients with dysesthetic vulvodynia can easily be differentiated from patients with localized vulvar dysesthesia, because they have less focal tenderness and complain less about dyspareunia. It has been hypothesized that this generalized vulvar hyperalgesia

163

is due to altered cutaneous perception, such as in other neuropathic pain syndromes, and that pudendal neuralgia should be considered if the hyperalgesia extends from the mons pubis to the upper inner thighs and posteriorly across the ischial tuberosities[20,21].

LOCALIZED VULVAR DYSESTHESIA

This subtype is typically localized to the vulvar vestibule and/or the clitoris. It is characterized by painful sensations when wearing pants, or with bicycle and horseback riding. Women with localized vulvar dysesthesia at the vulvar vestibule complain about entry dyspareunia and pain at the introitus of the vagina when inserting a tampon. On gynecologic examination there are varying degrees of vestibular erythema. Although histological studies have not yet been able to confirm an etiology of the erythema, it might possibly be the result of 'neurogenic inflammation'. This term is used to characterize reddening, edema and hyperalgesia of tissue that is not due to an infectious or allergic reaction but, arises as a result of a neurogenic mechanism. Such a mechanism has been postulated for 'inflammatory reactions of unknown etiology' in other chronic pain syndromes[22], including interstitial cystitis, irritable bowel syndrome, and prostatodynia ('prostatitis'). When sensory fibers are stimulated electrically near the spinal cord, electrical impulses travel from the site of stimulation in both directions: towards the spinal cord (the normal – orthodromic direction for sensory axons) and towards the periphery (the opposite to normal – antidromic direction). When the antidromic impulses arrive in the periphery in the area innervated by the activated primary afferent nociceptors, 'neurogenic inflammation' is produced, characterized by reddening (vasodilatation), edema (plasma extravasation), and hyperalgesia. The neurogenic inflammation is produced by diffusible substances or substances released from the terminals of primary afferent neurons. These include neuropeptides (e.g. substance P, calcitonin gene-related peptide, neurokinin A, neurokinin B) and probably other autoacoids.

TREATMENT APPROACHES

The first step in the treatment of vulvar dysesthesia is to identify and eliminate local irritants and potential allergens. A role of urinary oxalate excretion in vulvar vestibulitis has been considered[23], but this has not been confirmed by others and further research is necessary. Many patients presenting with vulvar dysesthesia can be helped with oral medications recommended for neuropathic pain management (**Table 20.1**), including

antidepressants, anticonvulsants, membrane-stabilizing agents, and opioids[1,11]. Although clinical trials and case reports on the pharmacological management of chronic pain syndromes provide general guidelines as to which drug to choose[24], there is currently no method to predict which drug is most likely to alleviate pain in an individual patient with vulvar dysesthesia.

Table 20.1 Treatment of Vulvar Dysesthesia.

A. PHARMACOLOGICAL

I. Oral Agents

Antidepressants

   Tricyclics (amytriptyline, nortriptyline, desipramine)

   Mixed reuptake inhibitors (venlafaxine, nefazodone, maprotiline)

   Selective serotonin-reuptake inhibitors (fluoxetine, trazodone, sertraline)

Anticonvulsants/Antiarrhythmics

   Sodium channel blockers (carbamazepine, phenytoin, lamotrigine, lidocaine, mexiletine)

   Other mechanisms of action (gabapentin, clonazepam, valproic acid)

Opioids

   Oral long-acting opioids

      Slow release opioids: preparations of morphine or oxycodone

      Opioids with a long half-life: levorphanol, methadone

   Transdermal (fentanyl patch)

   Epidural/intrathecal (morphine, fentanyl)

II. Topical Agents

Local Anesthetics (Lidocaine 5% ointment, EMLA cream)

Corticosteroid Ointments (triamcinolone, clobetasol)

Topical Estrogen (Premarin cream)

Topical Aspirin, Nonsteroidal Anti-inflammatory Drugs (must be compounded by pharmacy)

B. NONPHARMACOLOGIC TREATMENT OF VULVAR DYSESTHESIA

Biofeedback

Physical Therapy

   Kegel exercises

   Pelvic floor massage/relaxation

Acupuncture

Sexual counseling

The goal of pharmacotherapy is to find a medication that produces significant pain relief with minimal side effects for an individual patient suffering from vulvar dysesthesia. It is important for the patient to understand the limitations of this 'trial and error' method of prescribing drugs. Adequate trials should be performed for each drug prescribed, and only one drug should be titrated at a time, because obviously the effects of a particular drug on pain scores cannot otherwise be assessed. More than one treatment approach might be necessary to achieve pain improvement. The starting dose should always be the smallest dose available and titration should occur at frequent intervals guided by pain scores and side effects. This requires frequent contact between the patient and the healthcare provider during the titration period. Some side effects actually improve as the patient is taking the drug for several weeks and it is important, if they are not intolerable, that the patient is guided through this period. Common reasons for inadequate medication trials are failure to titrate to an adequate dose and early termination of treatment due to side effects produced by increasing the dose too rapidly, starting at a high initial dose, or starting multiple drugs at the same time[24].

In patients with localized vulvar dysesthesia with a small and specific area of pain, topical treatment regimens such as creams with local anesthetics, aspirin, steroids, or estrogen might be helpful, although these agents have had limited success for severe or extensive pain. Intralesional interferon α injections have been suggested as a treatment modality, with about 50% of patients reporting substantial or partial improvement[25]. Isoprenosine, another agent reported to enhance immune function, was found to improve pain in a small group of patients[26]. Glazer et al.[27] reported pain relief in over 80% of patients with vulvar vestibulitis using electromyographic biofeedback of the pelvic floor musculature.

Surgical procedures have been advocated to remove the hyperalgesic skin area in patients with vulvar vestibulitis[1]. The most commonly used procedure is perineoplasty. A simplified surgical revision, as an alternative to this extensive surgical intervention, has been advocated by Goetsch[13], in which the painful area is excised under local anesthesia.

PSYCHOLOGICAL ISSUES AND VULVAR DYSESTHESIA

The traditional psychosocial view of sexual pain disorders, including vulvar dysesthesia, has focused on sexual and marital issues, conflicts, and experiences. There has been a distinct attempt to dichotomize etiology between psychological and physiological factors. Recent psychological literature, however, has suggested a pain-centered approach, focusing on pain itself as the major symptom of these problems[28]. For the healthcare provider who is diagnosing and treating women with vulvar dysesthesia, it is important to recognize that location of pain is a significant predictor of appraisal of pain, affective response, and disclosure of pain. Klonoff et al.[29] demonstrated that subjects asked to imagine pain in their genital area appraised themselves as more ill and more likely to be having an emergency than if they were asked to imagine pain in other areas of the body. Vulvar dysesthesia has major implications on a woman's life, including effects on the lifestyle, relationships, sexuality, and self-image. These psychosocial aspects of the disease have to be addressed in a comprehensive treatment approach. For example, a woman who has not been able to have sex without severe pain for many years because of vulvar dysesthesia might need psychological support to resume a sexual life with 'less pain', once a treatment approach has been identified that is reducing the vulvar and vaginal discomfort. Considering the years of experiencing pain while attempting sexual intercourse, the woman might still remain quite anxious and apprehensive in her sexual life, even if the vulvar dysesthesia is improved.

CONCLUSIONS

In summary, vulvar dysesthesia is a recognized disease entity and a large body of literature has emerged over the past 15 years reporting the existence of this disease and suggesting causes and treatments. Further research is needed to identify the etiology of vulvar dysesthesia. To confirm the diagnosis of vulvar dysesthesia, excluding secondary causes such as dermatitis or gynecologic infections, and to design a treatment plan, a multidisciplinary approach involving the collaboration of gynecologists, dermatologists, neurologists, pain specialists, and psychologists is important. The first important step is to recognize that the patient is suffering from vulvar dysesthesia! Many patients with vulvar dysesthesia have remained undiagnosed and untreated, because the clinical presentation and treatment approaches are not widely known to healthcare professionals. Public information websites can be extremely helpful in assisting patients in finding specialists with an interest in treating vulvar dysesthesia (see Patient resources) and patient support groups offer emotional and informational assistance as well.

REFERENCES

1 Wesselmann, U., Burnett, A. L., and Heinberg, L. J. The urogenital and rectal pain syndromes. *Pain* 1997; **73**: 269–294.

2 De Groat, W. C. Neurophysiology of the pelvic organs. In: Rushton, D. N. (ed.) *Handbook of Neuro-Urology*, pp. 55–93. Marcel Dekker, New York, 1994.

3 Jänig, W. and Koltzenburg, M. Pain arising from the urogenital tract. In: Maggi, C. A. (ed.) *Nervous Control of the Urogenital System*, pp. 525–578. Harwood Academic, Chur, Switzerland, 1993.

4 Hilliges, M., Falconer, C., Ekman-Ordeberg, G., *et al.* Innervation of the human vaginal mucosa as revealed by PGP 9.5 immunohistochemistry. *Acta Anat. (Basel)* 1995; **153**: 119–126.

5 Thomas, T. G. (ed.) *Practical Treatise on the Diseases of Women*, p. 145. Philadelphia, Henry C. Leason, 1880.

6 Pozzi, S. J. *Traite de Gynecologie Clinique et Operatoire*. Masson, Paris, 1897.

7 Young, A. W., Azoury, R. S., McKay, M., *et al.* Burning vulva syndrome. Report of the ISSVD Task Force. *J. Reprod. Med.* 1984; **29**: 457.

8 McKay, M. Vulvodynia, a multifactorial problem. *Arch. Dermatol.* 1989; **125**: 256–262.

9 Laumann, E. O., Paik, A., and Rosen, R. C. Sexual dysfunction in the United States. Prevalence and Predictors. *J.A.M.A.* 1999; **281**: 537–544.

10 Jones, K. D. and Lehr S.T. Vulvodynia: diagnostic techniques and treatment modalities. *Nurse Pract.* 1994; **19**: 34–46.

11 Paavonen, J. Diagnosis and treatment of vulvodynia. *Ann. Med.* 1995; **27**: 175–181.

12 Goetsch, M. F. Vulvar vestibulitis: prevalence and historic features in a general gynecologic practice population. *Am. J. Obstet. Gynecol.* 1991; **164**: 1609–1616.

13 Goetsch, M. F. Simplified surgical revision of the vulvar vestibule for vulvar vestibulitis. *Am. J. Obstet. Gynecol.* 1996; **174**: 1701–1707.

14 Bergeron, S., Bouchard, C., Fortier, M., *et al.* The surgical treatment of vulvar vestibulitis syndrome: a follow-up study. *J. Sex. Marital Ther.* 1997; **23**: 317–325.

15 Fitzpatrick, C. C., Delancey, J. O. L., Elkins, T. E. *et al.* Vulvar vestibulitis and interstitial cystitis: a disorder of urogenital sinus-derived epithelium? *Obstet. Gynecol.* 1993; **81**: 860–862.

16 De Deus, J. M., Focchi, J., Stavale, J. N., *et al.* Histologic and biomolecular aspects of papillomatosis of the vulvar vestibule in relation to human papillomavirus. *Obstet. Gynecol.* 1995; **86**: 758–763.

17 Foster, D. C. and Hasday, J. D. Elevated tissue levels of interleukin-1 beta and tumor necrosis factor-alpha in vulvar vestibulitis. *Obstet. Gynecol.* 1997; **89**: 291–296.

18 Bohm-Starke, N., Hilliges, M., Falconer, C., *et al.* Increased intraepithelial innervation in women with vulvar vestibulitis syndrome. *Gynecol. Obstet. Invest.* 1998; **46**: 256–260.

19 Westrom, L. V. and Willen, R. Vestibular nerve fiber proliferation in vulvar vestibulitis syndrome. *Obstet. Gynecol.* 1998; **91**: 572–576.

20 McKay, M. Vulvodynia: diagnostic patterns. *Dermatol. Clin.* 1992; **10**: 423–433.

21 McKay, M. Subsets of vulvodynia. *J. Reprod. Med.* 1988; **33**: 695–698.

22 Wesselmann, U. Neurogenic inflammation and chronic pelvic pain. *World J. Urol.* 2001 (in press).

23 Solomons, C. C., Melmed, M. H., and Heitler, S. M. Calcium citrate for vulvar vestibulitis. *J. Reprod. Med.* 1991; **36**: 879–882.

24 Rowbotham, M. C. Chronic pain mechanisms and management. *Neurology* 1995; **45**(Suppl.9).

25 Marinoff, S. C., Turner, M. L., Hirsch, R. P., *et al.* Intralesional alpha interferon: cost effective therapy for vulvar vestibulitis syndrome. *J. Reprod. Med.* 1993; **38**: 19–24.

26 Petersen, C. S. and Weismann, K. Isoprenosine improves symptoms in young females with chronic vulvodynia. *Acta Derm. Venereol. (Stockh.)* 1996; **76**: 404.

27 Glazer, H. I., Rodke, G., Swencionis, C., *et al.* Treatment of vulvar vestibulitis syndrome with electromyographic biofeedback of pelvic floor musculature. *J. Reprod. Med.* 1995; **40**: 283–290.

28 Binik, Y. M., Meana, M., Berkley, K., *et al.* The sexual pain disorders: is the pain sexual or is the sex painful? *Annu. Rev. Sex Res.* 1999; **10**: 210–235.

29 Klonoff, E. A., Landrine, H., and Brown, M. Appraisal and response to pain may be a function of its bodily location. *J. Psychosom. Res.* 1993; **37**: 661–670.

PATIENT RESOURCES

American Pain Society
4700 West Lake Avenue
Glenview, IL 60025–1485, USA
Tel: 847–375–4715
Website: http://www.ampainsoc.org

International Association for the Study of Pain
909 NE 43rd Street, Suite 306
Seattle, WA 98105–6020, USA

Tel: 206–547–6409
Website: http://www.halcyon.com/iasp

National Vulvodynia Association
POB 4491
Silver Spring, MD 20914–4491, USA
Tel: 301–299–0775
Website: www.nva.org

21 Pigmented Lesions of the Vulva

Barbara E. McAlpine

INTRODUCTION

About 10–12% of women have pigmented vulvar lesions, as determined by a retrospective analysis of patients seen at a vulvar clinic[1] and a prospective study of a gynecologic practice[2]. Most of these lesions are benign lentigines. Only about 2% of patients have vulvar nevi, and this number decreases with age. Other discrete lesions that may be pigmented include seborrheic keratoses, vascular lesions, genital warts, and malignant tumors such as melanomas, basal cell carcinomas and squamous cell carcinomas. Diffuse hyperpigmentation may also be seen in inflammatory lesions such as lichen simplex chronicus and discoid lupus erythematosus, and in malignant lesions such as squamous cell carcinoma *in situ* and Paget's disease. In short, hyperpigmentation, including normal ethnic variation, is not unusual on the vulva, and differentiating benign from malignant processes is critical for appropriate patient management.

VULVAR NEVI AND MELANOMAS

There has always been particular concern about nevocellular nevi occurring in the vulva, because of the increased risk that a melanoma arising in the vulva seems to carry. Much of this risk is related to the depth, or Breslow level, of the melanoma at the time of diagnosis[3]. Vulvar melanomas tend to be more advanced (i.e. deeper) lesions at the time of diagnosis than melanomas found elsewhere on the body. The depth of the lesion is the single most important prognostic indicator for primary melanoma. Lesions less than 0.85 mm deep carry a 10-year survival rate of 95.7%, whereas lesions deeper than 3.6 mm are associated with a 10-year survival rate of 46.0%[4].

It is not yet known whether the differences in tumor thickness and prognosis of vulvar lesions are simply related to a delay in diagnosis because of the anatomic site, or whether there is a true difference in the biologic behavior of these lesions. There may be some differences in the molecular progression of melanoma from sun-protected sites such as the vulva, compared with sun-exposed parts of the body. In a recent report *ras* mutations were examined from melanoma tumor tissue from sun-protected areas and compared with mutations from sun-exposed areas. Some 32% of melanomas from sun-exposed head and neck areas contained mutations of the N-*ras* genes as detected by polymerase chain reaction analysis, whereas only 7% of tumors from sun-protected areas had such mutations[5]. The molecular genetics of melanoma were reviewed recently[6]. Approximately 2–5% of melanomas occur on the vulva, and approximately 8–11% of all vulvar cancers are melanomas[7–9]. Clinically, these lesions are usually deeply pigmented with irregular borders, and share the features of melanomas seen elsewhere on the body. They occur on mucosa as well as on hair-bearing skin of the vulva. Mucosal melanomas present as flat, very dark, irregularly shaped lesions. Eventually, they develop a nodular component, as seen in **21.1**.

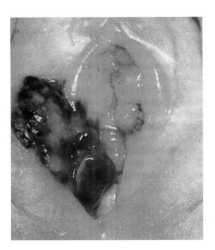

Fig 21.1 Melanoma (mucosal). Deeply pigmented and irregular nodules are seen on the labia minora. This is an advanced lesion and therefore the prognosis is grave.

Labia majora lesions tend to be of the superficial spreading type (**21.2**), which is the most common form of malignant melanoma. This type of melanoma often has a prolonged radial or horizontal growth phase, during which the lesion expands along the dermo-epidermal junction before developing a deep or vertical growth component. The fact that a lesion has been present for a long time is not necessarily reassuring, particularly if there are signs of enlargement or other change.

Mucosal melanomas may have a distinctive histologic appearance, and are referred to as mucosal lentiginous type. Nodular-type melanomas can also occur in both vulvar and mucosal areas, and carry the worst prognosis as they tend quickly to develop a deep component.

Benign nevi occurring on the vulva may be junctional (**21.3**), compound (**21.4**), or intradermal. Junctional nevi are typically small, darkly pigmented, slightly raised papules and are found on mucosal and keratinizing skin. They occur from childhood to young adulthood. At times they are indistinguishable from lentigines. Compound nevi contain both a junctional and intradermal component of nevus cells. They are benign lesions and are generally thought to be a progression from junctional nevi – nevus cells that have 'dropped down' or infiltrated the dermis. Compound nevi are small, dome-shaped, hyperpigmented papules. With time, these lesions tend to lose their junctional component and pigment, and become intradermal. Intradermal nevi are typically small, soft, skin-colored papules that may resemble a skin tag. In general, the morphologic and histologic characteristics of vulvar nevi parallel those of nevi on the torso, as shown in a retrospective histopathologic study comparing 59 vulvar nevi with 50 torso nevi[10].

ATYPICAL MELANOCYTIC NEVUS OF THE VULVA

There appears to be a group of young premenopausal women whose vulvar nevi have distinctive features.[10,11] These lesions (**21.5**) have been called 'atypical melanocytic nevi of the genital (vulvar) type'[12]. They are usually hyperpigmented, papular lesions with indistinct borders, but without the other clinical features of melanoma. Histologically, the lesions are quite unusual, with junctional melanocytic atypia overlying nests of dermal nevus cells. Differentiation from melanoma can be difficult, and evaluation by a dermatopathologist or pathologist with expertise in the diagnosis of melanocytic lesions is required.

A detailed study of the histopathologic findings of atypical melanocytic nevi of the genital tract (AMNGT) was reported by Clark *et al.*[13]. Stromal differences can be used to distinguish AMNGT from dysplastic nevi (discussed below). AMNGT are more common on

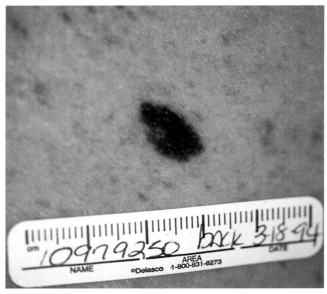

Fig 21.2 Melanoma. Typical superficial spreading melanoma with variation in pigmentation and irregular borders. The morphology of these lesions is the same on the skin of the trunk and the vulva.

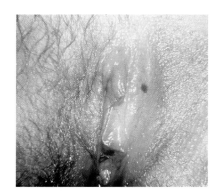

Fig 21.3 Junctional nevus. This benign lesion is composed of nevomelanocytes in nests at the dermoepidermal junction and is often associated with lentiginous melanocytic hyperplasia.

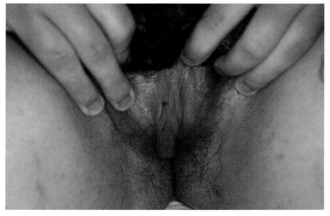

Fig 21.4 Compound nevus. Note: ungloved hands in these photographs are the patient's own.

mucosal surfaces, whereas dysplastic nevi are more common on the labia majora. Clinically these lesions are often distinguishable only by indistinct borders. The natural history of these lesions has not been determined, although complete excision is usually recommended.

DYSPLASTIC NEVUS

Dysplastic nevi occur sporadically and in patients with melanoma or a family history of melanoma (**21.6, 21.7**). The 'atypical mole' is one of several synonyms for dysplastic nevus. These lesions have irregular features compared with normal acquired nevi, including a larger size, a macular and papular component, asymmetry, irregular borders, pigmentation, and a distribution that includes sun-protected skin.

Dysplastic nevi are generally considered to be a marker for patients who are at increased risk of melanoma. These lesions can occur on the vulva, as well as on other areas of the body. When they occur on the vulva, they share some histologic features with atypical melanocytic nevus of the vulva (*see above*). Excisional biopsy is necessary in most cases to rule out melanoma.

CONGENITAL NEVUS

A congenital nevus (**21.8**) is one that is present at birth, or appears shortly thereafter. These lesions tend to be larger and more irregular in shape than acquired nevi. There is some evidence that the risk of developing malignant melanoma in larger congenital nevi is greater than that for acquired nevi, but this is not necessarily true for smaller lesions. Congenital vulvar nevi are rare and, consequently, little epidemiologic information is available.

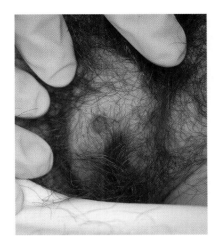

Fig 21.6 'Dysplastic' nevus. This lesion on the labia majora was excised and the diagnosis of dysplastic nevus confirmed.

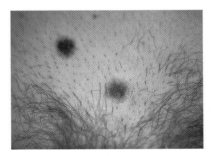

Fig 21.7 'Dysplastic' nevus. This patient has multiple dysplastic nevi over the trunk and extremities, as well as a history of malignant melanoma. These lesions resemble melanoma in that they are large and irregularly pigmented. Melanoma was ruled out in this case by excisional biopsy.

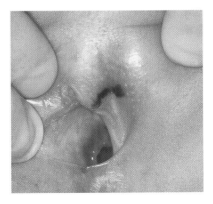

Fig 21.8 Congenital nevus.

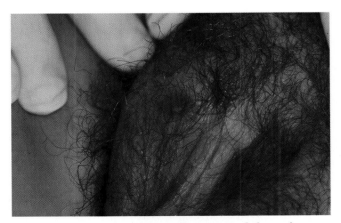

Fig 21.5 Atypical melanocytic nevus of the vulva. This lesion was approximately 1 cm in size, slightly hyperpigmented, and flat with a 3 mm papule in the central portion. The borders were somewhat indistinct, but the lesion was otherwise unremarkable. This patient had noted the growth of the papular component.

LENTIGINES AND VULVAR MELANOSIS

Lentigines (singular, lentigo) are small, less than 5 mm wide, hyperpigmented macules, which are found on vulvar skin and mucous membranes in 3.5–7% of patients (**21.9**). Histopathologic examination demonstrates increased pigmentation in the basal cell layer, lentiginous epidermal proliferation, and variable degrees of melanocytic hyperplasia.

The findings of vulvar melanosis (**21.10**) are similar, except that the lesions are larger and may be irregularly shaped, mimicking melanoma[14,15]. The lesions have similar, if exaggerated, histopathologic features to lentigines, with the additional feature of dermal melanophages. Atypical melanocytes suggestive of melanoma or melanoma precursors are not seen in either lesion. Adequate biopsy is necessary to differentiate vulvar melanosis from melanoma.

HYPERPIGMENTATION ASSOCIATED WITH NONNEVOMELANOCYTIC LESIONS

Any lesion or cutaneous eruption that has an inflammatory component can result in postinflammatory hyperpigmentation. Lichen simplex chronicus (**21.11**) is the classic example of this, but hyperpigmentation is also a feature of other inflammatory lesions, such as discoid lupus erythematosus (**21.12**). Lichen simplex chronicus is a form of chronic eczema that is often well circumscribed and characterized by lichenification and hyperpigmentation. Discoid lupus erythematosus is a form of cutaneous lupus, in which scarring, follicular plugging, and hypopigmentation or hyperpigmentation are common.

Similarly, some skin-derived, nonmelanoma tumors, such as basal cell carcinoma, squamous cell carcinoma, vulvar intraepithelial neoplasia, extramammary Paget's disease (**21.13**), and even benign seborrheic keratosis (**21.14**, **21.15**), contain melanocytes and may be pigmented. Seborrheic keratosis is a benign proliferation of keratinocytes and becomes more common with advancing age. Seborrheic keratoses and skin tags are also seen in conjunction with acanthosis nigricans. The sudden onset of multiple eruptive seborrheic keratoses (Leser–Trélat sign) may be associated with an internal malignancy, usually adenocarcinoma.

Hyperpigmentation is a fairly common characteristic of carcinoma *in situ*, and may in fact be the sole clinical clue (**21.16**).

Lastly, some lesions without melanocytes appear to be pigmented, such as vascular lesions and cysts (**21.17**) (*see Chapter 22*).

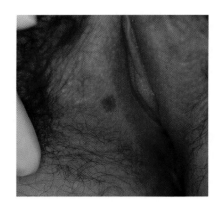

Fig 21.9 Lentigo. Typical small, flat, hyperpigmented macule.

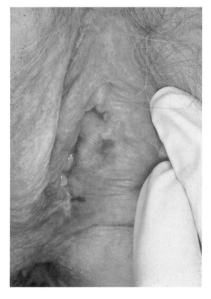

Fig 21.10 Vulvar melanosis. This irregularly pigmented lesion on the labia minora shares many clinical features with a dysplastic nevus or melanoma. A second irregularly shaped hyperpigmented lesion is also seen on the mucosa. A biopsy is necessary to confirm the diagnosis of vulvar melanosis.

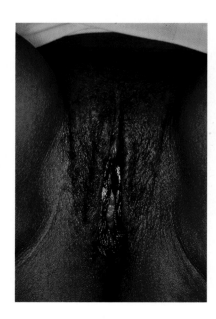

Fig 21.11 Lichen simplex chronicus. In this patient, the alteration of skin texture and hyperpigmentation is best seen along the mid-portion of the labia majora.

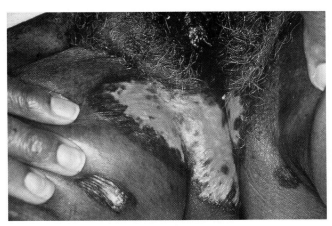

Fig 21.12 Discoid lupus. This patient had numerous discoid lesions over the trunk, face, and extremities.

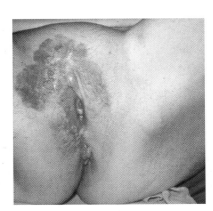

Fig 21.13 Extramammary Paget's disease. The less common clinical presentation of hyperpigmented, scaly plaques can be seen extending out from the typical, moist, macerated lesions of extramammary Paget's disease.

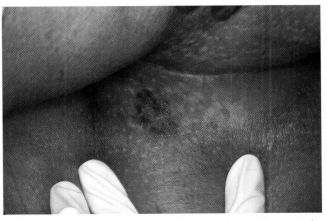

Fig 21.14 Seborrheic keratosis. This hyperpigmented, well circumscribed, 'stuck on' papule is sometimes confused with melanoma.

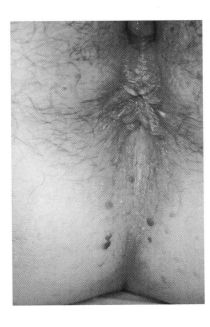

Fig 21.15 Multiple seborrheic keratoses. Seborrheic keratoses often occur in large numbers, particularly on the trunk. As in this case, they are benign.

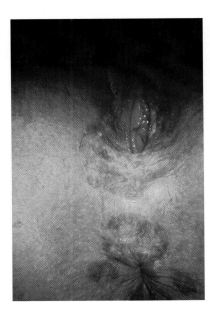

Fig 21.16 Carcinoma *in situ*. This patient also had areas of erythema and hyperkeratosis.

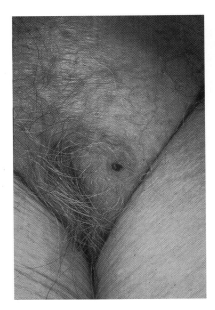

Fig 21.17 Epidermoid cyst (epithelial inclusion cyst). These benign cysts filled with necrotic desquamated keratinocytes are not unusual in the vulvar area. They may or may not have a connection to the skin surface. When they do, the cyst contents take on a dark appearance, as seen in this lesion.

REFERENCES

1 Friedrich, E.G., Burch, K. and Bahr, J.P. The vulvar clinic: an eight-year appraisal. *Am. J. Obstet. Gynecol.* 1979; **135**: 1036.

2 Rock, B. Hood, A.F. and Rock, J.A. Prospective study of vulvar nevi. J. Am. Acad. Dermatol. 1990; 22: 104.

3 Bradgate, M.G., Rollason, T.P., McConkey, C.C. *et al.* Malignant melanoma of the vulva: a clinicopathologic study of 50 women. *Br. J. Dermatol.* 1990; **97**: 124.

4 Friedman, R.J., Rigel, D.S., Silverman, M.K. *et al.* Malignant melanoma in the 1990s: the continued importance of early detection and the role of the physician examination and self examination of the skin. *CA Cancer J. Clin.* 1991; **41**(4): 201.

5 Jiveskog, S., Ragnarsson-Olding B., Platz, A. and Ringborg, U. N-*ras* mutations are common in melanoma from sun-exposed skin of humans but rare in mucosal membranes or unexposed skin. *J. Invest. Dermatol.* 1998; **111**(5): 757–761.

6 Piepkorn, M. Melanoma genetic: an update with focus on the CDKN2A(p16)/ARF tumor suppressors. *Am. Acad. Dermatol.* 2000; **42**(5): 705–722.

7 Karlen, J.R., Piver M.S. and Barlow, J.J. Melanoma of the vulva. *Obstet. Gynecol.* 1975; **45**: 181.

8 Morrow, C.P. and DeSaia, P.J. Malignant melanoma of the female genitalia: a clinical analysis. *Obstet. Gynecol. Surv.* 1976; **31**: 233.

9 Ronan, S.G., Eng, A.M., Briele, H.A. *et al.* Malignant melanoma of the female genitalia. *J. Am. Acad. Dermatol.* 1990; **22**: 428.

10 Christensen, W.N., Friedman, K.J., Woodruff, J.D. and Hood, A.F. Histologic characteristics of vulvar nevocellular nevi. *J. Cutan. Pathol.* 1987; **14**: 87.

11 Friedman, R.J. and Ackerman, A.B. Difficulties in the diagnosis of melanocytic nevi on the vulvae of premenopausal women. In: Ackerman, A.B. (ed.) *Pathology of Malignant Melanoma*, p. 119. Masson, New York, 1981.

12 Clark, W.H., Elder, D.E. and Guerry, D. IV. Dysplastic nevi and malignant melanoma. In: Farmer, E.R. and Hood, A.F. (eds) *Pathology of the Skin*, p. 742. Appleton & Lange, Norwalk, 1990.

13 Clark, W.H., Hood, A.F., Tucker, M.A. and Jampel, R.M. Atypical melanocytic nevi of the genital type with a discussion of reciprocal parenchymal–stromal interactions in the biology of neoplasia. *Hum. Pathol.* 1998; **29**(1 Suppl 1): S1–24.

14 Rudolph, R.I. Vulvar melanosis. *J. Am. Acad. Dermatol.* 1990; **23**: 982.

15 Lenane, P., Keane, C.O., Connell, B.O. *et al.* Genital melanotic macules: clinical, histologic, immunohistochemical, and ultrastructural features. *J. Am. Acad. Dermatol.* 2000; **42**: 640–644.

ACKNOWLEDGEMENTS

Figure **21.1** is reproduced from Tindall, V.R. *Colour Atlas of Clinical Gynaecology* (Fig. 84), Wolfe, London, 1981.
Figures **21.13** and **21.16** are reproduced by kind permission of J. Donald Woodruff.

22 Vulvar Tumors

Ira R. Horowitz,
John M. Monaghan,
Marilynne McKay

INTRODUCTION

The superficial vulva contains skin appendages and a small number of specialized glandular structures, each of which may develop tumors. The vulva has an excellent blood supply and a plethora of nerves. The outer part of the vulva (labia majora) is hair-bearing, with associated apocrine glandular systems. The inner part (labia minora) is covered by stratified squamous epithelium, which blends midway on the inner surface (Hart line) into a modification known as mucous membrane (vulvar vestibule) which lacks a granular layer. This nonkeratinized surface continues into the vagina. As vulvar tumors may be difficult to differentiate from one another, a biopsy is often necessary to establish the diagnosis.

BENIGN TUMORS

There is a variety of benign tumors (**Table 22.1**), of which one group – *the benign pigmented tumors* – has been discussed in *Chapter 21* and so will not be mentioned further.

CONGENITAL TUMORS AND CYSTS

ACCESSORY BREAST TISSUE

The breast line extends from the anterior border of the axilla, down the chest and abdominal wall, and ends on the vulvar labia majora on each side (**22.1**). Thus, swelling of the vulva, and even the secretion of breast

---

Table 22.1 Vulvar Tumors.

Benign tumors	Solid papules and tumors
Pigmented papules and nodules	Skin tag (acrochordon)
See Chapter 21	Fibroepithelial polyp
	Neurofibroma
Congenital tumors and cysts	Syringomas
Accessory breast tissue	Fox–Fordyce disease
Hernia	Hidradenoma
Mesonephric duct cyst	**'Potentially malignant' tumors**
Cyst of the canal of Nuck	Fibroma and fibrosarcoma
Cystic tumors	Lipoma and liposarcoma
Vestibular mucous cyst	Granular cell tumor
Pilonidal cyst, sinus, or abscess	Verrucous carcinoma
Bartholin cyst or abscess	Vulvar intraepithelial neoplasia (VIN)
Epithelial inclusion cyst	**Malignant tumors**
Lymphangioma	Squamous cell carcinoma
Vascular tumors and swelling	Melanoma
Hemangioma	Basal cell carcinoma
Cherry angioma	Adenocarcinoma
Angiokeratoma	Extramammary Paget's disease
Pyogenic granuloma	Adenoid cystic carcinoma
Endometriosis	Sarcoma
Hematoma	Metastatic tumors
Edema	

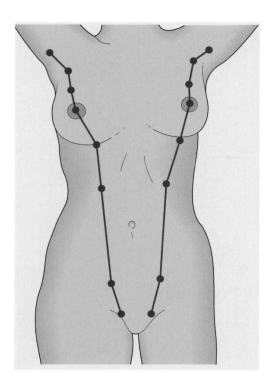

Fig 22.1 Breast line.

milk, may occur during the latter part of pregnancy and into the puerperium. Often, a vestigial nipple is present as a dark area or small swelling of the vulvar skin. However, fully formed nipples with significant amounts of breast tissue have been recorded. It is important to differentiate accessory breast tissue from hidradenoma, labial varicosities, fibroma, or lipoma. The accessory tissue may need to be excised if there are persistent problems. The potential for malignant change clearly exists, although most reports of breast cancer found on the vulva have been secondary from a primary in the breast[1].

HERNIA

Inguinal hernias are rare in women. Very rarely, an inguinal hernia may be found to pass down into the upper part of the vulva, where it presents as a small, elongated, unilateral swelling, which is compressible and soft. It is usually not painful, but may become tender due to strangulation or any of the common complications associated with inguinal hernias. It is imperative to rule out the presence of herniated bowel in large vulvar masses. Computed tomography with contrast, magnetic resonance imaging or ultrasonography may be utilized.

MESONEPHRIC DUCT CYSTS

During the development of the female fetus, the mesonephric (Wolffian) ducts lie lateral and parallel to the paramesonephric (Müllerian) system (*see Chapter 13*). Remnants of the mesonephric system may remain, resulting in cystic swellings anywhere from the introitus to the broad ligament. Although most commonly found in the upper vagina (Gartner cysts), it is not unusual to

find mesonephric duct cysts on the vulva. They tend to lie laterally, but can be located in various sites, and are commonly confused with the more common vestibular mucous cyst (*see below*). Paramesonephric duct cysts are found only in the vagina; the Müllerian system plays no part in the development of the vulva, but this is sometimes a misnomer given to vestibular mucous cysts (*see below*). Treatment is by simple excision if the lesion is symptomatic.

CYST OF THE CANAL OF NUCK

This rare problem may be mistaken for an inclusion cyst or even a hernia. The lesion is small and lies in the inguinal crease or the anterior labia majora, in the line of the round ligament remnant as it enters the upper part of the vulva on the lateral side. The diagnosis is usually made following excision of the cyst.

CYSTIC TUMORS

VESTIBULAR MUCOUS CYSTS

These are usually confined to the vestibular ring of the introitus and are probably more common than is thought. They are not infrequently seen in the newborn, but are less commonly diagnosed in the adult. These dysontogenetic cysts are usually asymptomatic and ignored by both patient and physician. The cysts lie between the hymenal ring and the outer part of the labia minora (**22.2**), and are thought to be caused by obstruction of the ducts of the small vestibular glands. They may be yellow, bluish, or skin-colored, and usually have a translucent appearance. Similar mucous cysts may also arise in close relationship to the urethra, where they may occasionally cause obstruction or diversion of urinary flow. Treatment is by simple excision if the cyst is symptomatic or the patient wants it removed.

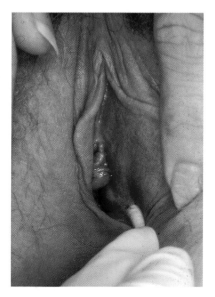

Fig 22.2 Vestibular mucous cyst. This asymptomatic lesion was found on incidental examination of a patient with recurrent candidiasis. Note: Ungloved fingers are the patient's own.

PILONIDAL CYSTS, SINUSES, OR ABSCESSES

These lesions begin as abscesses that develop from a foreign-body inflammatory reaction to hair within the dermis. The hair may be from a ruptured dermoid cyst or an ingrown follicle. The most common location is in the lower sacrococcygeal area, but the lesions may occur on the vulva, usually around the clitoris but sometimes on the mons pubis or perineum. Clinically, these are red papules that frequently erode and drain, forming a chronic sinus tract. The entire sinus tract must be excised to prevent recurrence. If an abscess is present, conservative management with Sitz baths and broad-spectrum antibiotics is recommended. When the mass is fluctuant, an incision and drainage should be performed. The wound should then be packed and permitted to heal by secondary intention.

BARTHOLIN CYST OR ABSCESS

Bartholin glands are bilateral and lie posterolaterally in the introitus at 5:00 and 7:00. The ducts secrete into the posterior vestibule at the base of the hymen, and provide a degree of lubrication, although most sexual lubrication in sexually experienced women is from vaginal secretions. Occasionally, the ostium of a Bartholin gland may become obstructed, causing the gland and duct to swell to a large size. The entire gland can be grasped between finger and thumb (**22.3**) when this occurs. If the gland is not infected, the swelling is painless.

The fluid contained within the Bartholin cyst may be released spontaneously, but it is often necessary to release the contents surgically. A standard procedure is that of marsupialization, whereby the cyst is deroofed (**22.4**) and the edges are carefully oversewn to generate a functioning duct (**22.5**)[2]. An alternative method is to make a small incision in the roof of the cyst and insert a Word catheter (or trimmed-off short pediatric Foley catheter), which is then inflated and allowed to remain in place for several weeks[2,3]. Failure to keep the cyst open will increase the risk of recurrence (**22.6**). Complete excision of the cyst is occasionally performed when there is recurrent painful obstruction. In cases where infection has been the cause of the obstruction, a combination of antibiotics and surgical drainage gives the best results.

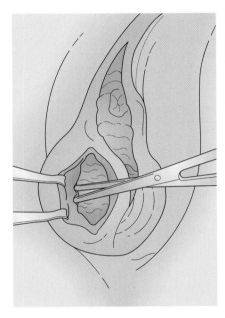

Fig 22.4 Marsupialization of a Bartholin cyst. The Bartholin cyst is being released from the overlying skin and excess skin removed.

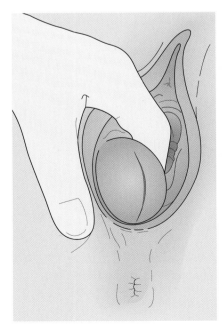

Fig 22.3 Marsupialization of a Bartholin cyst. A right-sided Bartholin cyst is shown being elevated by introducing the index finger into the lower vagina. The line of incision is shown.

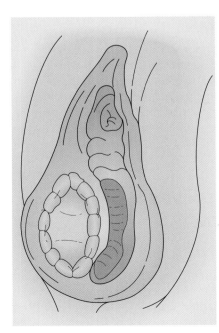

Fig 22.5 Marsupialization of a Bartholin cyst. The edges of the marsupialized cyst have been oversewn so that the secreting part of the gland can be preserved. Once healing is complete, the defect will remain as a small hole through which secretions can pass.

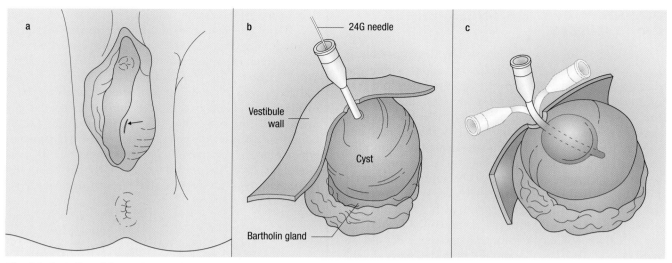

Fig 22.6 Inflatable catheter for a Bartholin cyst. This shows the inflatable bulb-tipped catheter used to treat Bartholin cysts and abscesses. (a) An arrow indicates the location for a stab wound in a cyst or abscess. (b) Insertion of the catheter in the stab wound. (c) Inserted catheter inflated with 2–4 mL of water.

EPITHELIAL (EPIDERMAL) INCLUSION CYSTS

Also called sebaceous, keratinous, or epidermoid cysts, these lesions are very common on the labia majora and sometimes minora (22.7). From time to time, they may become very extensive, making diagnosis more difficult (22.8). The cysts are lined by keratinizing squamous epithelium and are filled with a cheesy white accumulation of waxy secretions and cell debris. In contrast to large solitary lesions on the scalp, vulvar cysts tend to be small, multiple, and grouped. They may be recognized by a yellowish appearance and knobbly feel. If the patient is symptomatic or bothered by the appearance, simple excision is appropriate. Cysts will recur after incision and drainage unless the cyst wall is removed.

LYMPHANGIOMAS

These localized dilations and ectasias of lymphatic vessels may appear at any age, although one form – lymphangioma circumscriptum – typically develops in childhood. They usually appear as papules or nodules, from which a clear or milky fluid may drain. Diagnosis is made on biopsy and observation of the white lymphatic fluid (22.9, 22.10)

VASCULAR TUMORS AND SWELLING

HEMANGIOMAS

Three forms of hemangioma may be found on the vulva. The *cherry angioma* is extremely common and is a small, dark-red papule usually 2–3 mm in diameter (22.11). Cherry angiomas are discrete lesions which are

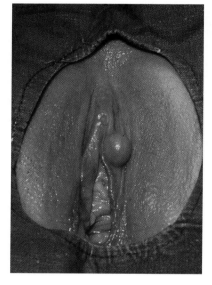

Fig 22.7 Epidermal inclusion cyst, 1 cm in diameter, in the left interlabial fold. Simple excision confirmed the diagnosis and treated the problem. Incision and drainage is not recommended, as the lesion usually recurs unless the cyst wall is removed.

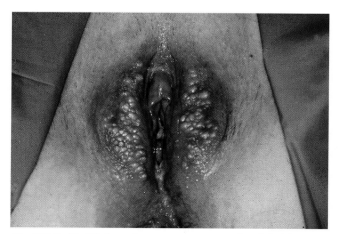

Fig 22.8 Multiple sebaceous cysts on both labia majora. The patient wished removal of the cysts, and a simple excision of both affected areas provided a satisfactory cosmetic result.

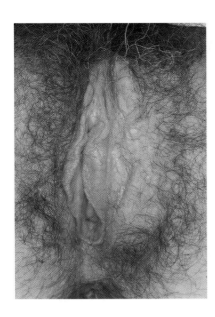

Fig 22.9 Lymphangiomas on the left labium majus. Note the white nodular lesions.

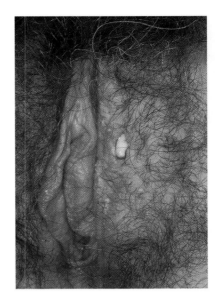

Fig 22.10 Biopsy of lymphangiomas. The lesions shown in **22.9** were easily compressible and drained typical white lymphatic fluid on biopsy.

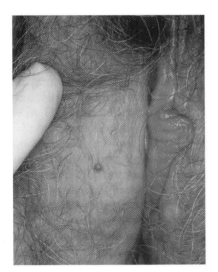

Fig 22.11 Cherry angioma, a common benign vascular tumor which can appear anywhere on the trunk.

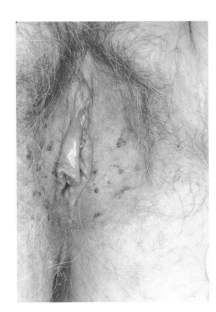

Fig 22.12 Angiokeratomas, commonly seen on the vulva or scrotum.

usually scattered over the trunk; they tend to increase in number with age and are most numerous in the fifth and sixth decades. Treatment is unnecessary.

Angiokeratomas are also fairly common, occurring mostly on the vulva (or scrotum in males). Lesions are usually multiple, dark red to almost black, and the diagnosis is confirmed when they blanch with pressure (**22.12**). They may be more prominent in pregnancy and with venous stasis. The histologic architecture shows interlacing layers of squamous cells with blood-filled spaces.

Pyogenic granulomas are capillary tumors that usually arise as the result of trauma. Oral gingival lesions are thought to be most common during pregnancy, but these tumors may arise at any time and at any location on the body (*see also* **3.15**, **3.16**). Excisional biopsy is recommended, as these lesions may mimic an amelanotic melanoma.

ENDOMETRIOSIS

Very rarely, ectopic endometrium may be found on the vulva, although it is seen more often on the cervix or in the vagina. The commonest etiology is for the endometrium to be implanted at the time of surgery on the perineum. It typically presents as a small mass which is cyclically uncomfortable. The surface appearance is often blue or darkly colored, but deep lesions may be flesh colored (**22.13**, **22.14**). Incision may occasionally produce old blood. Diagnosis and treatment are usually by local excision. Endometriosis may also present in an episiotomy site on the vulva.

HEMATOMA

Usually the result of trauma or intraoperative bleeding, ecchymoses can cause extensive purple-black discoloration of the vulva (**22.15**). Vulvar hematomas can

177

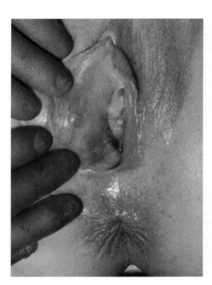

Fig 22.13 Endometriosis of the labium majus. There is a small nodule with a dimple on the right side.

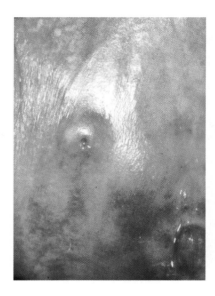

Fig 22.14 Close-up of nodule shown in 22.13, showing cyclic drainage site for blood-tinged fluid when ovulation was not being suppressed.

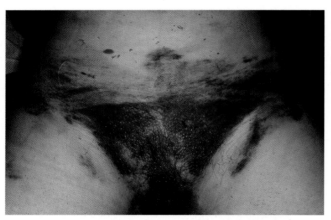

Fig 22.15 Ecchymoses and vulvar hematoma after abdominal liposuction (note bilateral sutures on incisions on lower abdomen). Extravasation of blood to dependent areas may cause marked discoloration even when vulvar trauma has not occurred.

Table 22.2 Causes of Contact Urticaria.

Medications
  Bacitracin
  Benzocaine
  Gentamicin
  Neomycin
  Penicillin
  Permethrin (Lindane)

Additives, preservatives, fragrances
  Acetic acid
  Many alcohols
  Balsam of Peru
  Benzoic acid
  Cinnamic aldehyde, acid
  Formaldehyde
  Lanolin
  Menthol
  Parabens
  Polyethylene glycol
  Polysorbate 60
  Sodium benzoate

Other
  Animal dander
  Hair
  Latex
  Nickel
  Placenta
  Saliva
  Semen

*From von Krogh, G. and Maibach, H.I. The contact urticaria syndrome. Semin. Dermatol. 1982; **1**: 59.*

also develop after operation if complete hemostasis has not been achieved; extravasation through the soft tissue occurs rapidly, often reaching on to the thigh. Hematomas of the vulva can also develop after relatively minor trauma. Accidents such as straddle injuries or split-legged falls will cause disruption of vulvar small vessels, particularly of the erectile tissue deep in the labia majora. The extravasated blood rapidly expands the loose areolar tissue of the labia, causing considerable swelling. The swelling ceases when the tension within it reaches that of the arterial blood supply; this tense swelling is exquisitely painful and often requires powerful analgesia.

Conservative treatment consists in the application of ice-packs as soon as possible. If this is not effective, surgical evacuation of the hematoma may then be necessary. A stable hematocrit and hematoma should not be evacuated. As it is often difficult to identify single bleeding points, insertion of a vacuum drain may be required. If swelling is extensive, urinary flow may be compromised; a urinary catheter provides relief and keeps the area clean.

EDEMA

An edematous vulva can reach remarkable proportions. The condition is most commonly found as a complication of generalized abdominal edema, such as that

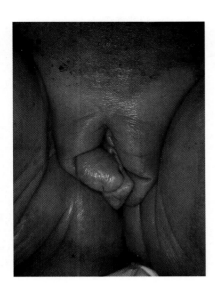

Fig 22.16 Vulvar edema in a nursing home patient with chronic intertrigo. Poor circulation contributes to chronic vulvar edema.

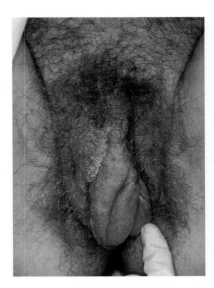

Fig 22.17 Chronic lymphedema after bilateral lymphadenectomy for cancer. This young woman suffered significant discomfort when sitting down, and distortion of the vulva made coitus difficult (gloved finger is at inlet). The papillary appearance of the anterior right labium majus is typical of chronic lymphedema (although the patient had been told this was genital warts). The area was easily traumatized; lymphatic drainage from abrasion sites had also been misdiagnosed as herpes simplex.

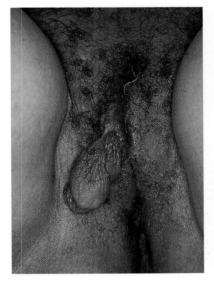

Fig 22.18 Skin tag. This skin tag demonstrates the typical pedunculated nature of this benign tumor.

associated with cardiac or liver failure. Obstruction of vulvar lymphatic drainage, due to surgical extirpation of the groin lymph glands or their massive involvement by tumor, will cause an irreversible enlargement of the entire vulva, often obstructing the entrance to the vagina.

Acute local edema or angioedema may be due to an immunologically mediated contact urticaria – the most important substance to consider is latex in examining gloves, condoms, and diaphragms (**Table 22.2**); anaphylaxis has been reported with severe sensitivity. Inflammation due to *Candida* infection can also produce an edematous appearance (**22.16**). The application of topical agents typically produces the complaint of burning on inflamed skin, but this is not an allergic reaction.

Chronic edema can cause the vulva to acquire a verrucous appearance which is sometimes mistaken for genital warts (**22.17**); lymphatic leakage may be mistaken for herpetic blisters. Crohn's disease of the bowel, hidradenitis suppurativa, and infestation of the lymphatics by filariasis may also present with vulvar edema.

SOLID TUMORS

SKIN TAGS AND FIBROEPITHELIAL POLYPS

Skin tags (acrochordons) are a common finding on almost any skin surface (**22.18**). They are small soft filiform papules, ranging from 1 to 2 mm in diameter and 3–5 mm in length in the anogenital region; they are smaller and more numerous in the axillae and around the neck. Pigmentation is variable, depending on the skin color of the patient. They have no medical significance, and are usually removed only for diagnosis or if they grow to any significant size. Management is essentially cosmetic, and excision using scissors or a no. 15 blade is effective.

Fibroepithelial polyps (soft fibromas) are more common in the anogenital region. The fibrofatty and muscular layers of the vulva and ischiorectal fossae can give rise to quite enormous fleshy soft tumours (**22.19**). Clinically, these are similar to neurofibromas; histologic examination makes the diagnosis. The stalk of a large polypoid lesion may become twisted, causing spontaneous necrosis with swelling.

NEUROFIBROMA

Solitary neurofibromas resemble fibroepithelial polyps (*see above*) and can be found anywhere on the body. Neurofibromatosis (von Recklinghausen's disease) produces the classic findings of café-au-lait spots, dermal neurofibromas, and subcutaneous nodules. Perineal and axillary freckling are virtually pathognomonic for neurofibromatosis and can be seen in childhood. Excision is required only when nodules interfere with urinary function or coitus owing to their position or size.

179

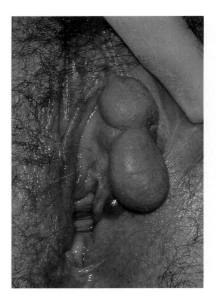

Fig 22.19 Bilobed fibrous lipoma of the left labium majus. Slow growth over many years suggested its benign nature, which was confirmed on excision. A small inclusion cyst is also present below the lipoma.

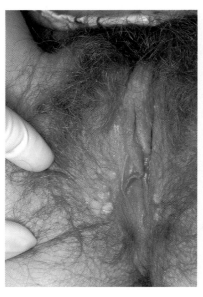

Fig 22.20 Multiple syringomata on both labia majora. The patient complained of itching and irritation from the larger lesions on the right, which were successfully excised under local anesthesia.

pruritic. High-potency topical steroids may be helpful in treating secondary lichen simplex chronicus. The condition regresses with menopause.

HIDRADENOMA

Hidradenoma papilliferum is a rare tumor of caucasian women, arising from the apocrine portion of the sweat glands. Although in the past it had been branded as malignant, it is in fact a benign tumor. The usual presentation is that of a small mass, 1 cm in diameter, arising from the labia or interlabial sulcus (22.21). The lesion surface is usually intact, but if ulcerated it can generate significant bleeding. Treatment is usually excision for diagnosis.

'POTENTIALLY MALIGNANT' TUMORS

The tumors listed below are most often benign, and it is difficult to distinguish malignant lesions without histologic confirmation. The examiner is advised to consider a biopsy for diagnosis when tumors are reported to be changing appearance or increasing in size.

FIBROMA AND FIBROSARCOMA

Two different types of these tumors may be seen on the vulva. The first type resembles a fibroepithelial polyp, but is firm rather than soft on palpation, while the second type is a sessile, firm nodule. Both are asymptomatic, flesh colored, and slow growing. Malignant lesions are not clinically different and may develop at any age. Excision is curative for benign lesions, but malignant lesions often recur.

SYRINGOMAS

These benign tumors of the eccrine sweat glands usually appear as clusters, especially on the face and lower eyelids. Vulvar lesions are smooth flesh-colored papules 2–5 mm in diameter. They occur on the hairy part of the vulva (22.20) and, because they are usually asymptomatic, the diagnosis may be missed, accounting for the rarity of reports in the literature.

FOX–FORDYCE DISEASE

These pruritic papules are related to the apocrine glands of hair follicles, and occur primarily on the mons pubis, labia majora, and axillae. The condition is more likely to occur in black-skinned individuals, and it develops after puberty. Fox–Fordyce papules resemble syringomas, but they are smaller, darker, and more

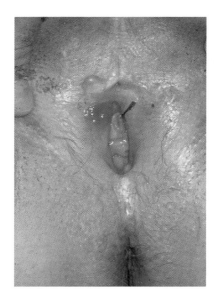

Fig 22.21 A small hidradenoma is seen at the right side of the vulva, which also shows marked atrophic change in a postmenopausal patient.

LIPOMA AND LIPOSARCOMA

These fatty tumors are hamartomas of the subcutaneous tissue. They are typically asymptomatic and slow growing; treatment is seldom necessary. Fast-growing lesions should be biopsied to rule out liposarcoma. The latter soft-tissue malignancy arises from intermuscular fascial planes rather than from a lipoma. Liposarcomas are more firm on palpation than lipomas.

GRANULAR CELL TUMORS

These rare neoplasms are more common in African American women. They are usually solitary and occur in early adult life. Most genital lesions that have been reported are on the vulva, usually the labia majora. They are round, firm lesions averaging 2–4 cm in diameter; they may be either smooth or hyperkeratotic. Histologic examination shows large cells containing granule-filled pale cytoplasm; the granules are periodic acid–Schiff (PAS) positive. Metastasis to sites such as the lung can occur with lesions that are histologically benign[4] as well as those with histologic atypia.

VERRUCOUS CARCINOMA

Although this tumor can grow to a remarkable size, it is commonly regarded as an essentially benign growth (22.22). In the past, the condition has been called 'giant condyloma of Buschke–Löwenstein' and it has been included here because of its propensity to spread by local 'pushing' margins and occasional reports of metastasis to regional lymph nodes. Some gynecologic oncologists believe that condylomas and verrucous carcinomas are separate lesions, although recent studies have found a close association with human papillomavirus type 6. In the spectrum of squamous cancer of the vulva, verrucous carcinoma lies toward the benign end. Although it has often been stated that verrucous carcinomas can become anaplastic if treated by irradiation, there have been few case reports.

TREATMENT

Wide local excision is required to treat these lesions. Margins should be evaluated to ensure complete excision. Lymphadenectomy is indicated for palpable and suspicious lymph nodes. Radiotherapy, as noted above, is unnecessary and inappropriate[6]. If lymph nodes are histologically positive, the lesion is probably an invasive squamous carcinoma.

VULVAR INTRAEPITHELIAL NEOPLASIA

Vulvar intraepithelial neoplasia (VIN) is categorized as mild (1), moderate (2), severe or carcinoma *in situ* (3)[7]. The VIN classification was introduced by the International Society for the Study of Vulvovaginal Disease to replace the many other names widely in use. Bowen disease, erythroplasia of Queyrat, and carcinoma *in situ* simplex are all included in VIN 3. Bowenoid papulosis, another form of VIN, is often characterized by pigmented lesions (22.23, 22.24). Both white and red lesions occur and resemble other neoplasias of the cervix, vagina, and perianal regions.

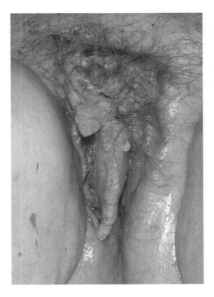

Fig 22.22 Verrucous carcinoma. A relatively small example of verrucous carcinoma showing the smooth pushing edge of the lesion. Excision biopsy was adequate therapy in this patient.

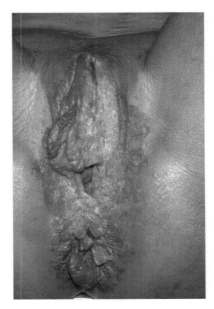

Fig 22.23 Widespread vulvar intraepithelial neoplasia (VIN) was found to hide multiple areas of early invasive cancer of the vulva. The patient also had cervical intraepithelial neoplasia (CIN) 3, and 10 years later she developed a primary invasive vaginal cancer. Multifocal disease of this type is not uncommon and may represent a 'field effect' of human papillomavirus (HPV) infection.

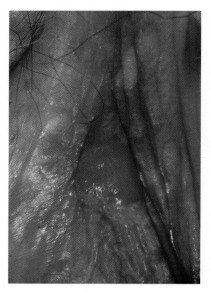

Fig 22.24 Vulvar intraepithelial neoplasia (VIN) A typical example of VIN of the 'red type'. The diagnosis can be made only on biopsy. Biopsy of the raised white area also confirmed VIN.

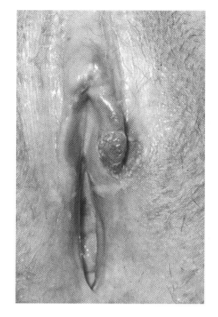

Fig 22.25 Small nodule of carcinoma at the lower part of the labia minora. Epithelial whitening, obliteration of the clitoral hood, and loss of vulvar architecture are consistent with the diagnosis of lichen sclerosus. Despite the size of this tumor, the lymph nodes in the groins contained carcinoma: the size of a tumor does not always reflect the extent of tumor spread.

Human papillomavirus infections have been associated with VIN[7,8]. It is controversial whether or not VIN is a precursor of vulvar carcinoma.

TREATMENT

If no evidence of an invasive lesion is present, VIN may be treated with the following modalities: simple vulvectomy, skinning vulvectomy, local excision, topical 5-fluorouracil, cryosurgery, carbon dioxide laser ablation, and ultrasonic surgical aspiration. The most commonly used and accepted techniques are wide local excision and carbon dioxide laser ablation.

MALIGNANT TUMORS

Invasive squamous cell cancer of the vulva represents between 5 and 8% of all female genital cancers; it is much less common than cervical cancer and occurs in older patients. In recent years, the proportion has been increasing due to a continuing decline in invasive cancer of the cervix and a steadily increasing proportion of elderly women in the population.

SYMPTOMATOLOGY

Most patients present complaining of itching, irritation, or soreness on the vulva, often of many years' duration. A lump (22.25) or slight bleeding may have been noticed, but these are less commonly reported than irritation or itching. The disease is commonly characterized by delay, both by the patient who self-medicates or ignores lesions, and by the healthcare provider who prescribes repeatedly without examining the patient. Embarrassment by one or both is often contributory. As a consequence, the cancer may sadly be well advanced by the time the patient presents (22.26).

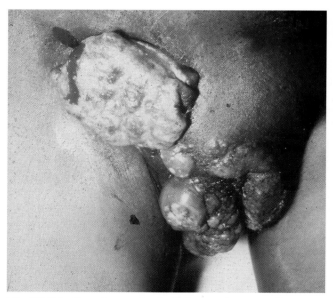

Fig 22.26 Massive metastasizing vulvar carcinoma in a young black woman. Palliative surgery was performed to improve the quality of life.

SQUAMOUS CARCINOMA

About 90–95% of cancers of the vulva are squamous. The mean age for presentation is in the late seventh decade, although the age range is wide, and patients may have vulvar cancers as early as the third decade (i.e. in their early twenties). Most squamous cancers presenting in older women are unifocal (22.25) and are often preceded by years of vulvar irritation or lichen sclerosus (*see Chapter 17*), although the latter condition is not strictly considered a precursor.

TREATMENT

Cancer of the vulva should be managed in a specialist center where a gynecologic oncologist can deliver the best-quality care for the patient. In the past decade there has been a trend towards conservative management of patients with vulvar carcinoma, with special consideration to cosmetic appearance and sexual function, especially in the younger patient.

Stage I (International Federation of Obstetricians and Gynecologists; FIGO) carcinoma, with lesions less than 2 cm in diameter and less than or equal to 1 mm stromal invasion, should be treated with a local wide radical excision. Lateral lesions with more than 1 mm stromal invasion should be treated with radical hemivulvectomy and ipsilateral inguinal femoral lymphadenectomy[9]. Midline lesions should be treated with radical vulvectomy and bilateral inguinal femoral lymphadenectomy. In stage I lesions, the bilateral lymphadenectomy can be performed through separate incisions rather than the *en bloc* resection described below.

For stages II and III (FIGO), the *en bloc*, 'butterfly', or three-incision approaches are effective methods of therapy. It is rare to perform a pelvic node dissection as part of primary therapy for vulvar carcinoma. Postoperative pelvic radiation has been proven effective in treating patients with positive femoral lymph nodes[10,11].

Radiotherapy to the groin and pelvic side wall is recommended where two or more nodes are involved, or where there is complete replacement of the node or capsular rupture. Cure rates for vulvar cancer in major medical centers are now extremely good, with node-negative and node-positive patients achieving a 94% and 62% 5-year survival rate, respectively.

Patients with FIGO stage IV disease have traditionally undergone radical vulvectomy, pelvic exenteration, and bilateral inguinal femoral lymphadenectomy. Patients with advanced stages are now offered neoadjuvant radiation or chemoradiation before surgical excision. This procedure has enabled oncologists to use less radical surgery[12–14].

MELANOMA

This rare condition is the second most common vulvar malignancy; it occurs predominantly in postmenopausal caucasian women[15]. Unlike the previous vulvar malignancies, melanoma is staged by the depth of the lesion[16] (*see Chapter 21*). Melanomas occur most often on the labia majora, clitoris, and labia minora. They can arise *de novo* or from a preexisting junctional nevus on the skin or mucous membrane. About 50% of vulvar melanomas are of the superficial spreading variety (**22.27**). Nodular melanoma is often a protuberant tumor, which often exhibits both melanotic and

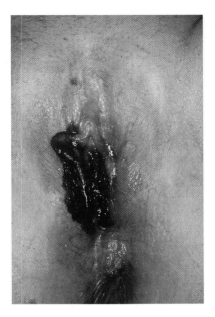

Fig 22.27 Vulvar melanoma. A very clear area of dense pigmented tissue with an irregular edge was in fact diagnosed as an '*in situ*' melanoma. Wide local excision produced a cure of the tumor.

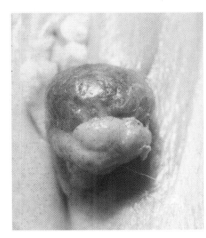

Fig 22.28 Vulvar melanoma. This unusual example of a combined melanotic and amelanotic melanoma was found to have extensive involvement of the inguinal nodes. The metastases represented both melanotic and amelanotic elements.

amelanotic elements (**22.28**). Amelanotic lesions are relatively more common on the vulva, and may present with ulceration, crusting, and bleeding[17,18].

TREATMENT

Lesions of less than 0.75 mm invasion should be treated with wide local radical excision with 2 cm margins. Lymph node excision is not required, as the 5-year survival rate is 98%. The outcome is directly related to the histologic depth of the lesion at the time of excision. A depth of invasion of less than 1.5 mm is associated with a good prognosis when wide local resection is performed. Small lateralizing lesions of more than 0.75 mm invasion must be treated with a radical hemivulvectomy, with ipsilateral inguinal femoral lymph adenectomy. Radical surgery for large lesions (*en bloc* radical vulvectomy and bilateral inguinal femoral lymphadenectomy)[19], although rarely curative, may increase survival time, and radiation may provide helpful palliative treatment.

BASAL CELL CARCINOMA

Accounting for less than 5% of vulvar cancers, basal cell carcinoma of the vulva has the same characteristics as tumors occurring in other parts of the body. Vulvar basal cell carcinoma is more prevalent in caucasian women over the age of 50 years, and lesions usually occur on hair-bearing skin. The presenting lesion is usually a dome-shaped nodule or plaque with a small rolled edge ('rodent ulcer'). There is surprisingly little pain and discomfort, but itching may be a complaint. Basal cell carcinomas are further discussed in *Appendix A*.

TREATMENT

Basal cell carcinoma is easily managed by wide local excision. An excision biopsy with good margins may not only be diagnostic, but curative as well. For elderly patients with large lesions, radiation therapy can be an effective modality[20].

ADENOCARCINOMA (BARTHOLIN GLAND)

This rare cancer is generally found in association with the Bartholin gland. It is characterized by the appearance of a relatively large mass lying deep to the vulvar and vaginal skin, often with only a small area of ulceration. The diagnosis is commonly made during the surgical treatment of a Bartholin cyst. Solid, suspicious material is found, which histologic examination proves to be an adenocarcinoma. Lymph node metastasis is found in 37% of Bartholin carcinomas[21,22]. The condition is treated in the same way as a squamous tumor, with great care being taken to achieve an adequate margin in resection of the vulva.

EXTRAMAMMARY PAGET'S DISEASE

This malignancy results from neoplastic secretory glandular adenocarcinoma cells arising in the vulvar epidermis. Vulvar Paget's disease may have migrated from a local tumor or be a metastasis from a distant neoplasm such as the breast. It is rare (less than 0.2% of all vulvar carcinomas), but, because of its similarity to benign vulvar dermatoses, it should be a diagnostic consideration when lesions fail to clear with appropriate therapy. The patient presents with a slowly growing, eroded, velvety plaque (22.29) which may be sore, but is rarely as itchy as typical dermatitic lesions. Histologic examination confirms the diagnosis, and a search for adjacent or distant neoplasm should be made.[23]

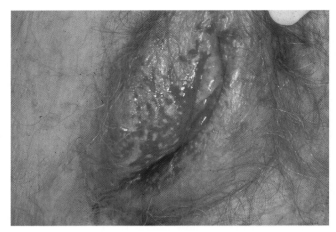

Fig 22.29 Vulvar (extramammary) Paget's disease. The similarity to vulvar eczema may delay diagnosis for months or years. No local or distant neoplasm was found in this patient.

TREATMENT

The preferred treatment is wide local excision with 3 cm margins and depth of resection to the Colles fascia. Recurrent *in situ* disease may be treated conservatively with topical bleomycin or 5-fluorouracil, carbon dioxide laser vaporization, or systemic retinoids[24].

If there is stromal invasion of underlying sweat glands, the surgeon should perform a radical hemivulvectomy and ipsilateral inguinal femoral lymph node dissection.

ADENOID CYSTIC CARCINOMA

This rare variant is characterized by a tendency to spread much more widely than at first appears by a process of subdermal infiltration (**22.30**). The normal margin for acceptable clearance of 1–2 cm may have to

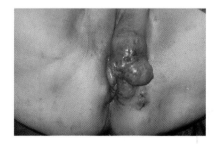

Fig 22.30 Adenoid cystic carcinoma. In contrast to the superficial lesions of Paget's disease, this adenoid cystic cancer undermines the epithelium to a far greater extent than is apparent. This lesion had invaded the pubic ramus as well as the bladder, and required exenterative surgery.

be significantly extended if the local disease is to be controlled effectively. The extent of this lesion is often underestimated. It is essential that a very wide excision is performed because there is a high risk of recurrent disease if this is not done. Survival is decreased compared with that of squamous cell carcinoma (5-year survival rate is 5.5%, compared with 62.3%, respectively[25]). Extensive surgery should consist of a radical vulvectomy and inguinal femoral lymph node dissection.

SARCOMA

Sarcomas of the vulva are extraordinarily rare, representing 1–2% of vulvar cancers. A wide variety of sarcomas has been described, including leiomyosarcomas, angiosarcomas, fibrosarcomas, neurofibrosarcomas, liposarcomas, and rhabdomyosarcomas. Wide local excision is the mainstay of therapy.

SECONDARY MALIGNANT TUMORS OF THE VULVA

Cancers may spread to the vulva from the anus, vagina, cervix, endometrium, ovary (22.31), breast, kidney, and thyroid.

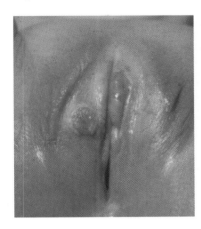

Fig 22.31 Secondary ovarian tumor. This small tumor occurred in a patient who had been treated 1 year previously for ovarian cancer. Although clinically it resembled a primary vulvar lesion, histologic examination revealed it to be identical with the previously resected ovarian primary.

REFERENCES

1 Garcia, J.J., Verkauf, B.S., Hochberg, C.J. *et al.* Aberrant breast tissue of the vulva. *Obstet. Gynecol.* 1978; **52**: 225–228.

2 Friedrich, E.G. Jr. *Surgical Procedures in Vulvar Disease*, 2nd edn. W.B. Saunders, Philadelphia, 1983.

3 Word, B. Office treatment of cyst and abscess of Bartholin's gland duct. *South Med. J.* 1968; **61**: 514–518.

4 Horowitz, I.R., Copas, P. and Majmudar, B. Granular cell tumors of the vulva. *Am. J. Obstet. Gynecol.* 1995; **173**: 1710.

5 Partridge, E.E., Murad, T., Shingleton, H.M. *et al.* Verrucous lesions of the female genitalia. II. Verrucous carcinoma. *Am. J. Obstet. Gynecol.* 1980; **137**: 419–424.

6 Kaufman, R.H. and Woodruff, J.D. The vulvar dystrophies, atypias, carcinomata *in situ*: an invitational symposium. Historical background in developmental stages of the new nomenclature. *J. Reprod. Med.* 1976; **17**: 132–136.

7 Crum, C.P., Braun, L.A., Shah, K.V. *et al.* Vulvar intraepithelial neoplasia: correlation of nuclear DNA content and the presence of a human papilloma virus (HPV) structural antigen. *Cancer* 1982; **49**: 468–471.

8 Gross, G., Hagedorn, M., Ikenberg, H. *et al.* Bowenoid papulosis: presence of human papillomavirus (HPV) structural antigens and of HPV 16-related DNA sequences. *Arch. Dermatol.* 1985; **121**: 858–863.

9 Stehman, F.B., Bundy, B.N., Dvoretsky, P.M. *et al.* Early stage I carcinoma of the vulva treated with ipsilateral superficial inguinal lymphadenectomy and modified radical hemivulvectomy: a prospective study of the Gynecologic Oncology Group. *Obstet. Gynecol.* 1992; **79**: 490–497.

10 Burrell, M.O., Franklin, E.W., III, Campion, M.J. *et al.* The modified radical vulvectomy with groin dissection: an eight-year experience. *Am. J. Obstet. Gynecol.* 1988; **159**: 715–722.

11 Cavanagh, D., Roberts, W.S., Bryson, S.C. *et al.* Changing trends in the surgical treatment of invasive carcinoma of the vulva. *Surg. Gynecol. Obstet.* 1986; **162**: 164–168.

12 Berek, J.S., Heaps, J.M., Fu, Y.S. *et al.* Concurrent cisplatin and 5-fluorouracil chemotherapy and radiation therapy for advanced stage squamous carcinoma of the vulva. *Gynecol. Oncol.* 1991; **42**: 197–201.

13 Horowitz, I.R. Neoplasms of the vulva. In: Rakel, R.E. (ed.) *Conn's Current Therapy*. W.B. Saunders, Philadelphia, 1999.

14 Horowitz, I.R. Gynecologic malignancies. In: Wood, W.C. (ed.) *The Anatomic Basis of Tumor Surgery*. Quality Medical Publishing, St Louis, 1999.

15 Ronan, S.G., Eng, A.M., Briele, H.A. *et al.* Malignant melanoma of the female genitalia. *J. Am. Acad. Dermatol.* 1990; **22**: 428.

16 Look, K.Y., Roth, L.M. and Sutton, G.P. Vulvar melanoma reconsidered. *Cancer* 1993; **72**: 143.

17 Dunton, C.J. and Berd, D. Vulvar melanoma, biologically different from other cutaneous melanomas. *Lancet* 1999; **354**: 2013.

18 Ragnarsson-Olding, B.K., Kanter-Lewensohn, L.R., Lagerlof, B. *et al.* Malignant melanoma of the vulva in a nationwide, 25-year study of 219 Swedish females: clinical observations and histopathologic features. *Cancer* 1999; **86**: 1273.

19 Podratz, K.C., Gaffey, T.A., Symmonds, R.E. *et al.* Melanoma of the vulva: an update. *Gynecol. Oncol.* 1983; **16**: 153–168.

20 Benedet, J.L., Miller, D.M., Ehlen, T.G. *et al.* Basal cell carcinoma of the vulva: clinical features and treatment results in 28 patients. *Obstet. Gynecol.* 1997; **90**: 765.

21 Leuchter, R.S., Hacker, N.F., Voet, R.L. *et al.* Primary carcinoma of the Bartholin gland: a report of 14 cases and review of the literature. *Obstet. Gynecol.* 1982; **60**: 361.

22 Copeland, L.J., Sneigen, W., Gershenson, D.M. *et al.* Bartholin gland carcinoma. *Obstet. Gynecol.* 1986; **67**: 794–801.

23 Sitaklin, C. and Ackerman, A.B. Mammary and extramammary Paget's disease (groin, vulva, perianal). *Am. J. Dermatopathol.* 1985; **7**: 335–340.

24 Stacy, D., Burrell, M.O. and Franklin, E.W., III. Extramammary Paget's disease of the vulva and anus: use of intraoperative frozen-section margins. *Am. J. Obstet. Gynecol.* 1986; **155**: 519–523.

25 Underwood, J.W., Adcock, L.L. and Okagaki, T. Adenosquamous carcinoma of skin appendages (adenoid squamous cell carcinoma, pseudoglandular squamous cell carcinoma, adenocanthoma of sweat gland of Lever) of the vulva. A clinical and ultrastructural study. *Cancer* 1978; **42**: 1851–1858.

ACKNOWLEDGEMENTS

Figures **22.13**, **22.14**, and **22.25** are reproduced from V.R. Tindall *Colour Atlas of Clinical Gynecology* (Figs 57, 58, and 90), Wolfe, London, 1981. Figure **22.6** has been reproduced with permission from B. Word. New instrument for office treatment of cysts and abscesses of Bartholin's gland. *JAMA* 1964; **190**: 777.

Appendix A

Differential Diagnosis of the Vulvar Ulcer

Marilynne McKay

The natural history of a cutaneous ulcer of any cause depends on many factors, including secondary infection, the patient's underlying immune status, systemic disorders, and dermatologic diseases – to mention just a few. In addition, the patient's history may be inaccurate. She may be unaware of how long an ulcer has been present, or whether any significant changes have occurred.

A biopsy is an important diagnostic test, especially for a chronic ulcer. The biopsy should be taken from the edge of the lesion rather than from its base. A wedge excision from normal skin to the ulcer base will provide the best information for the pathologist. If this is impractical, two or more punch biopsies, from opposite sides of the lesion, should be considered. Some infections may be recognized in biopsy tissue, but appropriate cultures should always be obtained before beginning therapy. With acute ulcers, a biopsy may not be necessary if bacterial, viral, and/or fungal cultures are performed promptly to establish the diagnosis before beginning treatment.

The most serious diagnostic error is to guess at the etiology of an ulcer and to treat it empirically before all the data have been gathered. This error is usually made when a vulvar ulcer is erroneously assumed to be a sexually transmitted disease. In general, noninfectious vulvar ulcers are due to primary dermatologic diseases, but secondary infection can occur in open lesions. Bacterial and candidal infections should be treated, but it should not be assumed that they are the primary cause of chronic ulcers.

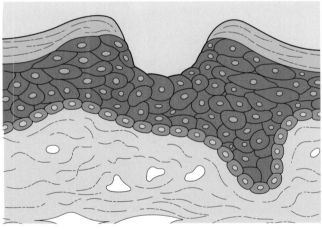

2 Erosion (this process involves the epidermis only).

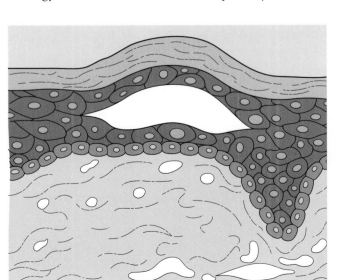

1 Blister (when the roof is lost, an erosion remains).

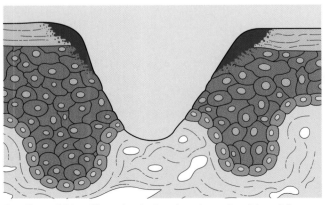

3 Ulcer (this affects both the dermis and epidermis).

Table 1 Differential diagnosis of vulvar ulcers[a].

Figure	Cause		DIAGNOSIS	DIAGNOSTIC TEST	ASSOCIATED FINDINGS
Solitary ulcer (usually)					
4	infectious	○	Chancroid	Culture	*Hemophilus ducreyi*
5	infectious	○	Syphilis	Darkfield	*Treponema pallidum*
6	noninfectious	●	Pyoderma gangrenosum	Biopsy	Systemic disease: myeloma, bowel disease
7	noninfectious	●	Urethral caruncle	Anatomic change	Atrophic epithelium reveals urethral mucosa
8	malignant	●	Basal cell carcinoma	Biopsy	Localized pearly translucent borders with telangiectasia
9	malignant	●	Squamous cell carcinoma	Biopsy	Human papillomavirus (HPV), lichen sclerosus, other chronic inflammation or scarring process
Multiple ulcers					
10	infectious	○	Herpes simplex, primary	Viral culture	Herpes simplex virus (HSV)
11	infectious	○	Herpes simplex, recurrent	Viral culture	HSV
12	infectious	○	Eczema herpeticum	Viral culture	HSV
13	infectious	○	Secondary syphilis	Darkfield	*T. pallidum*
14	infectious	○	Varicella-zoster	Viral culture	Varicella-zoster virus, unilateral distribution
15	infectious	○	Candidiasis	Fungal culture	*Candida albicans (C. glabrata, C. parapsilosis,* and others)
16	noninfectious	●	Trauma: factitia, excoriation	None	Application of erosive agents; linear excoriations, lichenification from scratching
17	noninfectious	●	Behçet's syndrome	Biopsy	Constellation of arthritis, uveitis, other signs
18	noninfectious	●	Epstein–Barr virus (EBV) secondary ulcer	Serum test for EBV, IgM	Prodrome of fever, fatigue, sore throat, oral ulcers, and swollen cervical glands
19	noninfectious	●	Aphthosis	Biopsy	Lesions recurrent, often occur in mouth also
Granulomatous (heaped up)					
20	infectious	○	Secondary syphilis	Darkfield, serology	Rising titer in serum, often generalized lesions
21	infectious	○	Granuloma inguinale (donovanosis)	Biopsy, special stains	*Calymmatobacterium granulomatis*
22	infectious	○	Lymphogranuloma venereum	Serum antigen tests	*Chlamydia trachomatis* (serotypes L1, L2, L3)
23	infectious	○	Diaper granuloma	Fungal culture	*Candida* spp.
24	noninfectious	●	Hidradenitis suppurativa	Biopsy	Often axillary lesions. Lack of bowel disease
25	noninfectious	●	Crohn's disease (ulcerative colitis)	Biopsy	Bowel disease
26	noninfectious	●	Lymphangiectasis	Biopsy	History of chronic vulvar edema. Rule out HPV
27	malignant	●	Vulvar intraepithelial neoplasia (VIN)	Biopsy	History of cervical dysplasia, infection with HPV
28	malignant	●	Leukemia or lymphoma	Biopsy	Other lesions on body

Table 1 Differential diagnosis of vulvar ulcers (continued).

Figure	Cause		DIAGNOSIS	DIAGNOSTIC TEST	ASSOCIATED FINDINGS
Recurrent ulcers[b]					
11	infectious	●	Herpes simplex	Viral culture	HSV, recurrent
15	infectious	●	Candidiasis	Fungal culture	*C. albicans (C. glabrata, C. parapsilosis*, and others)
17	noninfectious	●	Behçet's syndrome	Biopsy	Constellation of arthritis, uveitis, other signs
19	noninfectious	●	Aphthosis	Biopsy	Lesions recurrent, often occur in mouth also
Erosive (superficial)					
29	infectious	●	Inflammatory vaginitis	Wet smear, culture	*Trichomonas* spp., *Gardnerella* spp.
30	infectious	●	Candidiasis	KOH smear, culture	*Candida* spp., satellite pustules on skin
31	infectious	●	Impetigo (*Staphylococcus* spp.)	Culture	Follicular pustules, peeling
33	noninfectious	●	Lichen planus	Biopsy	Erosive mucosa, including oral mucous membranes
34	noninfectious	●	Lichen sclerosus	Biopsy	Not on mucosa, loss of vulvar architecture
35	noninfectious	●	Plasma cell vulvitis	Biopsy	Etiology not known, may be asymptomatic
36	noninfectious	●	Fixed drug eruption	Biopsy	Ingestion of tetracycline, laxatives, other drugs
37	malignant	●	Necrolytic migratory erythema (glucagonoma)	Alpha-cell pancreatic tumor	Periorificial and intertriginous dermatitis; resolves when tumor resected
32	malignant	●	Extramammary Paget's disease	Biopsy	Usually perianal, asymptomatic, chronic
Blisters and erosions					
38	noninfectious	●	Contact dermatitis	Biopsy, patch testing	Often due to neomycin, latex, preservatives in topical agents, perfumes
39	noninfectious	●	Erythema multiforme	Biopsy	Target lesions, especially palms and soles, mucous membranes; associated with HSV, drugs
Bullous diseases (autoimmune)					
40	noninfectious	●	*Bullous pemphigoid*		Immunoglobulin (Ig) G and C3 at dermoepidermal junction
41	noninfectious	●	*Pemphigus*		IgG between epidermal cells
	noninfectious	●	*Dermatitis herpetiformis*		IgA in papillary dermis
42	noninfectious	●	*Benign familial pemphigus (Hailey–Hailey disease)*		Negative immunoglobulin

[a]*Color code:* ● = *infectious;* ● = *noninfectious;* ● = *malignant.*

Erosive dermatoses may seem recurrent as they tend to flare and remit; see above.

SOLITARY ULCERS

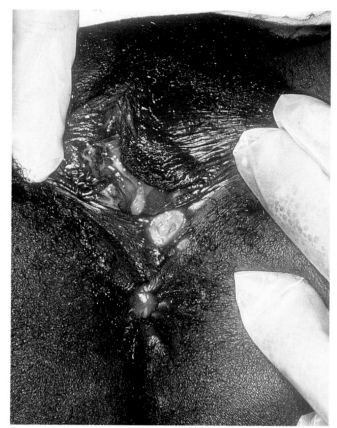

Color code for box outlines on pages 190–199:

☐ = *Infectious;* ☐ = *noninfectious;* ☐ = *malignant.*

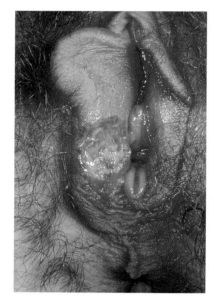

5 Syphilis. Primary syphilitic chancre is a painless button-like lesion, with a central shallow ulceration. Multiple lesions can occur, especially in immuno-compromised patients. Serum tests are usually not positive while the primary chancre is present.

4 Chancroid. Painful superficial ulcers may be seen in this sexually transmitted disease caused by *Haemophilus ducreyi*. Multiple lesions are usually contiguous, giving the appearance of a large irregular erosion with a granulomatous base. About 50% of affected women have inguinal adenopathy.

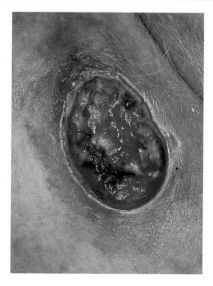

6 Pyoderma gangrenosum. The lesion of pyoderma gangrenosum is a deep necrotic ulcer with dusky overhanging borders. It is not infectious, and may occur in patients with various systemic diseases, especially inflammatory bowel disease.

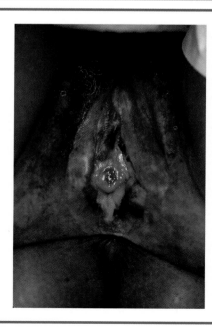

7 Urethral caruncle. This is a common finding in the hypoestrogenemic vulva. With shrinkage of the skin of the introitus, the distal urethral mucosa is everted and exposed. Despite the name, it is not an infection. It is sometimes mistaken for an ulcer or a cancer by inexperienced examiners.

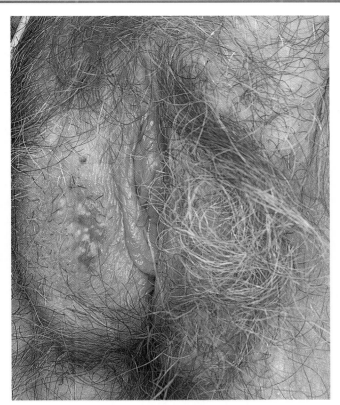

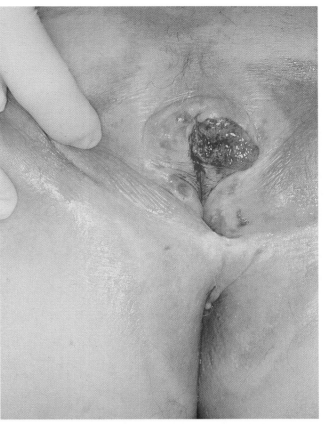

8 Basal cell carcinoma. The 'rodent ulcer', with its pearly telangiectatic border and necrotic center, is usually found on sun-exposed skin, although 10% of these lesions occur on covered portions of the body. Basal cell carcinomas rarely metastasize, but local invasion may cause significant tissue destruction.

9 Squamous cell carcinoma. Erosive or nodular lesions are often associated with chronic inflammation or scarring, such as in this patient with lichen sclerosus.

MULTIPLE ULCERS

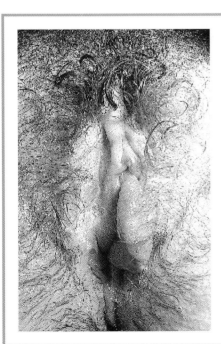

10 Primary herpes simplex virus (HSV). Primary HSV infections tend to be widespread and painful. Recurrences are usually localized and occur in variable sites within the area of the primary eruption.

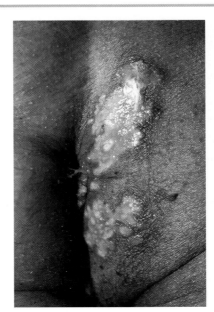

11 Multiple ulcers of herpes simplex. in a patient with acquired immune deficiency syndrome. These chronic and painful lesions did not resolve until the patient was given a fourfold increase in the usual dosage of acyclovir for several months.

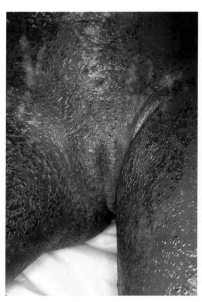

12 Eczema herpeticum. in a 4-year-old with atopic dermatitis. Typical umbilicated vesicles have unroofed, leaving uniform punched-out erosions that have become confluent over much of the body. This is a secondary infection of chronic dermatitis, not a sexually transmitted disease.

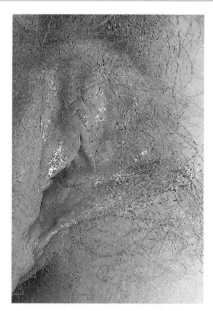

13 Secondary syphilis. Papular lesions of secondary syphilis typically generalize, usually involving the palms and soles. Lesions on mucous membranes in the mouth and vagina may ulcerate, forming 'mucous patches'. Serum tests for syphilis are strongly positive at this stage and moist lesions are highly contagious.

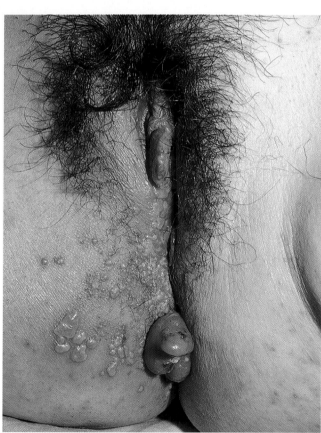

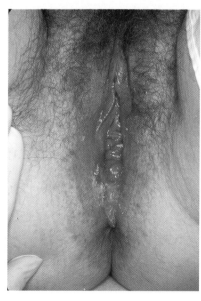

15 Candidiasis. Vaginal candidiasis is common, and lesions often spread to the vulva. Peeling and erosions occur in intertriginous areas, and satellite pustules are scattered at the periphery. In contrast, tinea infections do not have satellite lesions; tiny vesiculopustules occur along the lesional border.

14 Varicella-zoster (shingles). Groups of umbilicated vesicles localized to a dermatome are typical of herpes zoster; herpes simplex virus (HSV) is usually a single group of vesicles. Zoster is unlikely to recur; HSV typically recurs. Immunocompromised patients are more likely to develop both types of herpes infections; zoster may generalize to the entire body and HSV may become a large indolent ulcer. Treatment with acyclovir requires a fourfold dose increase for zoster, so it is important to differentiate the two conditions. This patient also has a rectal prolapse.

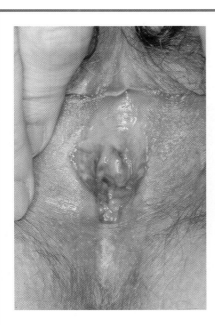

16 Trauma. In this case, the patient self-applied an alkaline household cleaner to her skin in an effort to 'get rid of germs'. Self-induced (factitial) ulcers may be induced by a variety of means, Shallow, linear erosions due to the patient's scratching are called excoriations.

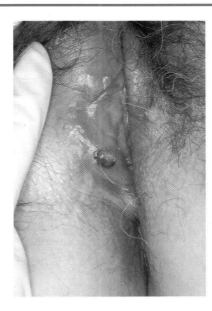

17 Behçet's syndrome. A relatively rare disorder, Behçet's syndrome is a complex multisystem disease. For a positive diagnosis, oral aphthae must be present, with at least two of the following: genital aphthae, synovitis, arthritis, cutaneous pustular vasculitis, posterior uveitis (retinal vasculitis), or meningo-encephalitis. The absence of inflammatory bowel disease and collagen vascular diseases must be documented. Lesions tend to be deep and may scar. Flares and remissions are typical.

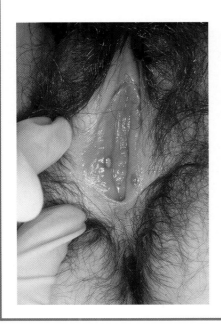

18 Second episode of vulvar ulcers after influenza-like syndrome in a 16-year-old. All tests for sexually transmitted disease were negative, but serology was positive for Epstein–Barr virus with an increase in IgM levels 2 weeks after lesions developed.

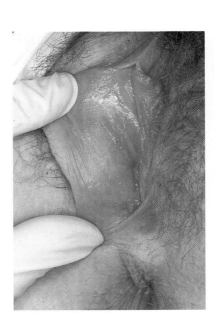

19 Aphthosis (canker sores). Patients with complex aphthosis have recurrent oral and genital aphthae which tend to be more frequent and more superficial than those of Behçet's syndrome. No other features of Behçet's syndrome can be identified. Treatment of early lesions with potent topical steroids can be very effective.

GRANULOMATOUS (HEAPED UP) LESIONS

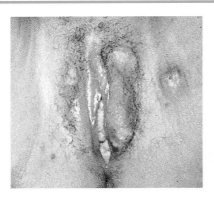

20 Secondary syphilis. Genital plaques of syphilis (condylomata lata) may resemble genital warts (condylomata acuminata), but the latter have a more verrucous appearance ('lata' means flat, 'acuminata' raised). The surface of these lesions is flat, clean, and moist; darkfield examination reveals swarms of treponemes. These are the most infectious lesions of syphilis.

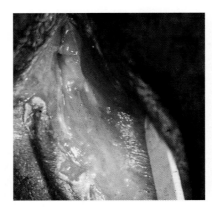

21 Granuloma inguinale (donovanosis). Necrotizing ulcerations in anogenital areas may be obscured by edema of the labia majora, as seen here. Early lesions are small eroded papules, which progress to hypertrophic, velvety, beefy-red, granulation tissue. Inguinal adenopathy does not occur unless secondary infection is present.

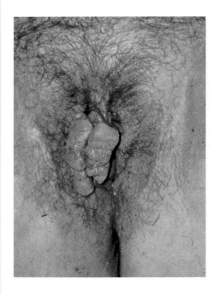

22 Lymphogranuloma venereum (LGV). Although ulcers are not typical of LGV, the diagnosis should be considered when edema of the labia is a prominent feature. The condition is most prevalent in tropical and subtropical areas, and usually presents with unilateral or bilateral enlargement of inguinal lymph nodes (buboes), which may mat together above and below the inguinal ligament (groove sign). Vulvar edema (elephantiasis) is known as esthiomène.

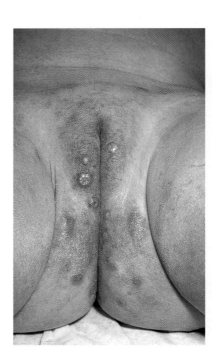

23 Diaper granuloma (granuloma gluteale infantum). These benign reddish-brown granulomatous nodules appear to be a cutaneous response to local inflammation, maceration, and secondary infection, usually with *Candida albicans*. Biopsy is helpful. Lesions of granuloma gluteale infantum resolve completely and spontaneously within several months after treatment of the inflammation and secondary infection.

GRANULOMATOUS (HEAPED-UP) LESIONS

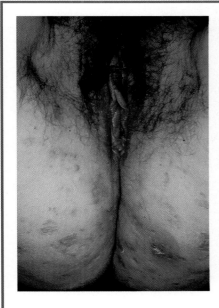

24 Hidradenitis suppurativa. Comedones, furuncles, sinus tracts, and scars are typical of hidradenitis suppurativa. Like cystic acne, this is a chronic scarring disease of the apocrine glands that occurs in the axillae and groin. Mild cases can be controlled with antibiotics, such as minocycline or trimethoprim–sulfamethoxazole (depending on which organisms are predominant). Oral retinoids, successful for facial acne, have been disappointing for hidradenitis. For severe cases, excision and grafting of the involved tissue is the treatment of choice.

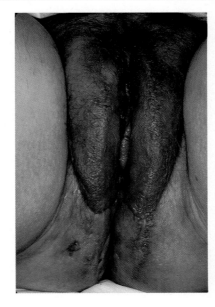

25 Crohn's disease, ulcerative colitis. Granulomatous nodules can give a cobblestone appearance to the mucosa in patients with Crohn's disease. A diffuse granulomatous thickening of the labia has also been reported in early inflammatory bowel disease. Rectal fissures and fistulas are often present, and deep 'knife-cut' ulcerations can occur in the inguinal folds.

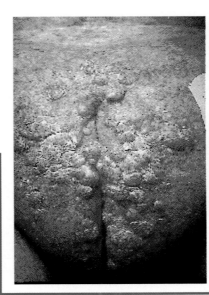

26 Lymphangiectasis. In patients with chronic vulvar edema, dilation of the lymphatic vessels can result in a verrucous surface, which may be difficult to distinguish from infection with human papillomavirus. In this case, the edema was due to chronic radiation dermatitis.

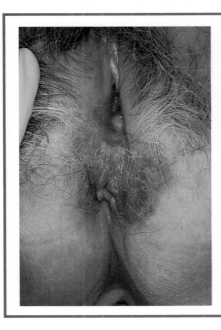

27 Vulvar intraepithelial neoplasia (VIN). Scaly, erythematous papules and plaques are typical of squamous cell carcinoma *in situ*, or VIN. Biopsies should be taken from the thickest parts of the lesion(s) and several areas should be sampled, as VIN is typically multifocal.

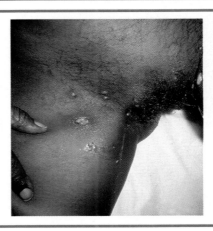

28 Leukemia, lymphoma. Cutaneous infiltrates are not uncommon in lymphomas; this is a case of chronic myeloid leukemia. Biopsy should be performed for diagnosis. These cutaneous lesions have ulcerated during chemotherapy.

SUPERFICIAL EROSIONS

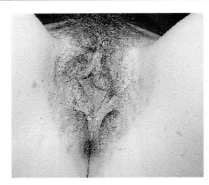

29 Inflammatory vaginitis. Although vulvar edema and inflammation is most often associated with candidal vulvovaginitis, other causes should also be considered. This is an example of trichomoniasis. Contact or irritant dermatitis to vaginal medication is another possibility.

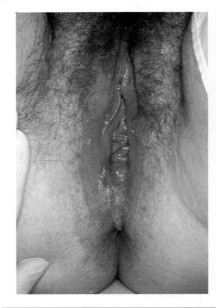

30 Candidiasis. Vaginal candidiasis is common, and lesions often spread to the vulva. Peeling and erosions are seen in intertriginous areas, and satellite pustules are scattered at the periphery. In contrast, tinea infections do not have satellite lesions; tiny vesiculopustules occur along the lesional border.

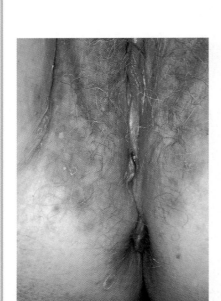

31 Impetigo (*Staphylococcus* spp.) Staphylococcal infection of the skin begins as follicular pustules, then spreads as thin-walled bullae that soon erode, leaving a moist superficial surface with peeling edges. Vulvar and perineal impetigo is particularly common in human immunodeficiency virus (HIV) infection and acquired immune deficiency syndrome (AIDS).

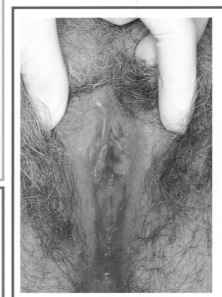

33 Lichen planus (LP). Erosions of LP are often limited to vaginal and introital mucosae. It is helpful to examine the gums and oral mucosa, as LP often affects both areas. Lesions are chronic and recurrent.

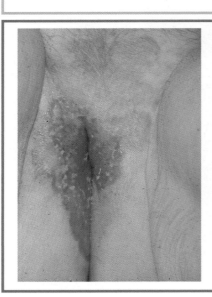

32 Extramammary Paget's disease. Diagnosis of this lesion depends on the examiner's index of suspicion and a biopsy. As it resembles dermatitis and grows slowly, it is not usually recognized for 1–2 years. It may be associated with an underlying apocrine, eccrine, or adenoid carcinoma.

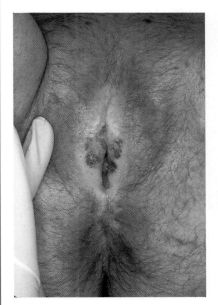

34 Lichen sclerosus (LS). In general, this is not as likely to erode spontaneously as LP. When the epithelium is damaged, it is usually the result of excoriation by the patient. In this case, a traumatic fissure in the posterior introitus has become secondarily infected with *Candida*. The diagnosis of LS was made by a biopsy of the whitened epithelium on the perineum.

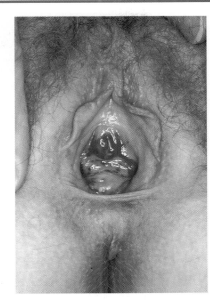

35 Plasma cell vulvitis. This bright red eruption (also called vulvitis circumscripta plasmacellularis) is limited to the mucous membranes and may be asymptomatic, although patients usually complain of tenderness. Lesions resolve slowly, leaving a rusty 'stain' on the skin as they disappear. Recurrences are common, and the etiology is not known. (A similar eruption may occur on the male glans penis, where it is known as Zoon balanitis.)

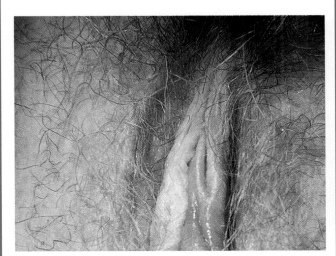

36 Fixed drug eruption. The erosion on the edematous labium minus will recur each time the patient ingests the medication responsible – in this case a combination of sulfamethoxazole and trimethoprim. Other areas on the body may also be affected, but the localized round, macular eruption does not involve the entire skin. When lesions resolve, the skin is often left hyperpigmented. Tetracycline and phenolphthalein are common offending agents.

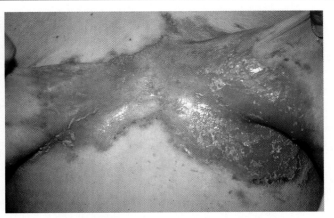

37 Necrolytic migratory erythema (glucagonoma). This unusual eruption typically involves the intertriginous areas, such as the inframammary folds (shown here), the axillae, and the groin. Lesions also occur around the mouth and the anus, as well as on the extremities. The patient has an alpha-cell tumor of the pancreas (glucagonoma) and serum levels of glucagon are markedly raised. Provided the examiner is familiar with this paraneoplastic syndrome, the eruption's peculiar nature is sufficiently characteristic to make the diagnosis possible.

BLISTERS AND EROSIONS

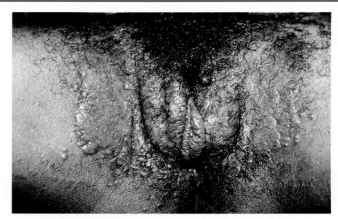

38 Contact dermatitis. Contact or irritant dermatitis may be caused by a medication or cleaning agent used by the patient because of an underlying problem, so infection should be considered in the overall evaluation. An irritant reaction typically causes immediate burning and stinging, usually because the agent has been applied to inflamed skin. A contact allergen does not initiate a dermatitis until about 2 days after application; the eruption lasts 2–3 weeks.

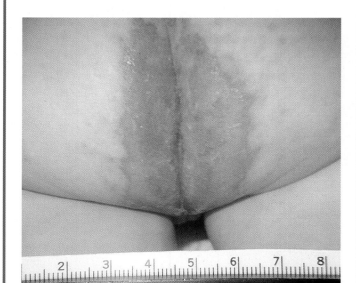

39 Erythema multiforme (Stevens–Johnson syndrome). Erythema multiforme (EM) is a cutaneous reaction pattern recognized in its early stages by target-shaped lesions on the palms and soles, as well as on the rest of the body. The most common causes are *Mycoplasma pneumoniae*, recurrent herpes simplex virus (HSV), in which EM follows each HSV outbreak, and various drugs. However, many cases are idiopathic.

IMMUNOLOGIC BULLAE

The immunologically mediated cutaneous blistering diseases have been studied extensively. Biopsies for routine histopathologic examination and immunofluorescent staining are recommended (the latter requires a special fixative). Lesions are rarely limited to the genitalia, and systemic immunosuppressive therapy is usually necessary.

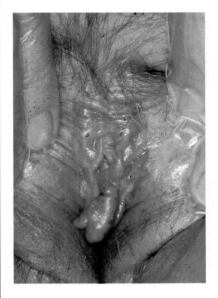

40 Bullous pemphigoid. This usually occurs in older patients and typically involves large tense bullae. Immunoglobulin is deposited along the basement membrane. A somewhat rarer form is cicatricial pemphigoid, which affects mucous membranes and causes scarring – eye lesions can cause blindness.

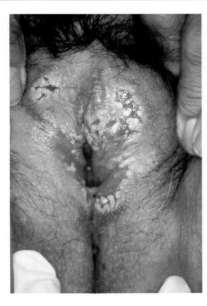

41 Pemphigus. This usually presents with thin-walled blisters, which are easily traumatized, leaving erosions. Immunoglobulin is deposited between epithelial cells, causing them to lose their adherence to one another. In this case, chronic *Candida* infection has caused itching and thickening of the involved skin.

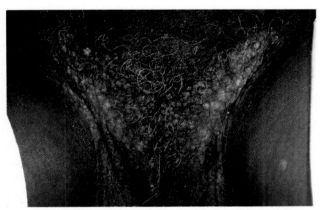

42 Benign familial pemphigus. This is a chronic and recurrent eruption of the axillae and groin; it usually occurs in several family members and has an equal predilection for males and females. The diagnosis is confirmed by an absence of immunoglobulins and by histopathologic findings.

Table 2. Differential diagnosis of vulvar itching[a].

Figure	Cause		Diagnosis	Diagnostic Test	Associated Findings
Red rash					
43, 44	infectious	●	Tinea cruris	KOH positive	Annular, clear centers
45	noninfectious	●	Tinea versicolor	KOH positive	Thin plaques, light scale, chronic
46	noninfectious	●	Intertrigo	KOH negative	Secondary to chafing from clothing, skin folds
47	noninfectious	●	Seborrhea	KOH negative	Erythematous plaques with greasy scale
48	noninfectious	●	Psoriasis	KOH negative	Annular, scaly plaques
49	noninfectious	●	Irritant dermatitis	None	Use of irritating topicals over days to weeks
50	noninfectious	●	Allergic contact dermatitis	Patch testing	Blisters, swelling; KOH-negative discharge
51	noninfectious	●	Steroid rebound dermatitis	None (KOH negative)	History of potent topical steroid use, resolves with discontinuation of steroid
White plaques					
52, 53	noninfectious	●	Lichen simplex chronicus	Biopsy	Thick, excoriated; may have *Candida* discharge
54	malignant	●	VIN	Biopsy	Thick, no response to topical steroid
55	malignant	●	Paget's disease	Biopsy	Mild or no itching, no response to topical steroid
56	noninfectious	●	Lichen sclerosus	Biopsy	Limited to vulvar skin; no vaginal involvement
57, 58	noninfectious	●	Lichen planus	Biopsy	Oral, vulvar, vaginal erosions
Vaginitis					
59	infectious	●	Bacterial vaginosis, trichomoniasis	Vaginal smear, wet mount	Vulvitis may be mild despite copious discharge
60	infectious	●	*Candida*	Vaginal smear, KOH	Swollen, scaly, fissured
Varicolored papules					
61	noninfectious	●	Syringoma	Biopsy	Skin-colored papules, usually bilateral
62	noninfectious	●	Fox–Fordyce disease	Biopsy	Follicular papules, may be dark due to rubbing
63	malignant	●	VIN	Biopsy	Itching may be first sign of recurrent disease
64	infectious	●	Condylomata acuminata	Biopsy	May be white, skin-colored, or dark
65	infectious	●	Molluscum contagiosum	Biopsy or crush preparation	Domed, umbilicated papules
66	infectious	●	Scabies	Oil preparation	Linear papules and nodules
Hives or wheals					
67	noninfectious	●	Contact urticaria (latex)		Recurrent, localized, last only hours
68	infectious	●	*Candida* hypersensitivity	Fungal culture	Postcoital swelling, may be cyclic
No rash					
69	noninfectious	●	Underlying disease	Serum tests	Generalized itching
70, 71	noninfectious	●	Factitial	Psychogenic	Localized excoriations, ulcers

[a] Color code: ● = infectious; ● = noninfectious; ● = malignant.

Differential Diagnosis of Vulvar Itching

RED RASH

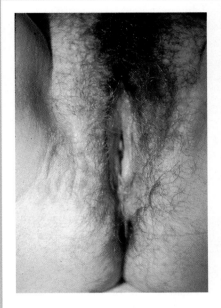

43 Tinea cruris, mistakenly treated with a topical steroid. This is sometimes called 'tinea incognito' because the steroid masks the scaling typical of tinea infections. The annular configuration of the plaque is a clue to the diagnosis and KOH smear of a skin scraping was positive.

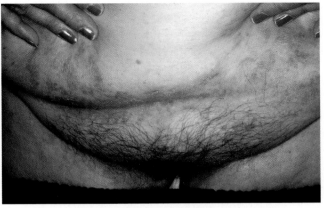

44 Tinea corporis in abdominal fold. The arcuate raised borders and clear areas of the rash distinguish tinea from intertrigo or seborrhea. KOH smear of scale was positive for dermatophyte.

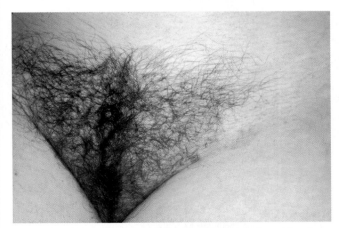

45 Tinea (pityriasis) versicolor of the vulva. The fine scale and salmon patches are very similar to seborrhea, but microscopic examination of lesional scale revealed spores and short hyphae of *Pityrosporum ovale*. The patient was only mildly pruritic, but also had involvement of the trunk.

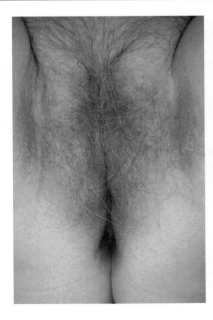

46 Intertrigo. The patient complained of irritation with heat and tight clothing. There was no evidence of *Candida* or tinea infection, and her condition improved with the use of drying powders and loose cotton underwear.

Color code for box outlines on pages 201–207:

☐ = *Infectious;* ☐ = *noninfectious;* ☐ = *malignant.*

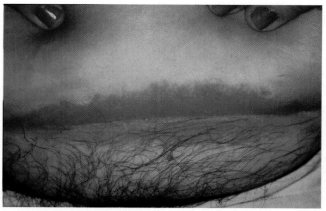

47 Seborrheic dermatitis in skin folds. Mild seborrhea often shows *Pityrosporum ovale* on KOH examination; severe involvement (shown here) may be an overlap with psoriasis (sebopsoriasis).

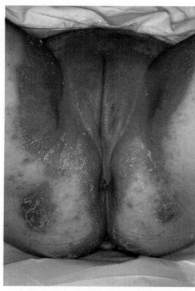

48 Psoriasis of the vulva in a patient with generalized disease. The intense erythema characteristic of psoriasis can be seen clearly.

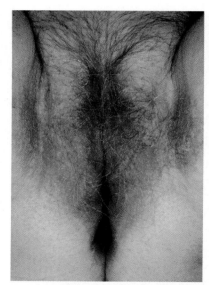

49 Irritant dermatitis to topical medication containing a relatively high concentration of propylene glycol, which was prescribed to be applied only once a day. The patient had been using it two or three times daily.

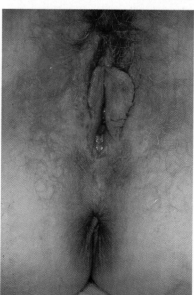

50 Allergic contact dermatitis of the vulva. The patient intermittently used a topical medication containing neomycin, to which she was allergic.

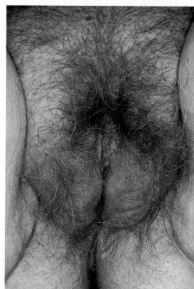

51 Steroid rebound dermatitis. There is an intense fine-textured papular erythema in the area where a class 1 topical steroid (fluocinonide 0.05% cream) had been applied for several months. The symptoms of itching and burning gradually cleared several weeks after discontinuing the steroid.

WHITE PLAQUES

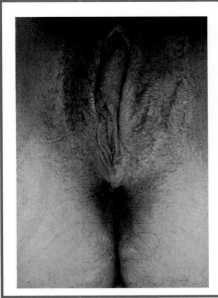

52 Lichen simplex chronicus (LSC). The typical findings of LSC anywhere on the body include leathery induration of the skin with accentuation of normal skin markings. Vaginal *Candida* colonization may trigger bouts of itching.

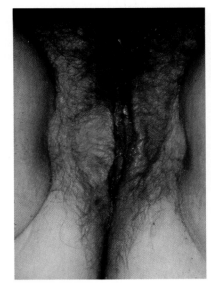

53 Localized plaque of lichen simplex chronicus. The patient admitted to scratching only this area and the lesion resolved after two intralesional injections with triamcinolone suspension (10 mg/mL).

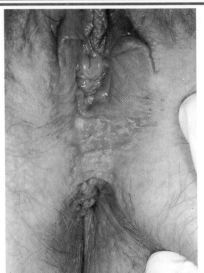

54 Vulvar intraepithelial neoplasia (VIN). Early lesion brought to the patient's attention by itching. In this case, there was no history of papillomavirus infection

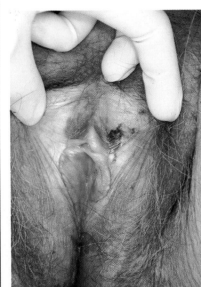

56 Lichen sclerosus (LS) of the vulva. LS is often extremely pruritic. The thin epidermis is easily traumatized by scratching, and petechiae and purpura are very characteristic findings in this disorder.

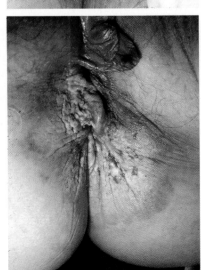

55 Extramammary Paget's disease, diagnosed by biopsy. The patient was aware of only minimal itching. This condition may be associated with an underlying apocrine, eccrine, or adenoid carcinoma.

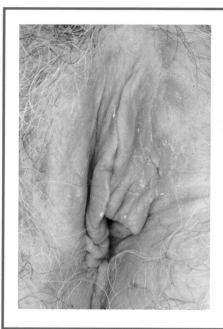

57 Lichen planus (LP) of the vulva. In this case, the vagina was not involved, but there were typical lesions on the wrists and shins. This type of LP is more pruritic than erosive mucosal LP, the more common vulvovaginal variant.

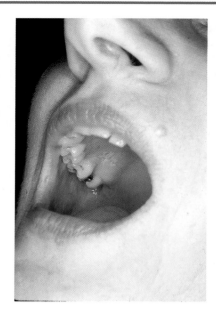

58 Lichen planus of the oral mucosa; same patient as in **57.** White reticulate plaques in the mouth may be seen in all varieties of LP and provide a helpful diagnostic clue.

VAGINITIS

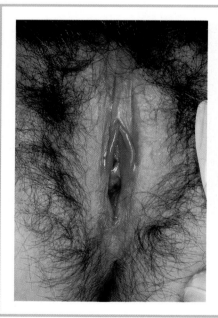

59 Pruritic vulvitis due to bacterial vaginosis and *Candida*. Although inflammatory vulvitis is not common with infectious vaginitis, patients may develop irritation from various over-the-counter agents used to treat discharge or odor.

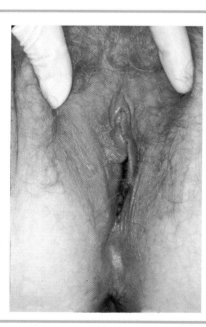

60 *Candida* vulvovaginitis with typical inflammation. Culture of the periclitoral skin was also positive for *Candida* in this patient with frequent recurrences of pruritic vulvovaginitis.

VARICOLORED PAPULES

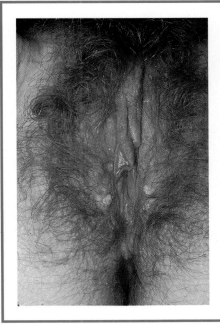

61 Multiple syringomas on both labia majora. This patient complained of itching and irritation from the larger lesions on the right, which were successfully excised under local anesthesia.

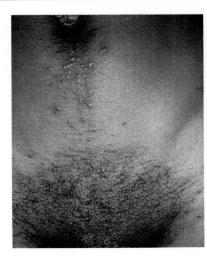

62 Fox–Fordyce disease on the vulva and periumbilical area. This intensely itchy disorder involves the apocrine gland-bearing skin and can also affect the axillae and areolae.

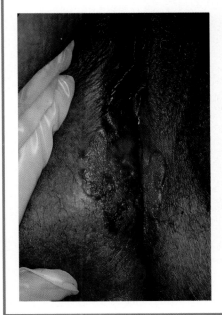

63 Confluent papules of vulvar intraepithelial neoplasia (VIN). diagnosed by biopsy. The patient had complained of itching for more than 8 months. In this case, there was a previous history of infection with human papillomavirus.

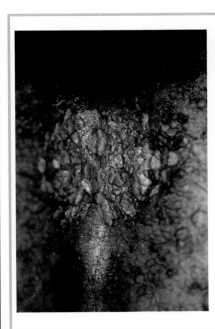

64 Condylomata acuminata on the perineum. This patient's lesions were chronic and recurrent, but there was no evidence of neoplasia on biopsy.

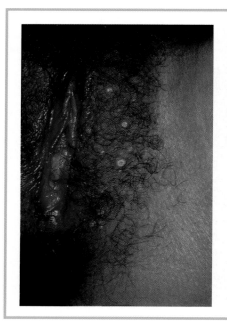

65 Molluscum contagiosum on the labia majora. The typical firm pink papules with a central umbilication are treated by mechanically disrupting the surface and extruding the white material containing 'molluscum bodies'.

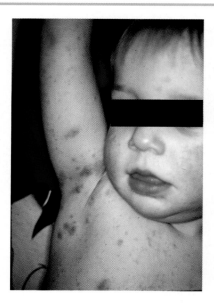

66 Scabies in an infant, showing the intertriginous nodular lesions typical of this infestation in childhood. It is unusual for scabies to localize to one area, such as the genitalia, without evidence of lesions elsewhere on the body, especially on the fingerwebs or wrists. Mites can sometimes be found by scraping underneath the fingernails.

HIVES OR WHEALS

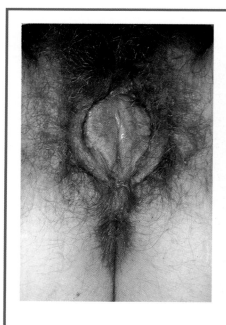

67 Vulvar edema can be seen with chronic trauma or inflammation, as seen in this patient who admitted to frequent rubbing to relieve itching. In some cases, acute edema may be due to latex sensitivity, a type of contact urticaria that occurs in individuals who have had long-term exposure to latex, such as healthcare workers and patients with spina bifida and chronic urethral catheters. Vinyl gloves should be used to examine patients with latex sensitivity, who may develop systemic symptoms such as difficulty breathing.

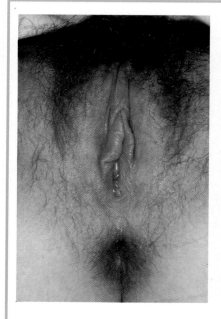

68 Postcoital edema of the labia minora. The patient also complained of burning with intercourse. Although she had no overt evidence of vaginitis, vaginal culture was positive for *Candida*. This is thought to represent a form of localized *Candida* hypersensitivity, and treatment with low-dose, long-term oral or topical anticandidal agents is usually effective. This patient's symptoms resolved after treatment with oral fluconazole, one dose weekly for 2 months, biweekly for 2 months, then monthly for 4 months.

NO RASH

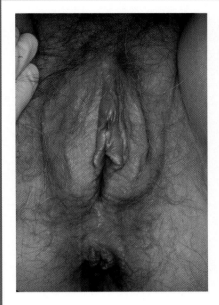

69 Lichen simplex chronicus of the vulva in a patient with diabetes. Generalized itching can occur with systemic problems such as diabetes, thyroid disease, renal failure, human immunodeficiency virus (HIV), lymphoma, and other cancers. Itching of this type is rarely localized to the vulva, but systemic disease should be considered in patients who do not respond to what should be appropriate therapy.

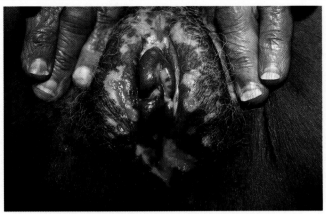

70 Factitial dermatitis of the vulva with linear erosions. This patient was a chronic picker and excoriator, and there were erosions and healed scars on her extremities. Scratch marks (excoriations) tend to be linear rather than round and flat like infectious ulcers. Patients may or may not admit to self-trauma, but chronic problems are usually psychiatric in nature. Patients with delusions of parisitosis should be treated with oral medications for obsessive–compulsive disorder.

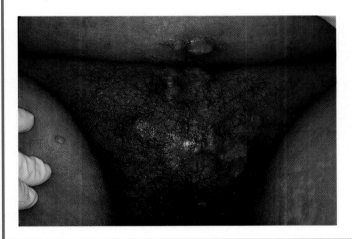

71 Vulvar erosions and ulcers in a patient with acquired immune deficiency syndrome (AIDS) These lesions were considered to be part of her immune deficiency state until a careful examination revealed one intact papule of molluscum contagiosum on her thigh (by the examiner's fingers). When asked, the patient readily admitted to 'digging them out' with her fingernails to stop the itching. As always, a careful history is invaluable to diagnosis.

ACKNOWLEDGEMENTS

Figure **4, 8, 9, 14, 22, 36** and **39** are reproduced from *Genital Skin Disorders: Diagnosis and Treatment.* Fisher, B. K. and Margesson, L. J. (eds), Mosby, St Louis, 1998 (Figs 14.13, 19.18B, 19,20B, 14.3A, 14.14B, 16.7 and 17.6A, respectively). Figures **10, 13, 23, 26** and **29** are reproduced from *Color Atlas of Clinical Gynaecology.* Wisdom, A., Wolfe Medical Publications Ltd, London, 1989 (Figs 306, 111, 114, 483 and 280, respectively). Figure **23** is reproduced from *Diseases of the Skin: A Color Atlas and Text.* White, G. M. and Cox, N. H. Mosby, 2000.

Appendix B

Topical Therapy of Gynecologic Skin Disorders

Marilynne McKay

For nondermatologists the factors determining the right choice of a topical steroid can be bewildering. Just as the obstetrician–gynecologist develops facility with the use of oral estrogen-containing preparations, the dermatologist must learn to choose the best topical steroid preparation for the patient and her problem. It is no more appropriate to ask a dermatologist for the 'best steroid' than it would be to ask a gynecologist for the 'best estrogen'. The answer always depends on many considerations, such as the condition being treated, the patient's age and reliability, the length of time for which the medication will be used, and the potential side effects.

Like oral estrogen preparations, some generalizations can be made about topical steroids:

- There are more kinds than you really need.
- The strongest is not necessarily the best.
- Side effects are often the limiting factor.
- The patient's preference may determine which medication you choose.
- They will not work if not used as directed.

Unlike drug combinations with oral estrogens, combinations of topical steroids with other drugs have not always been as effective as might be expected. A well-known combination of a potent topical steroid (betamethasone dipropionate) and an antifungal (clotrimazole) has been responsible for numerous instances of steroid rebound dermatitis and may even cause striae formation with prolonged use. For some reason, the antifungal does not seem to be as effective in this combination form either. The best advice is to learn to use a few topical steroids well and to know which conditions to treat with them.

HOW STEROIDS WORK

- Reduce inflammation
- Constrict cutaneous capillaries, directly decreasing erythema
- Decrease the mitotic rate of rapidly proliferating epidermis
- Decrease fibroblast proliferation

CHOOSING A TOPICAL STEROID: POTENCY AND VEHICLES

Topical steroids are ranked by classes (I–VII) based on their potency as measured by a standardized vasoconstrictor assay (**Tables 1 and 2**) Simply stated, this test measures how long blanching persists on the forearm after a measured amount of a steroid is applied. The longer blanching (vasoconstriction) persists, the more potent the steroid. Note that fluorination has nothing to do with the potency classification. The higher the potency, the more side effects, whether the corticosteroid is fluorinated or not. (When topical steroids were first developed, fluorination was linked to potency, but this is no longer a firm connection.)

Class VII topical steroids are relatively safe, even for children, and are now available in the United States without a prescription. They are effective anti-inflammatory and emollient agents, are safe to use in intertriginous areas (axillae and groin) as well as the face, and

Table 1 Topical Therapy of Gynecologic Skin Disorders.

Steroid Potency*	Condition	Action of Steroid	Benefit	Best dosage	Risk If Not Used as Directed
Super potent	Lichen sclerosus (LS)	Decreases inflammation leading to sclerotic process, thins scale, reduces scarring	Decreases itching, resolves scale and scarring	Super potent once daily for 4–6 weeks, then decrease frequency and potency	Overthinning of skin, steroid dermatitis (SRD) with burning, telangiectasia formation, gluteal and thigh striae, candida superinfection
Highly potent	Thick, scaly plaque (psoriasis, lichen planus, lichen simplex chronicus)	Decreases inflammation and mitotic rate, thins scale, reduces thickness	Decreases itching, resolves scale and thickness	Highly potent daily for 3–4 weeks, then decrease	1) Patient may become resistant to formulation (tachyphylaxis) 2) Continued use affects normal skin
Highly potent	Erosive dermatoses (erosive lichen planus, bullous diseases)	Reduces inflammation; suppresses immune-mediated process causing blister formation	Reduces blister formation; re-epithelializes erosions	Highly potent cream or ointment; begin daily, then decrease	Secondary candida infection of erosions, delayed healing when blisters controlled, telangiectasias, SRD, striae on buttocks, thighs
Potent	Acute local cutaneous inflammation (allergic, irritant, atopic eczema or dermatitis), oozy wet	Vasoconstriction, reduces inflammation	Resolves inflammation, controls dermatitis, prevents blisters	Potent for flare; moderately potent for maintenance	Skin atrophy and fragility, easy bruising, secondary infection (bacteria, candida, fungi), telangiectasia, depigmentation
Moderately potent	Symptomatic vulvar (or facial) skin with mild erythema but without scaling or plaques; may itch or burn	Vasoconstriction, reduces inflammation	Reduction of erythema, resolution of rash	Moderately potent; AVOID HIGHER POTENCIES	SRD and burning sensation when steroid discontinued; continued need for stronger preparations to control SRD; telangiectasia formation
Mild	Normal skin with patient complaint of burn, sting, irritation, rawness; NO VISIBLE RASH	Skin blanching from vasoconstriction	NONE	NONE	Skin atrophy and fragility, telangiectasia, rebound vasodilation and inflammation, secondary infection (bacteria, candida, fungi), bruising, depigmentation

High to moderate potency = class I–III
Moderate to mild potency = class IV–VII

Table 2 Topical Steroid Potency Ranking 2000.

Class	Generic Name	US Brand Name	UK Brand Name	France	Italy	Germany	Spain
Super potent	Clobetasol propionate	Temovate, oint 0.05%	Dermovate cr, oint 0.50%	Dermoval	Clobetasol Dermoxin	Clobate	
	Betamethasone dipropionate	Diprolene oint, AF cr 0.05%					
	Diflorasone diacetate	Psorcon oint 0.05%					
	Halobetasol propionate	Ultravate cr, oint 0.05%					
Highly potent	Amcinonide	Cyclocort cr, lot, oint 0.01%					
	Betamethasone dipropionate	Diprosone, Maxivate cr, lot, oint 0.05%	Diprosone cr, oint 0.05%	Diprolene	Diprosone	Diprosone	Diproderm
	Desoximetasone	Topicort cr, oint, gel 0.25%					
	Diflorasone diacetate	Maxiflor, Florene cr, oint 0.05%					
	Diflucortolone valerate		Nerisone cr, oily cr, oint 0.1%				
	Fluocinonide	Lidex cr, oint, gel, sol 0.1%	Metosyn cr, oint 0.05%				
	Halcinonide	Halog cr, oint, sol 0.1%	Halciderm cr 0.01%				
Potent	Betamethasone valerate	Valisone cr, lotion, oint 0.1%	Betnovate cr, lotion, oint 0.1%	Betnaval	Ecoval-70	Betnesol	Betnovate
	Beclomethasone dipropionate		Propaderm cr, oint 0.025%		Propaderm		
	Desonide	Tridesilon oint 0.05%					
	Fluocinolone acetonide	Synalar cr, oint 0.025%	Synalar cr, oint 0.025%	Synalar			Synalar
	Flurandrenolide	Cordran cr, oint 0.05%					
	Fluticasone propionate		Cutivate cr, 0.05%				
	Hydrocortisone butyrate	Locoid cr, oint 0.1%	Locoid cr, oint 0.1%				
	Hydrocortisone valerate	Westcort cr, oint 0.2%					
	Mometasone furoate	Elocon cr, lotion, oint 0.1%	Elocon cr, oint 0.1%	Kenacort-A	Kanacort	Volon-A	
	Triamcinolone acetonide	Aristocort, Kenalog oint 0.1%	Adcortyl cr, oint 0.1%				
Moderately potent	Aclometasone dipropionate	Aclovate cr, oint 0.05%	Modrasone cr, oint 0.05%	Aclosone	Legaderm	Delonal	Alcodal
	Betamethasone dipropionate		Stiedex oily cream 0.05%				
	Clobetasone butyrate		Eumovate cr, oint 0.05%		Eumovate	Eumovate	Eumovate
	Desonide	Tridesilon cr, 0.05%					
	Flumethasone pivolate	Locorten cr 0.03%					
	Fluocinolone acetonide	Synalar cr, sol 0.01%					
	Flurandrenolone		Haelan cr, oint 0.0125%				
	Triamcinolone acetonide	Aristocort, Kenalog cr, lot 0.1%, oint 0.025%					
Mild	Hydrocortisone	Cortdome, Eldocort, Dermacort, Hytone cr, oint, lot 1% and 2.5% Pramosone 1% and 2.5%	Dioderm, Efcortelan, Mildison Lipocream 1%	Hydrocortisone Astier	Algicortif Dermacoral	Hydrocortisone Wolff	Crema-Transcotanea-Asti
	Hydrocortisone acetate						

have a low risk of candida superinfection. For patients with chronic dermatitis (e.g. atopy) the class VII steroids can prevent flares that might occur if steroids were discontinued altogether.

Class IV midpotency topical steroids are actually 'full strength' medications which have been the dermatologic standard for years. Because vulvar skin absorbs steroids well (and is also an occluded area), these are the highest strength needed for most vulvar problems. They are considerably safer than the high-potency preparations, but still have significant side effects, so must be prescribed in judicious amounts.

Class I 'superpotent' topical steroids are remarkable medications[1,2]. Regular applications are equivalent to intralesional injections, but it is difficult to control the area treated. On the vulva, where several skin surfaces are in contact with one another, this can be a problem. There is significant systemic absorption with the class I steroids: studies have shown that 2 g (the size of a sample tube) per day of 0.05% clobetasol propionate can measurably suppress the hypothalamic–pituitary–adrenal axis[3,4]. It has been recommended that usage of clobetasol propionate 0.05% (Dermovate, Temovate) should not exceed 50 g per week[5]; this is approximately the size of a large prescription tube. The dosage should be tapered as soon as improvement is noted and should be discontinued after 2 weeks if there is no response. Class I steroids should not be prescribed for children under the age of 12 years[6] Medicolegal precedent in the UK and the USA has linked long-term class I steroid usage with aseptic necrosis of the femoral head[7], glaucoma and cataracts[8], and extensive irreversible striae formation.

SYSTEMIC COMPLICATIONS OF CLASS I STEROIDS

- Suppression of hypothalamic–pituitary–adrenal axis
- Aseptic necrosis of the femoral head
- Extensive irreversible striae formation
- Glaucoma and cataracts (with facial application)

COMPLICATIONS

In addition to the systemic effects described above, there are a number of local complications. Striae are particularly likely to occur on the thin skin of the inner thighs and abdomen, and topical steroids applied to the vulva almost invariably affect these areas due to anatomic contact. Bruising or petechial (nonblanching) erythema are the first signs of steroid side effects.

After use for more than 6 weeks, topical steroids with potencies of class V or higher can cause steroid rebound dermatitis to one degree or another when they are discontinued. Loss of steroid vasoconstriction results in rebound vasodilation of the cutaneous capillaries, often with burning discomfort which can be relieved only by reapplication of the topical steroid. The likelihood of this complication increases with the potency of the preparation, and patients who are prone to rosacea (those with fair skin and a tendency to flush easily) are particularly susceptible, whether the steroid is applied to the face or the vulva.

Local immunosuppression of vulvar skin with high-potency steroids may also potentiate acute outbreaks of recurrent herpes simplex and human papillomavirus. Concomitant therapy with topical steroids may also increase or sustain the severity of infections (candidiasis, tinea, staphylococcus) and infestations such as scabies[9].

STEROID SIDE EFFECTS WITH NORMAL USE

- Epidermal atrophy
- Dermal atrophy and striae formation
- Easy bruising
- Telangiectasias
- Steroid rebound dermatitis when discontinued

CREAM OR OINTMENT

Potency depends on the vehicle in which the steroid is mixed. Vehicles must carry the drug through the skin, which is a difficult task because a major function of the stratum corneum is to be a barrier to outside agents. Much research goes into developing vehicles that will be nonirritating, cosmetically elegant, and effective in maximizing delivery of the steroid to the dermis.

The basic principle is that when the stratum corneum is hydrated, medications penetrate better. This is why creams are so effective: as mixtures of water and oil, they hydrate the skin with water and 'seal in' the moisture with oil. Occlusion keeps the skin moist by retarding evaporation of water, so ointment bases (such as petroleum jelly) that are more occlusive allow medications to penetrate for a longer time, especially when they are applied to most skin immediately after a bath.

Ointment-based steroids are more potent than the same preparation in a cream or lotion base because ointments are more occlusive. Another advantage to ointments is that they are less likely to contain allergens such as preservatives, which are necessary in water-based creams. Unfortunately, many patients do not care for the 'greasy' feel of ointments, so they do not use them as often as they should. Gels also penetrate well, usually because they contain propylene glycol, a good vehicle for carrying drugs through the skin. Propylene glycol can be irritating, however, and patients with irritated mucosal surfaces (vulvar inflammation) often complain of stinging with gels.

Special 'optimized' vehicles can increase the potency of preparation by one or perhaps two classes, even though the concentration of drug is the same. This is how pharmaceutical companies constantly maneuver for position on the steroid potency chart, and why generic preparations are an unknown quantity. Some generic creams or ointments are significantly less effective because the vehicle does not deliver the drug as well as expected. There is no good way to predict this except by experience, because only brand-name drugs are included in the 'relative potency' evaluation. (Dermatologists who use these medications more frequently may have better experience with generic preparations, but many of them prefer specific brands because they are more predictable.) Mixing one's own steroid preparations is discouraged – these are even more unreliable than generic brands.

STEROID POTENCY DEPENDS ON

- Corticosteroid formula
- Concentration of steroid
- Vehicle
- Frequency of application and length of time used

WHEN NOT TO USE HIGH-POTENCY STEROIDS

Two questions should be asked when choosing a steroid: 'What am I treating?' and 'How long should it take to bring the condition under control?'. If you are unsure about either (or both) of these, then you should *not* prescribe a class I or II high-potency preparation. The patient is likely to develop side effects if a class I or II steroid is applied for too long a time. Likewise, if the steroid is not used long enough for an appropriate treatment trial, there will be minimal benefit and it will be unclear whether the medication has been effective. Do not use class I or II topicals for erythema alone, for vulvodynia (burning) or itching in the absence of skin disease, or for histopathology of nondiagnostic mild squamous cell hyperplasia.

STEROID-RESPONSIVE VULVAR DERMATOSES

- Thick, scaly lesions (usually pruritic)
  Lichen sclerosus (LS)
  Psoriasis
  Lichen simplex chronicus (LSC)
- Blisters and erosions
  Lichen planus (LP)
  Dermatitis/eczema
  Bullous diseases

OTHER TOPICAL MEDICATIONS

Faced with a skin disorder of any kind, the first topical medications that most care providers consider is a topical steroid or an antifungal agent. Acute outbreaks of dermatitis should be evaluated carefully to determine the correct diagnosis, as indiscriminate treatment may confuse the issue. In many cases, treatment with wet compresses and a bland emollient may be all that is required to dry and sooth a wet, oozy dermatitis, to prevent infection, and to make the patient more comfortable. (*See also Chapter 10*, Eczema in Pregnancy.)

BUROW'S SOLUTION COMPRESSES

For open, oozing dermatitis, Burow's solution (aluminum acetate) is an excellent astringent and antiseptic. It is somewhat anesthetic as well, and is particularly effective in treating primary herpes simplex infections. Tablets or powder packets may be obtained at the pharmacy; one packet dissolved in one pint of water makes a 1 : 40 solution, which is recommended for topical application. The patient should mix the solution fresh daily, but it can be used throughout the day. A washcloth or soft gauze should be saturated with the solution and applied to the vulva and left in place for 20 minutes three or four times daily. The patient may sit on a folded towel to absorb excess moisture, or may find it more convenient to sit in a dry bathtub. The compress should be kept moist and not allowed to dry; rinsing is not necessary.

SEA WATER SITZBATHS

The main benefit of this preparation over self-mixed salt solution is the relatively constant concentration of ingredients; in addition to sodium chloride, magnesium sulfate and other salts are also included. Packets of powdered salts may be found where aquarium supplies are sold, and mixing instructions are usually by the gallon. This makes preparation of a Sitzbath more convenient, and this solution has been recommended for pain relief and healing after laser or electrosurgical procedures.

TOPICAL ACYCLOVIR OINTMENT

Although this medication has been shown to decrease viral shedding when used in combination with oral acyclovir in primary herpes simplex (HSV) infections, it has not been proven efficacious in recurrent HSV. There does not, however, appear to be any justification in the use of topical acyclovir ointment as a therapeutic agent in recurrent HSV.

EURAX–VALISONE CREAM

Eurax (crotamiton) is a scabicide and antipruritic cream that is not as effective for scabies as lindane (Kwell) or permethrin (Elimite). The antipruritic effect is achieved by mild skin irritation which distracts from the sensation of 'itch'. The late vulvologist, Dr Eduard G. Friedrich, Jr., recommended mixing 3 parts Eurax with 7 parts betamethasone valerate 0.1% cream (Valisone) for pruritic vulvar dermatoses. The reasoning for this mixture was that the antipruritic effect of the crotamiton would provide immediate relief of itching, while the topical class V steroid would gradually treat the underlying skin condition. There are two problems with this mixture: (1) crotamiton is an irritant, and causes marked stinging on skin that is already inflamed; (2) a mixture is significantly more expensive than two tubes of medication. There is nothing particularly 'scientific' about the 3 : 7 mixture; equal parts could be used for intense pruritus and the steroid could be tapered gradually in favor of the crotamiton for persistent or occasional itch. The topical steroid is the most important ingredient and it should be prescribed as noted below. Crotamiton may be considered an 'anti-itch' cream which the patient may apply whenever she wishes, but it should be used only on thickened, scaly lesions where pruritus is the major complaint.

TOPICAL TESTOSTERONE OINTMENT

Two per cent testosterone propionate in petrolatum was long considered the mainstay of treatment for lichen sclerosus. Topical testosterone was never recommended for vulvar dermatoses other than lichen sclerosus, although it was widely used as a 'treatment trial' when gynecologists were unsure why patients had symptomatic vulvar itching or burning. It was thought that the androgenic effect served somehow to 'toughen' vulvar skin in opposition to the influences of estrogen. This has not been found to be the case; improvement with topical testosterone has probably been due to the conversion of androgenic steroid to glucocorticoid within the skin itself. Testosterone ointment has not been found to be as effective as topical steroids for vulvar dermatoses, and new data have shown the class I steroids to be more effective in the treatment of lichen sclerosus[10–12]. Side effects of topical testosterone include clitoral hypertrophy, increased libido, local hair growth, deepening of the voice, and other signs of masculinization which patients often find unpleasant.

HOW MUCH TO PRESCRIBE

Thirty grams is about one ounce. In the US, topical medications are dispensed by the ounce, so multiples of 30 are common (along with 15 g and 45 g tubes). Sixty grams (2 oz) will cover the whole body twice. A 30 g tube of cream, rubbed in well, will be enough for a patient to apply to the entire vulva three times daily for a week. (Applying medication more than that is probably wasting it. Twice daily is generally enough, and tapering to once daily or every other day is a good way to decrease usage as the patient improves.) Patients sometimes think they have to reapply creams to the entire vulva each time they wipe after using the toilet, but this is not necessary. If a medication has been rubbed in well, it will be absorbed in about 30 minutes to the point that reapplication is not necessary.

It is important to explain to the patient how much medication to use. Patients who expect a medication to stop the sensation of itching, for instance, may apply a thick layer of cream several times a day and protest that 'it's not working' when they are still itching a week later (see below). Patients who are concerned about the cost of medication may not use enough cream to treat the condition. Always ask how much cream ('how many tubes?') the patient has used since the last visit and counsel her accordingly. The patient information sheets in Appendix D are helpful for specific disorders.

SUMMARY

Review the actual cost to the patient of topical steroids. While money can be saved by prescribing generic preparations, some of these are not nearly as effective because the vehicle is not as good at delivering the drug. (See **Table 2** for brand names and variations in potency between cream, ointment, and optimized cream.) Choose an ointment-based steroid in class I or II to use as a 'strong medicine' (write that on the prescription so it will appear on the label that the patient will see – don't count on her to remember which cream is the most potent.) An ointment base is less pleasant to use, so a high-potency ointment will be more likely to be put aside in favor of a lower-potency class IV 'maintenance cream' (also written to appear on the prescription label). If a patient tells you that a topical preparation is irritating, make a note of it. If you hear it from several patients, stop using this product and choose another. Ointments and water-based creams are usually well tolerated on the vulva.

Do not write unlimited refills or refill these by telephone. A flare of symptoms may be superinfection with candida or recurrence of herpes simplex because of steroid immunosuppression. Steroid rebound dermatitis may cause the patient to use the topical steroid well beyond the time it should have been discontinued.

Skin problems take time to resolve, and the physician should counsel the patient accordingly. Patients are often confused about causes and effects of genital symptoms; they do not understand that damaged skin may itch or burn until it heals. They demand 'tests to find out why I have this' and expect relief within a few days. This confusion may be worsened when the provider does not realize that symptomatic dermatoses typically take weeks to resolve. Changing prescriptions after only a few days makes the patient think that whatever

disease she has cannot be treated. Often the best therapy is persistent use of bland emolients or mild topical steroids, and gentle but firm reassurance that no infection or malignancy has been discovered. With skin conditions, successful treatment gradually results in symptom improvement as therapy is continued, so treatment protocols should be continued for a fair trial of 6–8 weeks.

> **REMEMBER:**
>
> - Topical steroids are not a 'cure'.
> - Use the lowest steroid potency that will control the problem.
> - Chronic skin diseases require long-term therapy.
> - Topical steroids can potentiate coinfections with candida, tinea, bacteria, and scabies.

REFERENCES

1 Olsen, E. A., and Cornell, R. C. Topical clobetasol-17-propionate: review of its clinical efficacy and safety. *J. Am. Acad. Dermatol.* 1986; **15**: 246–255.

2 Harris, D. W., and Hunter, J. A. The use and abuse of 0.05 per cent clobetasol propionate in dermatology. *Dermatol. Clin.* 1988; **6**: 643–647.

3 Anonymous. Clobetasol proprionate (Temovate by Glaxo). *Drug Newslett.* 1986; **5**(3): 24.

4 Ohman, E. M., Rogers, S., Meenan, F. O., *et al.* Adrenal suppression following low dose topical clobetasol propionate. *J. R. Soc. Med.* 1987; **80**: 422–423.

5 Carruthers, J. A., August, P. J., and Staughton, R. C. Observations on the systemic effect of topical clobetasol propionate (Dermovate). *B.M.J.* 1975; **4**(5990): 203–204.

6 Stoppolini, G. Potential hazards of topical steroid therapy. *Am. J. Dis. Child.* 1983; **137**: 1130–1131.

7 Hogan, D. J., Sibley, J. T., and Lane, P. R. Avascular necrosis of the hips following long-term use of clobetasol propionate. *J. Am. Acad. Dermatol.* 1986; **14**: 515–517.

8 Katsushima, H., Souma, K., Nishio, C., *et al.* Glaucoma and posterior subcapsular cataract after long-term use of corticosteroid lotion in a case with photodermatitis. *J. Clin. Ophthalmol.* 1986; **40**: 1345–1349.

9 Millard, L. G. Norwegian scabies developing during treatment with fluorinated steroid therapy. *Acta Dermatovenereol.* 1977; **57**(1): 86–88.

10 Dalziel, K. L., Millard, P. R., and Wojnarowska, F. The treatment of vulval lichen sclerosus with a very potent topical steroid (clobetasol propionate 0.05%) cream. *Br. J. Dermatol.* 1991; **124**: 461–464.

11 Bracco, G. L., Carli, P., Sonni, L., *et al.* Clinical and histologic effects of topical treatments of vulval lichen sclerosus. A critical evaluation. *J. Reprod. Med.* 1993; **38**: 37–40.

12 Cattaneo, A., De Marco, A., Sonni, L., *et al.* Clobetasolo vs testosterone nel trattamento del lichen scleroso della regione vulvare. Minerva Ginecol. 1992; **44**: 567–571.

Diagnostic Techniques: Clinical Evaluation of Patients with Vulvovaginal Complaints

Marilynne McKay, Lynette J. Margesson

Although a number of skin diseases may be recognized by a characteristic clinical appearance, simple diagnostic techniques readily provide confirmation of a first impression. These may be performed quickly in the office setting, and are often the definitive method of differentiating between morphologically similar skin problems. Reliable diagnosis means appropriate therapy – a benefit to patient and physician alike.

Patients with vulvar disease take time. Most patients have had chronic symptoms and multiple, often ineffective, treatments. For each patient, start from the beginning. It is important that the course of each patient's disease be accurately documented. This must be carried out in a nonjudgemental and a very supportive environment. *Take the time to listen.*

New or changing symptoms require a new physical examination. Scabies or squamous cell carcinoma in a patient with vulvar lichen sclerosus is not just a worsening of the lichen sclerosus. High-potency topical steroids may encourage secondary candida infection. Resist using the telephone for either diagnosis or therapy.

HISTORY

A fresh general, medical, social, and family history should be obtained from the patient and should include details of all the following subjects:

- Menstrual
- Gynecologic
- Obstetric
- Sexual – sexual practices, sexually transmitted diseases (STDs), treatments
- Previous treatments with responses (positive and negative)
- Prescription medications, 'natural' and 'alternative' preparations
- Over-the-counter products, past and present
- A review of old records

SPECIFIC SYMPTOMS

The most common complaints in vulvar disease are itch and pain. These may stand alone or in combination, and vary in their description and localization. Complaints of burning or irritation are often heard. Characteristics to be defined for each symptom include the following:

- Episodic pattern
- Time of day or month
- Menstrual association
- Factors that relieve or worsen
- Degree of incapacity

PHYSICAL EXAMINATION

Examine all surfaces of the external genitalia and do a vaginal examination as needed. Problems with dermatoses, blistering diseases, or infections may involve other body areas. Examine other body surfaces, including scalp and nails, and the oral mucosa. The diagnosis may be more obvious elsewhere (e.g. scalp in psoriasis).

VISUALIZATION

Proper lighting for the physical examination is imperative. The light should be bright but without glare. Full-spectrum incandescent lighting provides the red needed to discern subtle color variations. Magnification needs to be available with special eyeglasses, loupes, or a magnifier–light source combination. Colposcopy can be very useful.

Skin signs of vulvar disease include the following:

- Crusting
- Discharge
- Erosion
- Erythema
- Excoriations
- Exudation
- Lichenification

217

- Loss of architecture
- Maceration
- Purpura
- Scaling
- Ulceration
- Whiteness

Note: Look for related cutaneous physical signs (e.g. pitted nails and papulosquamous rash on the scalp or body in psoriasis).

EXAMINATION OF THE VAGINA

Vaginal infection cannot be diagnosed properly without a thorough clinical examination. For this, the clinician needs an examination room with a suitable couch, a good light, and privacy. A female chaperone is essential for a male clinician performing a vaginal examination.

The decision as to how far to go with laboratory tests in individual cases must be based on sensitive but thorough history taking, epidemiologic knowledge, and common sense. Although not essential, a colposcope does make vaginal examination easier, as there are some situations in which a magnified view of the vagina is helpful.

The vulva and vestibule are first inspected for signs of infection and other disease, and the inguinal areas are palpated for clinically apparent lymph nodes. An unlubricated (or water-lubricated) bivalve vaginal speculum is passed into the vagina and opened to expose the uterine cervix. If the patient's legs are supported in stirrups or footrests, the speculum is best inserted handle downwards. However, if the patient is lying flat on the couch it is best to insert the speculum with the handle upwards.

The lateral vaginal walls are exposed, together with the fornices. Vaginal discharge may have collected in the posterior blade of the speculum. (*See* **Table 1** for the tests that should be performed on a sample of this discharge if it is thought to be pathologic). The vagina is then cleared of discharge, and the cervix wiped clean. If there is a significant risk of sexually transmitted infections, tests for pathogens (*Neisseria gonorrheae*, *Chlamydia trachomatis*, and possibly herpesvirus) should be performed on smears taken from the endocervix. A cervical smear is usually stained by the Papanicolaou method, to test both for the presence of premalignant change (cervical endothelial neoplasia; CIN) and for cellular marks of infection.

The visible portion of the vagina and the cervix are now carefully inspected, under magnification if a colposcope is available. A washout with normal saline may be necessary to obtain a proper view and, if premalignant change of the cervix or vagina is suspected, colposcopic examination should be repeated after the application of 5% acetic acid.

Table 1 Laboratory Evaluation of Acute Vaginal Symptoms.

Test	Technique	Points to remember	Result
Vaginal pH	Touch swab with vaginal secretions to pH paper with a range of 3.5–5.5	Swab the middle third of the vagina, as fluid from from pool at the posterior fornix includes cervical secretions and may not be accurate	Normal pH excludes bacterial vaginosis; pH >4.5 see **Table 12.1**
Amine (whiff) test	Place a drop of 10% KOH on swab with vaginal secretions; check for fishy odor	FemExam diagnostic card combines pH and amine tests (available from Cooper Surgical, Shelton, CT, USA)	Amine test is positive in bacterial vaginosis; may also be positive with trichomoniasis
Potassium hydroxide (KOH) smear	Place a drop of 10% KOH on swab with vaginal secretions; roll swab on to microscope slide	Use same swab as for amine test; check for odor before applying swab to slide. Always use coverslip for best viewing	KOH lyses epithelial cells and makes it easier to find candidal pseudohyphae
Saline smear	Roll swab with vaginal secretions in drop of saline on microscope slide; add coverslip	Use nonbacteriostatic saline to maintain motility of trichomonads	View trichomonads, clue cells, ratio of polymorphonuclear leucocytes (PMNLs) to epithelial cells, overall bacterial flora
Adjunctive tests (not routine)			
Culture for yeast	Apply swab of vaginal secretion to culture plate or send to laboratory	For patients with a history suggestive of candida, but with negative KOH exam	Speciation may help with selection of antifungal therapy
Culture for herpes simplex	Swab base of ulcer or open vesicle to obtain fluid	Special viral culture medium is required; rapid diagnostic tests are also available	

The inspection is continued by gradual withdrawal and partial closure of the speculum, which will reveal the previously concealed parts of the anterior and posterior walls of the vagina. The overall picture of the vaginal wall is noted, together with specific features such as ulcers, warty lesions, or keratin plaques.

As the speculum is finally withdrawn, it will have 'milked' the urethra to reveal any discharge. This discharge may need to be tested for infection. Skene and Bartholin glands should be palpated and the entrances to their ducts inspected for discharge. Finally, a bimanual examination should be carried out, with full palpation of the upper pelvic organs.

OFFICE TOOLS AND EQUIPMENT

EQUIPMENT FOR VULVAR DIAGNOSIS

Ten per cent potassium hydroxide (KOH) for microscopic diagnosis of dermatophyte, yeast Litmus paper for pH determination (pH 4–5 in candidiasis, 5–7 in trichomoniasis, > 4.5 in bacterial vaginosis)

Microscopic slides and cover slips
Microscope
Magnifying glass or specialized eyeglasses/loupes
Culture media for bacteria, fungi and yeast, and herpes simplex (have access to special media for STDs such as chlamydia and gonorrhea)
Bivalve vaginal speculum (Cusco pattern) – various sizes
Vinegar for aceto-whitening
Normal saline (non bacteriostatic) and test tubes for wet mounts

EQUIPMENT FOR LOCAL ANESTHESIA

Lidocaine 2% with and without epinephrine
30-gauge needles
3 mL syringes
Topical lidocaine/prilocaine cream (EMLA) or 5% lidocaine cream (ELA-MAX 5)
Plastic wrap

EQUIPMENT FOR BIOPSY

Disposable skin biopsy punches: (3 mm and 4 mm)
Cervical biopsy forceps
Small iris scissors
Needle driver
Mosquito hemostat
No. 15 scalpel blades plus handle
Monsel solution
Absorbable suture material – polyglactin (Vicryl) or chromic
Formalin and specialized transport media (Michel solution) for immunofluorescence

Note: For interpretation of histopathology, a dermato-histopathologist is invaluable. It may be necessary to mail specimens or slides to a specialist laboratory for accurate interpretation.

EQUIPMENT FOR THERAPY

Liquid nitrogen and cotton-tipped applicators, probes, and spray units for cryotherapy.
Triamcinolone acetonide for intralesional treatment (Kenalog 10) and for intramuscular treatment (Kenalog 40)
Normal saline for injection
Hyfrecator for electrodesiccation
Trichloroacetic acid

MISCELLANEOUS EQUIPMENT NEEDED

Gauze
70% isopropyl alcohol
Cotton-tipped applicators and cotton balls
Gloves

OPTIONAL EXTRAS

Colposcope
Camera
Patient information sheets

TOPICAL ANESTHETIC

Topical anesthesia is very useful before any intralesional injections including infiltration anesthesia for biopsy, wart destruction, removal of small tumors, etc. Use either a mixture of lidocaine–prilocaine cream (EMLA) or 5% lidocaine cream (ELA-MAX 5). The lidocaine–prilocaine cream must be applied generously under plastic wrap occlusion. The 5% lidocaine cream needs no occlusion. They both may sting for a short period on initial application. For optimal effectiveness, the cream must be left in place for 10–15 minutes for the skin of the vulvar trigone and in the labia minora. For the thicker epithelium, an hour is more appropriate.

VULVAR BIOPSIES

Although it does not qualify as a quick 'office' diagnostic technique, a biopsy actually shows the pathologic processes underlying a skin lesion. Skin biopsies provide a great deal of information, especially when read by a dermatopathologist or someone with special expertise in vulvar cutaneous pathology. Findings on biopsy can confirm some office tests (fungal hyphae may be seen in infected stratum corneum, for example), but bacterial infections can be difficult to diagnose and scabies mites may be missed.

If possible, preanesthetize with a topical anesthetic; see description above. Warm the anesthetic up to body temperature. Infiltrate the area with a mixture of lidocaine 1–2% plus epinephrine to limit bleeding. Inject slowly with a 30-gauge needle to minimize pain. Buffering the lidocaine with sodium bicarbonate is another way to decrease discomfort with injection.

A standard 3 mm or 4 mm punch is good, but tissue should be handled gently to avoid 'crush artifacts' from forceps.

For superficial biopsies, gently 'tent' or 'spear' the area to be sampled using the 30-gauge needle, and use fine iris scissors or a no. 15 scalpel blade to undercut the specimen. Avoid crushing the tissue with forceps. For some locations, the cervical biopsy forceps are very useful. For thicker areas of skin, a punch biopsy may be more appropriate. An excisional biopsy may be necessary for certain types of lesions. The no. 15 or 15C scalpel is used to carry out an elliptical excision. For the majority of vulvar biopsies, Monsel solution and pressure are all that are necessary to stop bleeding. For a deeper biopsy, a suture may be necessary. For the patient's comfort and healing, consider avoiding the suture or choose the more comfortable polyglactin (Vicryl) suture material.

TZANCK SMEAR

Tzanck smear is used for the diagnosis of herpes simplex or herpes zoster. In both conditions, the viral infection creates multinucleated giant keratinocytes that can be seen with appropriate stains. This technique is useful only on fresh blisters. A no. 15 scalpel blade is used to scrape the base of the blister. The material is smeared on to a glass slide, briefly immersed in a cytology fixative (Pap smear solution), air dried and stained with Wright, Giemsa, Gram or Sedi stain to demonstrate the giant cells. If the test is negative, it does not rule out a herpes infection. A culture should always be done at the same time to determine the viral type. Using the same no. 15 blade, scrape the base of the lesion and send that material for culture for optimal results.

When examining a dry stained smear, put a thin layer of *immersion oil* on the specimen, even though you are using only the high dry objective. The cells will be much clearer and easier to see.

MINERAL OIL PREPARATION

Ectoparasites such as lice may be immobilized in a drop of immersion or mineral oil for examination under the low-power microscope. A drop of oil is placed on the slide and the mite is put in the oil under a coverslip.

Lice: phthiris pubis (crab louse)
pediculus humans humanus (body louse)
pediculus humanus capitis (head louse)
Lice all have three sets of legs, but the crab louse has enlarged posterior claws which grasp larger diameter body hairs (pubic, axillary, beard, eyelash); it looks like a little crab, hence the name. Head and body lice have smaller claws and are found at the base of head hairs and inside clothing seams respectively. Look for nits and empty egg cases on hairs.

Scabies: sarcoptes scabiei

These mites are microscopic and live in the topmost skin layer. Mites have a rounded body and four pairs of legs.

The secret to finding the scabies mite is in knowing where to look for likely burrows. The finger webs are the classic location, but the wrists, elbows, areolae, and umbilicus are other fruitful regions where the small linear papules may be found. Only the top of the papule is scraped: mites live in the superficial stratum corneum, and drawing blood means that the blade is going too deep. Many papules should be scraped at one time to increase the chances of a positive preparation. Mineral oil is applied to the glass slide and the blade is tapped in the oil before scraping the skin; this makes the specimen stick to the blade for easy transfer to the slide. Methodically scan the entire field under the coverslip – mites and eggs may not be in a 'clump' of debris. *Note*: Scabies mites will be intact, not in scattered pieces. Some practitioners prefer to mount the scraping in KOH (see below).

An alternative technique, using magnification and a no. 15 blade, involves picking the solitary mite out of its burrow. The tiny grayish-tan speck is examined on a glass slide, with or without oil or KOH.

POTASSIUM HYDROXIDE PREPARATION

The most common office diagnostic technique used by the dermatologist is probably a KOH preparation. A 10% solution of KOH added to epithelial scrapings dissolves keratin. After adding KOH, wait for 5 minutes for the keratin to 'clear'. Faster clearing is obtained by using KOH in dimethylsulfoxide (DMSO). Visualization of fungal hyphae is diagnostic. (KOH examination only confirms presence of hyphae: Candida pseudohyphae and short sticks of *Pityrosporum ovale* and their spores can be distinguished by their appearance, but identification of other tinea species requires fungal culture.)

When examining KOH preparations, the substage condenser should be racked down to its lowest position, and the light intensity should be decreased. Hyphae are refractile and show up best in indirect light.

Candida

Budding filamentous pseudohyphae and egg-shaped to round yeast cells may be observed in a candida wet preparation. Heating will help to dissolve epithelial cells faster and show hyphae better. Heat gently because boiling destroys the preparation. (Gram stain can also be used to demonstrate candida; for skin lesions, Gram stain of a pustule gives a better yield of budding yeast forms than KOH.)

Tinea

The border of the lesion should be scraped gently with a no. 15 blade. Only scale is necessary, and no blood should be drawn. If blisters are present (acute tinea), trim off the blister roof and apply it to the slide with KOH solution. If blisters have resolved (chronic tinea), scrape the dried 'collarette' of scale for high fungal yield. The KOH may need to be heated slightly for thick scale of tinea corporis or cruris, but this is probably not necessary for the powdery scale of tinea versicolor. Fungal hyphae are thin, refractile, cylindrical, and uniform in diameter. Branching may be seen. Irregular 'thick and thin' strands are probably artifacts but may be dying fungus in a previously treated case. Epithelial cell borders in hexagonal patterns can look like branched hyphae to the inexperienced.

Scabies: sarcoptes scabiei

These mites or ova can be demonstrated easily with the KOH preparation. KOH with DMSO will permit dissolution of thick keratin and visualization of mature mites, nymphs, eggs, and mite feces. *See* Mineral oil preparation above.

DARKFIELD MICROSCOPY

The darkfield microscope is used to visualize *Treponema pallidum* in a serum sample (usually taken from a scraped and oozing syphilitic skin lesion). Light rays strike the objects in the field obliquely so that the only light rays seen are reflected from the surface: the organism shines luminously against a dark background. *T. pallidum* must be distinguished from nonpathogenic spirochetes living in the mouth or genital region. Its size, shape, and movements are characteristic. Treponemes are shaped like corkscrews and rotate spirally as well as bending or twisting from side to side. This examination is done routinely only in STD clinics, because it takes experience and skill to set up and standardize the darkfield scope.

SALINE WET PREPARATIONS

Examining the vaginal secretions microscopically with a drop of saline on a glass slide under a coverslip allows one to evaluate the patient for infection and judge the maturity of vaginal epithelium. A cotton-tipped applicator is used to collect vaginal secretions or is rolled against the vaginal wall for assessment of vaginal cell maturity. The material is smeared on a glass slide, a drop of saline added, and a coverslip placed gently on top. Lactobacilli, candida and trichomonas can be seen directly. When bacteria cling to the edges of the epithelial cells, the cell's borders are obscured, creating the 'clue cell' found in bacterial vaginosis. This diagnosis can be further supported with a pH greater than 4.5 and a positive 'whiff' test. For the latter, a drop of KOH is added to vaginal secretion and this results in the typical fishy odor (*see* **Table 1**).

PATCH TESTING

There are two different types of contact dermatitis: allergic and irritant. *Allergic* contact dermatitis is a cell-mediated (type IV) allergic reaction; the rash develops 48–72 hours after the exposure. Only someone sensitized to a substance will develop allergic contact dermatitis, and it happens every time the patient is exposed. *Irritant* reactions, on the other hand, occur only if the skin's barrier function is compromised (like the stinging of vinegar on chapped hands.) When the skin heals, the irritant reaction is reduced or eliminated. Allergic contact dermatitis itches, swells, and blisters; the rash lasts 2–3 weeks. Outbreaks lasting only a few days are more likely to be eczema; if episodes seem continuous, *patch testing* may be necessary to discover the allergen.

When a patient has developed an itchy rash possibly due to a topically applied product or material, patch testing with components of that material or product can be carried out to define the allergen. The common allergens are available individually or on prepared strips as in the 'True Test'. These chemicals are taped onto the patient's back and left in place for 48 hours. They are then removed and the area is examined, preferably at 72 hours. Dermatologists routinely do this procedure and are knowledgeable as to which products should be chosen for testing and how to interpret the tests and educate the patient accordingly. Candidates for patch testing include women with sudden onset of a very itchy vulva, particularly if the vulvar rash appears after the use of a new topical product, or those with long-term itchy rashes that are nonresponsive to treatment.

Note: Any topically applied material, including topical steroids, may result in an allergic reaction.

BIBLIOGRAPHY

Lynch, P. J. and Edwards, L. Diagnostic procedures. In: Lynch, P. J. and Edwards, L. (eds) *Genital Dermatology*, pp. 7–10. Churchill Livingston, New York, 1994.

Fisher, B. K. and Margesson, L. J. *Genital Skin Disorders: Diagnosis and Treatment*. Mosby, St Louis, 1998.

PATIENT INFORMATION – LICHEN PLANUS (like-in plane-us)

Lichen planus (LP) is a skin condition very familiar to dermatologists. The typical skin rash of LP has itchy, purple red bumps on the shins, inner wrists and ankles. It can less commonly involve the vulva and/or the vagina.

WHAT IS THE CAUSE OF LICHEN PLANUS?

The exact cause is unknown. It is believed to be an autoimmune disease in which the body has developed antibodies that attack the skin and mucous membrane. The triggering factor may be an infection or foreign chemical. Lichen planus is not contagious. It is not related to hormones or aging.

WHAT CAN LP LOOK LIKE ON THE VULVA OR IN THE VAGINA?

There is a white, lacy, or 'confetti-like' pattern on the vulva and around the vagina. In the erosive form there is redness, sometimes with moist, open ulcers. Scarring can smooth over the clitoris and the labia minora. Ulcers in the vagina may produce a white or yellow discharge. Vaginal erosions on opposing surfaces may 'heal together' and form ribbons of scar tissue that can make the vagina very narrow or close it partially or (rarely) completely.

HOW IS LP DIAGNOSED?

A biopsy is necessary to rule out other scarring or blistering skin diseases. This is usually a minor procedure done in the office under local anesthetic – a small plug of skin can answer many questions for you and your doctor.

WHAT KINDS OF PROBLEMS MAY I HAVE WITH LP?

Lichen planus on the skin can be very itchy but itchy LP is not often found on the vulva. The vulva can be very red and sore, especially if there are open areas or ulcers. Vaginal LP can feel very raw and intercourse may be uncomfortable if not impossible. Vaginal discharge can be heavy. Associated mouth LP can show sores on the gums, inner cheeks or tongue.

CAN LP BE TREATED? IS IT CURABLE?

Lichen planus can be treated and controlled in most cases but not always cured. Treatment is directed at stopping the body's immune system from destroying the skin. Various forms of corticosteroids (cortisone) are commonly used to do this. They decrease inflammation, help itching and heal skin ulcers. Careful use of these strong medications is necessary to make sure the treatment is effective and side effects few. Along with the cortisone, antibiotics and anti-yeast treatments may be used. Dermatologists generally know most about the new treatments for LP. Patients who do not respond well to topical steroids may need other, more aggressive treatments.

ARE THERE OTHER MEDICATIONS TO TREAT LP?

There are many medications that can be used to alter the immune response. Medications normally used for infections that can also do this are tetracyclines, metronidazole or antimalarial drugs. Immunosuppressive drugs like azathioprine and cyclosporine are also being used, and some new drugs and creams are being tested. Frequently, combination therapy is necessary. If there is scarring of the vagina a vaginal dilator will be needed.

Ulcerated LP can be difficult and can require multiple visits, but most patients improve and are well controlled.

From Black, M. M. and McKay, M. (eds): *Obstetric and Gynecologic Dermatology*, 2nd edition.
© Mosby International Limited 2002.

PATIENT INFORMATION - LICHEN PLANUS
continued

WHAT CAN I DO TO HELP?
Anything that irritates you must be avoided. Soaps, cleansers and lubricants must be mild, such as Cetaphil® cleanser or unscented Dove® cleansing bar. As a lubricant, use olive oil or plain petrolatum, so that the vulva does not dry out. Treatment will take time and may require trial and error with different medications. Have patience as you learn what you can use that does not irritate you.

DO I NEED ADDITIONAL HELP?
Surgery is best avoided because the trauma can activate or flare LP. Counseling, sexual or psychological, may be a great help to deal with the stress. You will need an understanding partner.

IS THERE A CHANCE THAT LP CAN TURN INTO CANCER?
Lichen planus scars the skin, and scars do carry a very small risk of developing cancer. The signs of skin cancer are similar to those on other parts of body: a sore or ulcer that does not heal in a few weeks, a lesion that continues to bleed easily, a bump or a raised lesion that is getting progressively larger. If you have any of these, see your doctor. A biopsy may be necessary. You should have regular (at least yearly) visits to a gynecologist or dermatologist who knows about LP.

From Black, M. M. and McKay, M. (eds): *Obstetric and Gynecologic Dermatology*, 2nd edition.
© Mosby International Limited 2002.

PATIENT INFORMATION - LICHEN SCLEROSUS (like-in skler-o-sus)

Lichen sclerosus (LS) is a common genital disease involving the skin around the vulva and anus in women (and more rarely, the penis of men). It can occur at any age but is more common around 40–50 years. The skin around the vagina and anus becomes thin, white, and fragile. Scratching causes the skin to become thick and it may split or bleed. Some patients have only a few areas of LS while others may have the whole vulva involved. Some have itching and/or burning. And others few to no symptoms. If untreated, LS may scar the vulvar skin.

HOW DID I GET LICHEN SCLEROSUS?

Lichen sclerosus is not an infection, and we know that you did nothing to cause it. You cannot give this to anyone. It can sometimes develop in sisters or in mother and daughters, so there is an inherited factor. Patients with LS sometimes have other diseases that have antibodies to the body's own tissue, such as thyroid disease or diabetes. These conditions, however, do not cause LS.

CAN LS BE TREATED? IS IT CURABLE?

There is excellent treatment available to improve the symptoms and to heal the open lesions of LS, but there is currently no cure. Treatment will control LS but it must be ongoing and carefully monitored indefinitely. Sometimes surgery will be needed to widen a shrunken vaginal opening. Even with good treatment, the skin may not entirely return to its normal appearance.

HOW IS LS TREATED?

First the diagnosis must be confirmed with a biopsy. Then treatment is started with a high potency topical steroid. These ointments are especially helpful if the skin is thick and/or there is intense itching. Early lesions of LS often heal completely, while older lesions are more resistant. The cortisone may be combined with anti-candida treatment for associated yeast. The ointment is usually applied nightly for about 2–3 months and then 1–3 times a week as needed. Your doctor will recommend the best program for you. To improve itching, use a mild soap or cleanser. Avoid using panty liners or anything that may rub or irritate the area. Long-term follow-up is important.

CAN LS DEVELOP ON OTHER PARTS OF MY BODY?

The most common place for LS is around the genitals and anus, but in 10–20% of patients it involves other parts of the body. Patients who get widespread LS usually have it on the other parts of the body, usually the trunk, from the beginning. Patients who have only genital lesions for years are less likely to develop LS elsewhere. The typical skin lesions are flat, white, or pale 'confetti' spots that may gradually come together to enlarge.

WHAT WOULD HAPPEN IF I GOT PREGNANT? COULD I HAVE A VAGINAL DELIVERY?

Lichen sclerosus behaves differently in different patients during pregnancy: some have few symptoms and others report marked itch and discomfort. Lichen sclerosus should not prevent a vaginal delivery. Stitches heal in that area as well as in other areas. Strong topical corticosteroids may be used in limited amounts during pregnancy and breastfeeding.

IS THERE A CHANCE THAT LICHEN SCLEROSIS MAY TURN INTO CANCER?

Lichen sclerosus scars the skin and this increases the risk of a local type of skin cancer. (This happens in about 5% of cases.) The signs of a developing skin cancer are similar to those in other parts of the body: a sore or ulcer that does not heal in a few weeks, a lesion that continues to bleed easily, a bump or a raised lesion that is getting progressively larger. If an area does not heal despite regular use of your prescribed medication, you should insist that your doctor examine the area. It may be that your topical ointment needs to be changed, but a biopsy may be needed to tell what is happening. A biopsy is a minor procedure usually done in the office with a local anesthetic – a small plug of skin can answer many questions for you and your doctor. Usually cancer develops in patients who have untreated LS for many years.

IS THERE ANY RISK WHEN USING THE STRONG CORTISONE RECOMMENDED?

Strong cortisone can thin the skin, particularly the skin of the labia and inner thighs. This thinning may result in stretch marks. Extensive use can result in a burning sensation and increases the chance of associated yeast infection. Rarely, a patient may be allergic to the steroid cream or ointment, which causes itching and irritation every time it is applied. This ointment should be used in strictly limited areas, as directed, for limited periods of time. You should have regular, at least yearly, visits to a gynecologist or dermatologist who knows about LS.

From Black, M. M. and McKay, M. (eds): *Obstetric and Gynecologic Dermatology*, 2nd edition. © Mosby International Limited 2002.

PATIENT INFORMATION – LICHEN SIMPLEX CHRONICUS (like-in sim-plex kron-i-cus)

Latin for 'long-standing simple thickening' caused by chronic scratching. There are several vulvar conditions that begin with the word 'lichen'. They are all different, but each may have areas of white, thickened skin. Lichen simplex chronicus (LSC) is the one that itches the most.

WHAT CAUSED MY ITCHING? DO I HAVE AN INFECTION?

Many things can cause itching (such as skin allergy, eczema or psoriasis), but usually the itching stops when the skin heals. If you have scratched for several weeks, the itching can sometimes continue on its own. Scratching the skin makes the itching worse – this is called the 'itch-scratch-itch cycle'. With continued rubbing and scratching, the skin gradually becomes thick and leathery, a change called lichen simplex chronicus (LSC). The nerve endings in the skin signal 'itch' more easily in LSC than in normal skin. Over time, it becomes impossible to tell whether scratching triggers itch or vice versa. Your problem is not from an infection but chronic scratching can open the skin to secondary infection from bacteria and/or yeast that will need treatment. Itching and scratching often worsen with stress, heat and humidity. Vigorous scratching gives pleasure and relief, and you may even scratch while you are asleep.

IS THERE SOMETHING ELSE WRONG WITH ME?

Lichen simplex chronicus develops more easily in patients with other skin diseases, especially atopic dermatitis (eczema), psoriasis or rashes from topical products that irritate the skin or cause an allergic reaction (contact dermatitis). The continued scratching of chronic yeast infections or LS can cause LSC on top of the original problem. Thus, there may be several factors working together, such as an irritating soap and a tendency to eczema. Any products (creams, cleansers, antiseptics etc.) you use on this irritated skin may further worsen the problem. You will need to work with your doctor to find what factors are contributing to your problem and to diagnose any underlying condition. Patch testing by a dermatologist may reveal specific allergies. You must tell your doctor everything you have used, past and present. A skin biopsy may help your doctor to diagnose your problem.

WHAT DO I FEEL AND WHAT DOES IT LOOK LIKE?

The vulvar skin is sensitive and extremely itchy. You may wake up at night scratching. When you scratch, the skin will become wounded, raw, burning and sore. The area looks pink to dusky red, even purple. There is swelling and thickening so that the skin feels leathery. There may be open weeping, bleeding or dried crusts depending on the scratching.

CAN LSC BE CURED? HOW IS TREATED?

The goal in LSC is to stop the itch-scratch-itch cycle, because if you can stop the scratching the skin will eventually heal and stop itching. It takes a long time to develop LSC, so do not expect to improve overnight. Therapy consists of avoiding harsh, irritating soaps, lotions, moisturizers and other products. The area must be kept cool and ventilated. No tight or synthetic clothing is permitted. Mild to moderate strength corticosteroid creams and ointments are used for children, and more potent medium strength to superpotent corticosteroid ointments are used in adults, for limited periods of time. Antihistamines or sedatives may relieve itching at night. Oozing or moist lesions of LSC may be infected, so you may need oral antibiotics and/or oral or vaginal anti-candida medications to allow healing. A cool water compress or sitz bath with Burow's solution may be helpful for open, oozing, itchy vulvar skin. Following this, a steroid ointment may be applied in a reducing regimen over a couple of months to control inflammation. Strong cortisones may cause skin thinning and redness if used too long, so your doctor will supervise and limit your prescriptions and follow you carefully. If the skin remains thick and uncomfortable, a few injections of cortisone into the area of severe itching can help bring things under control. Surgical procedures and alcohol injections are not necessary for LSC.

Do not be discouraged if improvement takes several weeks or even months. It is typical for itching to flare up from time to time. As the skin improves, your doctor will prescribe less frequent applications of the strong ointments or switch to a milder one. You must be careful to avoid any irritation that can trigger a relapse.

From Black, M. M. and McKay, M. (eds): *Obstetric and Gynecologic Dermatology*, 2nd edition.
© Mosby International Limited 2002.

PATIENT INFORMATION – VULVAR ITCH THERAPY

When you are itchy you will be in tempted to scratch, or even use products that will further irritate your skin, making the problem worse.

HOW DO YOU STOP THE ITCHING?

Avoid irritating soaps, feminine deodorant products, any perfumed products, disposable wipes, and regular use of panty liners, girdles, tight synthetic clothing and pantyhose. Stop any clothing or activity that makes the area warm and/or sweaty.

Use only detergents free of enzymes, dyes and perfumes

- Use no fabric softeners
- Do not douche
- Wear loose cotton underwear
- Use loose clothing
- Consider using:
  - Thigh high 'stay-up' hose
  - Garter belt and stockings
  - Pantyhose with cutout crotch

TO CLEANSE

Regular cleansing:
- Use a mild liquid cleanser (Cetaphil®) or an unscented cleansing bar (Dove®). Do not use a facecloth. Use bare hands only. Never scrub. Rinse thoroughly and gently pat dry. Never use 'wipes'.

For severe itch:
- Use Burow's solution 1 : 40. Mix one packet or tablet of Domeboro or Bluboro in 500 mL (1 pint) of cool water in a sitz bath for 5–10 minutes, 2 or 3 times per day. Plain water may be used.

TO DECREASE SWELLING AND ITCH

- Use cold packs (plastic picnic or freezer packs) kept in a self-sealed plastic bag in the refrigerator. These can be covered with thin dry cotton and applied directly to the vulva and used as needed.
- Ice, chopped up in a plastic bag, can be applied to the itchy area.
- A plastic dishwashing soap bottle can be partially filled with water and frozen in the freezer. It may be left at the bedside when retiring and used during the night, wrapped in a thin dry cotton towel for relief as needed.
- Plain, cold yogurt from the refrigerator can be spread on a sanitary napkin and applied directly to the raw, itchy vulva as needed.
- For thick itchy rashes you will need a cortisone ointment from your doctor. You may also need treatment for secondary bacterial and yeast infections.

Note: Ice packs or frozen items should not be placed directly on the skin. Use with a dry cloth as a barrier to prevent frostbite.

- If you are waking at night scratching, you may need an antihistamine such as diphenhydramine or hydroxyzine 25–75 mg taken at 6–7pm.
- For a sexual lubricant, try olive oil or vegetable shortening.
- Use unscented 100% cotton menstrual pads and tampons.

Note: If you scratch, you will wound the area further and it will take longer to heal.

PATIENT INFORMATION – EROSIVE OR ULCERATIVE VULVAR THERAPY

GENERAL INSTRUCTIONS FOR WEEPING, BLISTERING, OR RAW AREAS OF THE VULVA

Open, weeping areas of the skin are very tender and easily irritated. Avoid irritating soaps, feminine deodorant products, any perfumed products, disposable wipes, and regular use of panty liners, girdles, tight synthetic clothing and pantyhose. Stop anything that makes the area warm and/or sweaty.

- Use only detergents free of enzymes, dyes and perfumes
- Use no fabric softeners
- Do not douche
- Wear loose cotton underwear
- Loose clothing
- Consider using:
    Thigh high 'stay-up' hose
    Garter belt and stockings
    Pantyhose with cutout crotch

TO CLEANSE:
For open raw areas:

- Soothing compress:
  – Mix a packet of Burow's solution (Domeboro, Bluboro or Pedi-Boro) in 1 pint (500 mL) of lukewarm to cool water. This should be mixed fresh daily. Plain water may also be used. Refrigerate if desired.
  – Moisten a thin cotton handkerchief or soft cloth in the solution and lay the cloth over the vulva for 1–2 minutes, then remove and let the solution evaporate for 1–2 minutes. Repeat 5–10 times each treatment session. (Sit in an empty bathtub to avoid dripping.)
- Sitz bath (2–3 inches of lukewarm to cool water in a shallow pan or plastic basin): soak for 10 minutes 3–4 times a day and air dry afterward.

For gentle cleansing, if the area is not very open or raw:

- Use a mild 'no-soap' liquid cleanser such as Cetaphil® or an unscented cleansing bar (Dove®). Never use a facecloth. Never scrub. Always rinse thoroughly. Gently pat (do not rub) dry.

TOPICAL PAIN CONTROL:

- Anesthetic creams such as EMLA® or Xylocaine® (lidocaine) can be applied in a thick layer under plastic wrap for 30 minutes to numb the area for 1–2 hours. This initially stings, but stops in 4–5 minutes.
- If the area is open and raw after the sitz bath or compress, use a protective barrier such as Ihle's paste (25% zinc oxide, 25% starch, 25% anhydrous lanolin, 25% petrolatum) or zinc oxide ointment (25% zinc oxide in petrolatum). Apply in a thick layer over the open areas once or twice a day. To remove the paste, liberally soak several cotton balls with light mineral oil, apply the oil to the paste, and gently dab it away. The mineral oil will melt the paste. Pat, do not rub.
- Anti-inflammatory ointments. Your physician may prescribe strong topical steroids. Oral antibiotics may be needed for infection.

From Black, M. M. and McKay, M. (eds): *Obstetric and Gynecologic Dermatology*, 2nd edition.
© Mosby International Limited 2002.

PATIENT INFORMATION - VULVAR PAIN, VULVODYNIA (vul-vo-din-ee-ah) OR DYSESTHESIA (dis-ess-thee-sha)

Vulvodynia is chronic (long-term) vulvar pain with burning, stinging, irritation, itching and rawness that causes physical, sexual and psychological distress. The new term for this is vulvar dysesthesia and it replaces the older terms burning vulva syndrome and essential vulvodynia. The two most common forms of chronic vulvar pain are vulvar dysesthesia and vestibulodynia (also called vestibulitis), a local form of vulvar dysesthesia. Vulvar pain can be caused by a chemical irritation, like a harsh soap. A yeast infection causes vulvar burning and pain. Herpes simplex infection also causes vulvar pain. But these are all known causes and are not referred to as vulvar dysesthesia/vulvodynia.

This term is used when the cause of the pain is not known.

WHY DO I HAVE THIS?

The pain and discomfort is probably due to altered sensations in the nerves to the vulvar area. It happens when the nerve is damaged and it continues to send pain signals even when the original injury is healed. Any inflammation in the back, pelvis, muscles, tendons or nerves can create such a 'pain loop' in which the pain sensation feeds back, resulting in more pain. This exaggerated pain response can cause pelvic floor muscle spasms, leading to more pain. The nerve could have been injured by one of many possible insults, including bony injuries or surgery to the back, hips or pelvis; repetitive musculoskeletal injury or postural stresses. Back problems such as a ruptured disk or spinal arthritis are other examples. A viral injury from shingles (Herpes zoster) or genital cold sores (Herpes simplex) can cause nerve injury with resulting long term pain. These viral infections may occur unrecognized.

WHAT DID I DO TO START THIS?

You may not have done anything you can pinpoint. Possibly, you had an injury to your back or pelvis, such as a fall. You may have had a difficult delivery or a surgical procedure. An infection like yeast or an irritation may have worsened your problem.

HOW IS IT DIAGNOSED?

A thorough review of your problem must be done. All organic causes of burning and pain must be ruled out, as this is a diagnosis made by excluding other causes. During the physical examination all will look normal. Touching the area may be very uncomfortable, even with very light touch, because the sensation is abnormal.

WHAT OTHER PROBLEMS MIGHT I HAVE WITH THIS?

When you have chronic pain for a long time, it is tiring. You may be fatigued and depressed, with loss of energy. Chronic pain can be demoralizing and exhausting. Remember that this is not a contagious condition and is not due to poor hygiene. Some patients have associated pain conditions such as inflammatory bowel disease, fibromyalgia, and interstitial cystitis.

PATIENT INFORMATION – VULVAR PAIN, VULVODYNIA OR DYSESTHESIA continued

CAN VULVAR DYSESTHESIA BE TREATED? IS IT CURABLE?

This condition can be treated with significant improvement. All irritants should be avoided. Loose ventilated cool clothing is best. Mild cleansers, cotton sanitary napkins along with bland emollients such as plain petrolatum should be used. Topical estrogen cream can be useful if there is any atrophy. For local pain a topical anesthetic can be useful.

Specific treatment is aimed as breaking the pain loop. Oral medications are used to calm the 'sore nerves'. Tricyclic anti-depressant drugs in low doses are frequently used as they block pain fibers and help disrupt the pain message loop. There are several types from which to choose and you may respond to one better than another, as the side effects are individual and variable. These include amitriptyline, nortriptyline, desipramine and doxepin. Side effects such as dry mouth, constipation and drowsiness are not uncommon. These medications work slowly. They can be used alone or with other pain-modulating medications such as anti-convulsant drugs like gabapentin. The doses are low at first and are gradually increased. Treatment will vary according to your tolerance and response. You may need these medications for a long period of time.

Other helpful treatments include massage, stress management, support for depression, and counseling for sexual difficulties. A diet low in calcium oxalate (which can be discussed with your physician) may be useful. A pelvic floor physiotherapist can assist in a biofeedback program to break the muscle pain and spasms. This chronic pain problem will need time and the help of several specialists. Improvement is gradual.

WHAT CAN I DO TO HELP?

Understand that this will take time. Do talk to other people about this. You will need support from friends and family. If you are very down and angry, you may need a trained counselor to help you through this time. Stress management and relaxation are very important. Sexual counseling may be helpful. Keep your spirits up. Maintain your ability to manage and overcome the pain. Accept small steps. Do not expect an 'instant cure.'

From Black, M. M. and McKay, M. (eds): *Obstetric and Gynecologic Dermatology*, 2nd edition. © Mosby International Limited 2002.

VESTIBULITIS/VESTIBULODYNIA (ves-**tib**-you-**lite**-iss, ves-**tib**-you-low-**din**-ee-ah)

Vestibulitis (vestibulodynia) is one of the chronic vulvar pain disorders (vulvar dysesthesia or vulvodynia). The pain is localized to the opening of the vagina. The primary symptom of vestibulitis is pain when the opening to the vagina is touched or entered with a finger or tampon; during intercourse; or with your doctor's vaginal speculum examination. Some patients have pain even wiping the area with toilet tissue, wearing tight clothing, or riding a bicycle. The pain may be severe enough that it causes involuntary tightening of the muscles of the vagina, causing muscular spasms that make the pain worse.

WHAT ARE THE CAUSES OF THIS CONDITION?

Around the entrance to the vagina is a little rim of tissue called the hymenal ring. Just outside the ring are tiny glands that produce fluid to keep the area moist. These little glands become inflamed, red and very tender, but the triggering factors for this condition are not known. Different factors may cause the problem in different patients. Yeast infections, trauma at delivery or during pelvic surgery, and even back injuries have been implicated. In some cases, there may be a genetic predisposition. Some think that high levels of calcium oxalate in the urine may irritate the vulvar tissue, but this association has not been confirmed. The initial inflammation associated with these conditions seems to start an abnormal feedback loop leading to chronic pelvic muscle tension, which keeps the pain going. You try to protect yourself by tensing up the pelvic floor muscles (or this happens as a reflex) and so, even when the pain stimulus is gone, the tension remains, leading to more pain.

HOW IS THE DIAGNOSIS MADE?

To make the diagnosis of vestibulitis/vestibulodynia, a thorough history and physical must be carried out to rule out other causes of vulvar pain such as infections (herpes, candida, etc.), allergic reaction, skin rashes, tumors, etc. The diagnosis is made by excluding those problems, by obtaining a history of pain and by confirming pain when the area is touched with a cotton swab. Usually there is no visible skin problem. A biopsy is usually neither necessary nor helpful.

HOW IS THIS TREATED?

So far, there is no magic 'cure' and treatment takes time. You will need to work closely with your doctor, physiotherapist, and pelvic floor specialist. A sexual counselor may be needed.

1 Avoid irritants. Cleanse gently with plain water or a soap substitute such as Cetaphil® cleanser.
2 If the area feels dry, use a bland lubricant such as plain olive oil as needed.
3 Topical estrogen cream (estradiol 0.01%) may be used 2–3 times daily.
4 A low oxalate diet may remove calcium oxalate from the urine. Such a diet is outlined in appropriate cookbooks or from a local dietician. To this is added 400 mg calcium citrate, three times a day.
5 Medications for nerve pain are often prescribed to modify the pain loop. Amitriptyline may be started with 10 mg at bedtime and gradually increased over weeks to months. The effect of these medications is slow and gradual. Dry mouth may occur and there may be some dizziness and/or fatigue.
6 Biofeedback and pelvic floor physiotherapy: by relaxing and strengthening pelvic floor muscles, the pain can be reduced. A knowledgeable pelvic floor specialist must assess you and start you on a home program. This takes time.
7 Topical anesthetic cream can blunt the pain triggered by touching the area so that sexual penetration may be possible. Lidocaine (Xylocaine®, Ela-Max®) 5% or lidocaine-prilocaine (EMLA®) cream may be used, in a thick layer covered with plastic wrap, under a sanitary napkin for 10–15 minutes. These creams sting and burn at first.
8 Surgery: for the occasional resistant case there is a surgical procedure to remove the offending inflamed tissue in the hymenal area. This can be discussed further with your doctor.

From Black, M. M. and McKay, M. (eds): *Obstetric and Gynecologic Dermatology*, 2nd edition.
© Mosby International Limited 2002.

VESTIBULITIS/VESTIBULODYNIA continued

WILL I BE CURED?

Most patients do well, with sufficient improvement in the discomfort that they can resume normal sexual relations. There may be some residual or intermittent discomfort. Patients with severe pain problems that are generalized or associated with other problems such as irritable bowel syndrome or interstitial cystitis may have more difficulty.

WHAT IS THE DIFFERENCE BETWEEN VULVODYNIA AND VESTIBULODYNIA?

These are both chronic vulvar pain conditions and they can overlap in the same patient. Vulvar vestibulitis is a subset of vulvodynia. The pain is limited to the hymenal ring area and occurs only when it is touched or pressed. The pain in vulvodynia is constant.

WHERE CAN I GET MORE INFORMATION?

The National Vulvodynia Association
PO Box 4491
Silver Springs
MD 20914-4491
USA
Tel. (301) 299 0775

From Black, M. M. and McKay, M. (eds): *Obstetric and Gynecologic Dermatology*, 2nd edition. © Mosby International Limited 2002.

VULVAR SELF EXAMINATION

You should be familiar with your own vulva. You can learn to examine it just as you do your skin and breasts. With regular self-examination you will recognize whether there is a change. If there is a sore, itchy, or bleeding area, do look at it, noting the changes so that you can discuss these with your physician. With regular examination, you will be able to detect problems at an early stage.

You will need a good light, such as a gooseneck or desk lamp, plus a hand mirror with a regular and a magnified side for best visualization. Wash your hands.

Find a comfortable position. You can stand with one leg up on a chair, squat, kneel, or lie down and prop yourself up with your elbows, cushions, and/or both. Adjust the light and mirror so that you can easily see your vulva, perineum, and anus.

With reference to the figure, first locate the bigger structures: the thick vulvar lips (labia majora), the thin lips of the vulva (labia minora), the clitoris, the opening to the vagina, the skin area between the back of the vagina and the anus (perineum), and the anus.

Gently separate the small lips (labia minora) and familiarize yourself with the vulva from the clitoris to the vaginal opening. Note the colors and texture. Look at the clitoris by gently pulling back the clitoral hood. Look at the opening of the vagina. Familiarize yourself with the area around the outside of the vulva and the anus. If you see any unusual change over time, see your physician.

Any new lesions should be evaluated by your doctor. Most vulvar diseases are easily, successfully and safely treated when diagnosed early. Just as you do your regular breast examination also examine your vulva. This is another healthy habit.

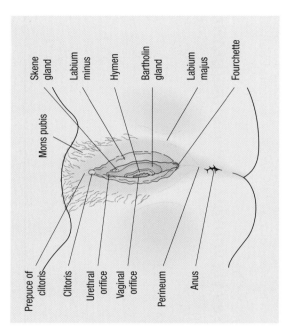

Schematic diagram of the vulva

Prepuce of clitoris — Clitoris — Urethral orifice — Vaginal orifice — Perineum — Anus

Mons pubis — Skene gland — Labium minus — Hymen — Bartholin gland — Labium majus — Fourchette

Index

233

Page references in *italics* refer to Figures; those in **bold** refer to Tables

Page references in *italics* refer to Figures; those in **bold** refer to Tables

Page references in *italics* refer to Figures; those in **bold** refer to Tables

Page references in *italics* refer to Figures; those in **bold** refer to Tables

Page references in *italics* refer to Figures; those in **bold** refer to Tables

Page references in *italics* refer to Figures; those in **bold** refer to Tables

239

Page references in *italics* refer to Figures; those in **bold** refer to Tables

Page references in *italics* refer to Figures; those in **bold** refer to Tables